100 Top Consultations in Small Animal General Practice

100 Top Consultations in Small Animal General Practice

Peter Hill
BVSc, PhD, DVD, DipACVD, DipECVD, MRCVS, MACVSc
*Senior Lecturer in Veterinary Dermatology and
Immunology, The University of Adelaide, South
Australia, Australia*

Sheena Warman
BSc, BVMS, DSAM, DipECVIM-CA, PGCert(HE), MRCVS
*Clinical Fellow in Small Animal Medicine, University
of Bristol, Bristol, UK*

Geoff Shawcross
BVSc, Cert SAO, MRCVS
General Practitioner (retired), Liss, Hampshire, UK

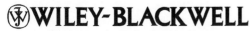

A John Wiley & Sons, Ltd., Publication

This edition first published 2011
© 2011 Blackwell Publishing Ltd

Blackwell Publishing was acquired by John Wiley & Sons in February 2007. Blackwell's publishing programme has been merged with Wiley's global Scientific, Technical, and Medical business to form Wiley-Blackwell.

Registered office
John Wiley & Sons Ltd, The Atrium, Southern Gate, Chichester, West Sussex, PO19 8SQ, United Kingdom

Editorial offices
9600 Garsington Road, Oxford, OX4 2DQ, United Kingdom
The Atrium, Southern Gate, Chichester, West Sussex, PO19 8SQ, United Kingdom
2121 State Avenue, Ames, Iowa 50014-8300, USA

For details of our global editorial offices, for customer services and for information about how to apply for permission to reuse the copyright material in this book please see our website at www.wiley.com/wiley-blackwell.

Library of Congress Cataloging-in-Publication Data

100 top consultations in small animal general practice / edited by Peter B. Hill, Sheena Warman, Geoff Shawcross.
       p. ; cm.
   One hundred top consultations in small animal general practice
   Includes bibliographical references and index.
   ISBN 978-1-4051-6949-3 (pbk. : alk. paper)   1. Pet medicine.   I. Hill, Peter B. (Peter Barrie)   II. Warman, Sheena.   III. Shawcross, Geoff.   IV. Title: One hundred top consultations in small animal general practice.
   [DNLM: 1. Dog Diseases.   2. Cat Diseases.   3. Professional-Patient Relations.   4. Veterinary Medicine—methods. SF 991]
   SF981.A55 2011
   636.089—dc22

                                                    2010040961

A catalogue record for this book is available from the British Library.

This book is published in the following electronic formats: ePDF [ISBN 9781444393347]; ePub [ISBN 9781444393354]

Set in 9/11 pt Calibri by Toppan Best-set Premedia Limited
Printed and bound by CPI Group (UK) Ltd, Croydon, CR0 4YY

C9781405169493_190224

Contents

Miscellaneous   Specific conditions   **Differential diagnosis**   Appendices

List of contributors

Editors

Peter Hill
BVSc, PhD, DVD, DipACVD, DipECVD, MRCVS, MACVSc
Senior Lecturer in Veterinary Dermatology and Immunology, The University of Adelaide, School of Animal and Veterinary Sciences, Roseworthy Campus, Roseworthy, SA 5371, Australia

Sheena Warman
BSc, BVMS, DSAM, DipECVIM-CA, PGCert(HE), MRCVS
Clinical Fellow in Small Animal Medicine, Division of Companion Animal Studies, Department of Clinical Veterinary Science, University of Bristol, Langford House, Langford, Bristol BS40 5DU, UK

Geoff Shawcross
BVSc, Cert SAO, MRCVS
General Practitioner (retired), Shrublands, St Patrick's Lane, Rake, Liss, Hampshire GU33 7HQ, UK

Additional authors

Jon Bowen, BVetMed, MRCVS, DipAS(CABC)
Behavioural Medicine Referral Service, Queen Mother Hospital for Small Animals, Royal Veterinary College, Hawkshead Lane, Potters Bar, North Mymms, Hatfield, Herts AL9 7TA, UK

Jim Carter, BVetMed, DVOphthal, MRCVS
RCVS Recognised Specialist in Veterinary Ophthalmology, South Devon Referrals, The Old Cider Works, Old Cider Works Lane, Abbotskerswell, Devon TQ12 5GH, UK

Mark Goodfellow, MA, VetMB, CertVR, DSAM, DipECVIM-CA, MRCVS
European Recognised Specialist in Veterinary Internal Medicine, Molecular Oncology Laboratories, Weatherall Institute of Molecular Medicine, John Radcliffe Hospital, University of Oxford, Oxford, UK

Andrea Harvey, BVSc, DSAM(Feline), DipECVIM-CA, MRCVS
RCVS Recognised Specialist in Feline Medicine, Feline Advisory Bureau, Taeselbury, High Street, Tisbury, Wiltshire SP3 6LD, UK

Peter Holt, BVMS, PhD, DipECVS, CBiol, FSBiol, FHEA, FRCVS
Emeritus Professor of Veterinary Surgery, Division of Companion Animal Studies, Department of Clinical Veterinary Science, University of Bristol, Langford House, Langford, Bristol BS40 5DU, UK

Norman Johnston, BVM&S, FAVD, DiplAVDC, DiplEVDC, MRCVS
RCVS American and European Recognised Specialist in Veterinary Dentistry, DentalVets, 31 Station Hill, North Berwick, Lothian EH39 4AS, UK

Martin Owen, BVSc, BSc, PhD, DSAS (Orth), DipECVS, MRCVS
ECVS Recognised Specialist in Small Animal Surgery, RCVS Recognised Specialist in Small Animal Surgery (Orthopaedics), Dick White Referrals, Six Mile Bottom Veterinary Specialist Centre, Station Farm, London Road, Six Mile Bottom, Suffolk CB8 0UH, UK

Sharon Redrobe, BSc(Hons), BVetMed, CertLAS, DZooMed, MRCVS
RCVS Recognised Specialist in Zoo and Wildlife Medicine, Clinical Associate Professor in Zoo, Wild and Exotic Animal Medicine, Director of Life Sciences, Twycross Zoo, School of Veterinary Medicine and Science, University of Nottingham, College Road, Sutton Bonington, Leicestershire LE12 5RD, UK

Sue Shaw, BVSc (Hons), MSc, Dip ACVIM, Dip ECVIM, FACVSc, MRCVS
Senior Lecturer in Dermatology and Applied Immunology, Division of Companion Animal Studies, Department of Clinical Veterinary Science, University of Bristol, Langford House, Langford, Bristol BS40 5DU, UK

Paul Smith, BVetMed, DVC, MRCVS
RCVS Recognised Specialist in Veterinary Cardiology, East Anglia Cardiology Ltd, The Bakers Cottage, Church Street, Buntingford, Hertfordshire SG9 9AS, UK

Acknowledgements

Peter Hill would like to thank Sarah, his wife, for her constant support during the writing of this book.

Sheena Warman would like to thank her husband Adrian for his patience and support whilst this book has been written. She would also like to thank colleagues and students, past and present, who have provided inspiration and helpful suggestions.

Geoff Shawcross would like to take this opportunity to thank all the professional colleagues with whom he has had the pleasure to work during his career for their unstinting support and advice, without which his contribution to this book would not have been possible.

Dedication

This book is dedicated to all the animals we have treated over the course of our careers. Without them, we would have known nothing.

About this book

This multidisciplinary text begins with a comprehensive guide to the consultation process in small animal practice. Within this section, clinicians will find highly practical, invaluable tips about history taking, physical examination and diagnostic approaches.

The book then covers 100 of the most common scenarios that a small animal practitioner will have to deal with in the consulting room. These chapters are of three main types:

1) *Presenting-sign-based chapters* – These chapters, coloured blue, cover an important symptom, listing the common differential diagnoses, outlining the diagnostic approach for its investigation and indicating how the case should be treated. These chapters inform clinicians about what to tell clients before a diagnosis has been made.
2) *Diagnosis-based chapters* – These chapters, coloured purple, cover important diseases and describe how clinicians should diagnose and treat them. These chapters inform clinicians about what to tell clients after a diagnosis has been made.
3) *Miscellaneous chapters* – These chapters, coloured red, cover various topics that are rarely found in veterinary texts, such as annual health checks, neutering, oestrus control and euthanasia.

Within the first two types of chapter, there are three unique 'boxed' sections covering 'What if it doesn't get better?', 'The low-cost option' and 'When should I refer?', which can be quickly identified by their colour (red, orange and purple, respectively). This type of information is rarely taught at veterinary school and practitioners usually have to learn it the hard way, by trial and error.

There are then five appendices covering the use of antibiotics, glucocorticoids and non-steroidal anti-inflammatory drugs, as well as information on obesity control and the interpretation of laboratory tests.

Never before has such practical information been put together in a single text. When grouped together, these chapters provide a comprehensive guide to the vast majority of consultations undertaken in small animal general practice. It's like having an experienced or specialist clinician standing by your side in the consulting room.

This book will be invaluable to:

* Undergraduate veterinary students
* Newly graduated veterinarians
* Experienced veterinarians who are looking for an up-to-date refresher on small animal practice
* Veterinarians who are returning to the profession after a leave of absence
* Veterinarians who are converting from large animal to small animal practice, or for whom small animal consulting constitutes only a small part of their duties.

Introduction: Diagnostic and therapeutic approaches in small animal general practice

Peter Hill

In order to treat diseases of small animals, clinicians must adopt a systematic approach that leads to a diagnosis and specific treatment. This process typically involves the following steps:

1. Obtaining a history.
2. Performing a physical examination.
3. Making a diagnosis or generating a list of differential diagnoses.
4. If necessary, performing tests to rule in or out differential diagnoses.
5. Determining a prognosis.
6. Prescribing treatment.

In general practice, this whole process has to be orchestrated around a consultation that typically lasts around ten to fifteen minutes. In order to achieve this, clinicians have to develop and hone their skills so that they can deliver competent medicine without compromising patient care, as well as appearing unhurried in front of the client. The basic structure of a typical consultation is illustrated in Figure 0.1.

Prior to seeing a case, the clinician should know the signalment of the animal (age, breed and sex) and be aware of its vaccination and worming history. This information should be in the animal's medical records, but if it is a new client, it can be obtained by the reception staff. Other information that should be in the animal's records includes dietary, foreign travel and previous medical history.

History taking

Taking a history is a process in which a veterinarian listens to, and questions the owner of a pet, in order to determine what abnormalities or signs have been observed. Typically, the owner is first asked what the problem is, and then allowed to describe the problem in more detail. The clinician can supplement the information obtained by asking specific questions.

To be good at history-taking, clinicians must learn to get the right balance between listening and questioning. This

is an important aspect of the veterinarian's 'bedside manner' and is essential if the appropriate information is to be gathered. Too much listening can lead to incomplete or confusing histories; too much questioning can come across as an interrogation. Mastering this important skill requires practice and students should observe a number of experienced practitioners to determine the optimal balance.

When asking questions, it is important that clinicians do not speak to clients using technical terminology that is not widely understood. Veterinarians must become 'bilingual', using plain language for clients, and veterinary terminology for professional colleagues and medical records. As an example, 'Is he pruritic on his ventral abdomen?' should become 'Is his tummy itchy?' Clinicians should also

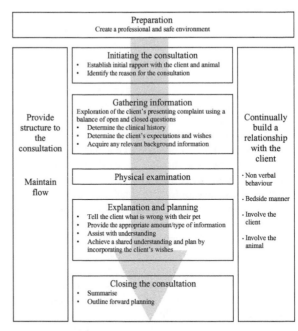

Figure 0.1 An overview of the consultation process, modified from a system known as the Calgary–Cambridge Model Framework. This approach is commonly taught in medical and veterinary schools. In general veterinary practice, some of the 'information gathering' may take place during, or after, the physical examination

100 Top Consultations in Small Animal General Practice, First Edition
By Peter Hill, Sheena Warman and Geoff Shawcross
© 2011 Blackwell Publishing Ltd

be aware of regional variation in the use of terminology (such as use of the term 'jags' to signify injections in Scotland) and the various terms that can be used by owners to describe symptoms.

In addition to keeping the questions simple, clinicians must be logical and objective when questioning clients. They need to extract information from the client that might not otherwise be forthcoming. Clients may not mention important facts because they are not aware of their relevance. They may also be embarrassed at disclosing information about previous home remedies or conditions involving neglect. If the clinician is not entirely convinced by a particular response, it is often helpful to repeat the question in a slightly different way to determine if the answers are consistent. Useful information can also be obtained by listening to other people in the examination room such as the client's partner or children.

When obtaining a history, clinicians should first ascertain what the owner's complaint is and how long it has been present. An immediate assessment should be made at this stage to determine if the animal looks well enough to continue with history taking. Seriously ill animals (e.g. road accidents, haemorrhage, collapse) may need urgent hospital treatment and should be admitted for physical assessment and stabilisation.

The length of time devoted to obtaining histories will depend on the nature and severity of the presenting problem. In some cases, the owner may provide very specific information that clearly refers to a single organ system and progression to a physical examination can occur after one or two answers. For example, 'I've found a lump on my dog's leg' or 'My dog was running around and suddenly started limping.' In such cases, further questioning is likely to arise during and after the examination, in order to find out if there are any related symptoms. In other cases, the owner may report a specific problem that warrants further questioning to clarify its nature. For example, if the owner says 'My dog has diarrhoea', the clinician should ask for further details about the nature of the stools, such as consistency, frequency, smell, colour, presence of blood or mucus and whether there are any associated signs of straining or difficulty defecating.

If animals are presented with non-specific problems, appear very unwell or clearly have a serious condition, it is necessary to obtain a more complete medical history. Four questions are particularly valuable in characterising an animal's general health:

- Any changes in appetite?
- Any changes in thirst?
- Any changes in weight?
- Any changes in behaviour or activity level?

If none of these parameters has altered, it can be assumed that the animal feels well in itself. If changes have been observed, an approach to investigating the problem can be found later in this book. Further questions that provide specific information about various organ systems include:

- Any vomiting or diarrhoea?
- Any coughing, sneezing, or changes in breathing?
- Any problems with urination?
- Any sign of lameness?
- Any problems with sexual activity or heat cycles?
- Any fits, seizures, 'funny turns' or strange behaviour?
- Any skin or coat problems?

Whether or not a clinician needs to ask all these questions will depend on how specific or vague the initial information is, and the index of suspicion for a multi-systemic disorder versus an organ-specific disorder.

During recheck examinations, it is not necessary to obtain the same type of history as in the initial consultation. The clinician should focus on the following aspects:

- Is the treatment working, i.e. is the animal better, worse or unchanged?
- Are there any new problems?
- Have there been any problems or adverse effects associated with the treatment?

Physical examination

The aim of the physical examination is to evaluate an abnormality that an owner has noticed, or to determine if there are any detectable abnormalities that may account for a problem revealed in the history. When performing a physical examination, a clinician can use the senses of vision (direct observation), hearing (listening or auscultation), touch (palpation) and smell. An ability to perform a physical examination requires knowledge of normal topographical and organ anatomy.

A physical examination can be partial or complete. A partial examination is when only a particular part of the body or one organ system is examined. Normally, this would be an area that the owner has identified as being abnormal, such as a limb or the skin. A complete examination involves examining the whole animal. However, an examination is rarely truly 'complete' because there would rarely be sufficient time to evaluate all the organ systems in detail. In reality, a routine 'complete' physical examination normally refers to examination of the head, chest, abdomen, lymph nodes, genitalia, legs and skin, and measuring the animal's temperature, pulse and respiratory rate (see Table 0.1).

The order in which a complete physical examination is performed is at the discretion of the clinician. Some clinicians like to record the temperature, pulse and respiratory rates first, followed by a systematic examination of the organ systems. Other clinicians (the author included)

Table 0.1 The components of a routine 'complete' physical examination.

	Normal findings	Abnormalities
General appearance	Bright Alert Responsive General symmetry	Lethargic Depressed Collapsed Hyperactive
Body weight and condition	Normal for breed	Too fat or thin
Eyes	Bright Clear Moist Normal pupil size	Discharge Redness Opacities Abnormal mucous membrane colour Anisocoria
Nose	Moist Cobblestone appearance	Discharge Lesions
Mouth	Clean teeth Healthy gums Pink mucous membranes CRT < 2 seconds Normal tongue and palate Normal pharynx	Tartar Periodontal disease Abnormal mucous membrane colour CRT > 2 seconds Inflammation Ulceration Foreign bodies Swollen tonsils
Ears	Clean	Inflammation Discharge Odour
Lymph nodes: submandibular, prescapular and popliteal	Normal size (prescapular may not be palpable in normal animals)	Enlarged Painful
Larynx and trachea	Normal shape on palpation Cough not induced by gentle palpation	Cough induced by gentle palpation
Thorax (assess by auscultation)	Normal heart sounds Normal heart rate (correlate with pulse rate) Normal heart rhythm Breathing pattern normal Normal respiratory rate Normal breath sounds	Murmurs Tachycardia Bradycardia Abnormal rhythm Laboured breathing Increased respiratory rate Increased lung sounds or audible crackles/wheezes
Abdomen (assess by palpation)	Normal size Liver not palpable Stomach not palpable Spleen not palpable Intestines feel like squelchy tubes Normal kidneys (easier to palpate in cats) Normal bladder No abnormal masses	Distended or pendulous abdomen Hepatomegaly Stomach enlarged with food or gas Splenomegaly Can palpate intestinal gas, thickening, foreign bodies, constipation, pain Enlarged or painful kidneys Bladder distended or painful Abnormal mass palpable

(Continued)

Table 0.1 (*Continued*)

	Normal findings	Abnormalities
Perineum/genitalia	Normal anus Normal vulva Normal/absent testicles Normal penis/prepuce	Masses or lesions Swelling Discharge (pus or blood)
Limbs	Normal musculature Normal joints	Lameness/abnormal gait Swollen or painful joints Limited range of movement Atrophy
Skin	Shiny coat Healthy skin Normal elasticity	Skin lesions Parasites Skin tenting (dehydration)
Rectal temperature	Normal	Elevated Decreased

CRT = capillary refill time.

prefer to conduct the examination from the front of the animal to the rear. The advantage of starting at the front end first is that the clinician can interact with the animal and put it at ease as the examination begins. Putting a thermometer into the rectum initially might not be the best way to make friends! Whichever way it is done, a skilled clinician should develop a routine that becomes second nature, allowing a complete examination to be performed in less than five minutes.

There has been a traditional view amongst educators in veterinary schools that a complete physical examination is mandatory in every case. The reality is that this is neither practicable (due to time constraints) nor necessary in order to deliver good quality medicine. Clinicians need to use their clinical skills and experience to determine what level of physical examination is required, based on the nature and severity of the illness that is presented. A partial examination can be appropriate for many problems seen in general practice such as lameness, skin problems, ocular problems, dental disease, minor external trauma or mild medical disorders. For example, a dog presenting with fleas does not need to have its abdomen or limbs palpated; a dog with a mild case of diarrhoea does not need a full dermatological or thoracic examination; a cat with ear mites does not need to have its temperature, pulse and respiration recorded.

In other situations, a detailed assessment of multiple parts of the animal would be indicated, without necessarily performing a full examination. For example, prior to general anaesthesia, an animal should have its temperature, hydration status and cardiac, respiratory and circula-

tory systems assessed in detail, but examination of the skin or limbs would not be necessary. Despite this, there are many situations where a complete examination should be considered essential, including:

- When a diagnosis is not obvious based on history and partial physical examination
- When an animal hasn't responded to treatment as expected
- When an animal presents with vague clinical signs such as lethargy, inappetence or weight loss
- When an animal presents with serious symptoms such as anaemia, jaundice, severe depression or collapse
- When an animal appears very unwell
- When an animal is pyrexic and there isn't an immediately obvious cause
- When an animal has symptoms that may indicate a systemic cause
- When a neoplastic disease is suspected or confirmed
- When puppies and kittens are checked prior to vaccinations
- When an animal is having an annual health check.

A complete examination may be initiated immediately after the history has been obtained, or it may follow on from a partial examination. If an owner has pointed out a particular area of concern, it is most appropriate to examine that part first. For example, if an animal is presented with a cutaneous mass or is limping on one leg, the owner will expect those areas to be examined first.

The clinician can then decide if a complete examination is warranted. If it is deemed necessary, the clinician can say 'We'll just check him all over to make sure there's nothing wrong anywhere else.' Some clinicians suggest that a complete examination should take place first, followed by a more focussed examination, but it may seem strange to a client when a veterinarian starts to examine the teeth of a dog that presents for lameness.

In addition to the partial and routine complete examinations described above, there are additional examination techniques that may be necessary in particular circumstances. These include ophthalmoscopic examination, otoscopic examination, detailed examination of the skin, in-depth orthopaedic palpation and assessment (e.g. flexing and extending every joint), thoracic percussion, neurological examination and behavioural assessment. Clinicians only need to employ these techniques when there is a specific clinical requirement.

Making a diagnosis or generating a list of differential diagnoses

Based on the history and physical examination, a clinician will arrive at one of four possible outcomes.

1. It may be possible to make a definitive diagnosis and recommend specific treatment. This ability is derived from clinical knowledge and experience and is known as **pattern recognition**. This approach is based on the fact that many diseases produce a characteristic pattern of historical and clinical features that the clinician can recognise. Many common conditions in small animal practice can be diagnosed in this way (e.g. abscesses, flea allergy, dental disorders, some lameness, superficial ocular problems, traumatic injuries). Pattern recognition is a very cost-effective approach which can save the owners money and time, avoid unnecessary tests, and allow the animal to get the most appropriate treatment quickly. However, it takes time for new graduates to gain the necessary experience to be fully confident with this approach.
2. It may be possible to make a tentative diagnosis and provide empirical treatment. This approach is similar to pattern recognition but differs in that the history and physical examination do not allow a definitive diagnosis to be made. With this approach, the clinician is basing the diagnosis on **probability**. Probability diagnosis requires the clinician to choose the most likely possibility for a set of clinical signs, based on the premise that 'common things occur commonly'. As with pattern recognition, this approach is used widely in small animal practice, and is appropriate for conditions such as gastritis,

sarcoptic mange, kennel cough and certain forms of lameness. It is essential when using this approach that the animal is re-evaluated if the clinical signs do not respond to treatment as expected. By definition, this approach implies that other differential diagnoses could be causing the signs and these need to be investigated if the initial outcome is not satisfactory.

3. In some cases it is only possible to generate a list of differential diagnoses. This is the case in animals presenting with general signs of illness such as polydipsia, weight loss or jaundice, but also with many organ-specific signs that either do not allow a precise diagnosis to be made, or have not resolved following treatment based on pattern recognition or probability diagnosis. In order to differentiate between multiple possible causes of a condition, clinicians need to use a **problem-oriented approach**. In this approach, the predominant problem is determined from the initial history and physical examination (e.g. pruritus, vomiting, diarrhoea, coughing, lameness, haematuria) allowing a list of prioritised differential diagnoses to be generated. If there is more than one problem, multiple differential lists can be generated. A diagnostic plan is then formulated which involves tests and investigations to rule in or out the conditions on the list(s). The tests may all be carried out at one time, or they may be staggered so that the most common or potentially serious conditions are investigated first (a sequence known as a diagnostic algorithm). In general practice, the tests are often staggered, but the final decision will be determined by the severity of the presenting problem, the likelihood of the various differentials, and the wishes and financial circumstances of the client. A fundamental principle of the problem-oriented approach is that only tests which relate to conditions on the differential list should be performed. Clinicians should not perform a standard set of tests (a 'workup') in the hope that a diagnosis will emerge from the laboratory. Failure to observe this principle will result in unnecessary tests being performed on a frequent basis. The only exception to this rule is the performance of haematological and biochemical tests, which are often more economical when run as a panel. However, clinicians should not use this as an excuse to avoid the initial thought processes that lead to a differential list.

    The problem-oriented approach can be used by students and new graduates for all cases before they have the necessary experience to utilise pattern recognition and probability diagnosis. However, it can lead to long differential lists and excessive use of tests that might not be required. Experienced clinicians can also use this approach for complicated cases and those that are not responding to treatment as expected.

4. In some cases, clinicians may not be able to think of any differential diagnoses for the condition they are faced with. This can happen with recent graduates who lack experience, but it can also occur with experienced practitioners when uncommon or rare entities are presented. When this happens, clinicians should first seek a second opinion from someone else within the practice. If the condition still remains an enigma, the most appropriate option is to recommend referral to a specialist. Specialists can apply any of the three diagnostic approaches outlined above to conditions that may be rarely seen in general practice. In some cases, pattern recognition may be possible, saving the owner and animal a prolonged series of investigations. Unless enforced by the client, it is not appropriate to perform an extensive set of tests when the clinician does not know what they are looking for.

Throughout this book, the appropriate use of these various diagnostic approaches is highlighted.

Performing diagnostic tests

Diagnostic tests are an essential component of the investigation of many cases in small animal practice. As described above, they are an integral part of the problem-oriented approach. However, there has been a trend in veterinary medicine for tests to be over-used when not needed (e.g. running blood tests on young, healthy animals prior to anaesthesia for routine procedures), under-used when they are needed (e.g. not performing cytology on ear infections and cutaneous masses), or used to replace a sound clinical approach (e.g. performing skin biopsies on a chronically itchy dog).

It is crucial that clinicians do not transfer the responsibility for making a diagnosis onto laboratories and pathologists. The clinician has the benefit of a full history and the findings from a thorough physical examination, and these go a long way towards establishing a diagnosis. Sending small pieces of the animal away for analysis can be a very valuable adjunct to this clinical process, but it must never replace it. Some of the pitfalls in diagnostic testing that clinicians must be aware of are:

- *The meaning of a normal range:* Normal ranges are established to include 95% of the healthy population. This means that 5% of the population would be outside the normal range, and could be misdiagnosed as having a disease

- *Tests are rarely 100% sensitive:* This means that an animal could have a disease and the test would not detect it
- *Tests are rarely 100% specific:* This means that the test may say the animal has the disease when in fact it doesn't
- *Many tests have a grey zone:* This means that there can be overlap between what is considered normal and abnormal
- *Some tests require interpretation:* This means that the clinician has to employ clinical skills to determine if a test result is abnormal or not
- *Some tests require specialised skills to perform:* This would include procedures such as ultrasonography and endoscopy
- *Some tests require skilful sample collection:* This applies to samples such as skin biopsies, CSF collection or bone marrow aspirates. If good quality samples are not submitted, it will be impossible to obtain meaningful results.

To overcome these problems, the use of diagnostic tests must always be focussed and not indiscriminate. They must be based on a previously generated list of differential diagnoses, and 'standard workups' should be avoided. Each test must answer the specific question – will this test help me decide if the animal has this disease? Finally, the results of diagnostic tests must always be interpreted in the context of clinico-pathological correlation. This means that the results can only be interpreted in conjunction with the clinical findings, whether they are blood tests results or biopsy reports. As it is only the clinician that has access to all the clinical and laboratory data, it is the clinician who has to perform the clinico-pathological correlation and make the final diagnosis. If the case appears too complex for all these principles to be adhered to, referral to a specialist should be recommended.

Determining a prognosis

The prognosis is a critical factor in veterinary medicine. In humans, appropriate treatment is given regardless of the prognosis. However, in animals the cost of treatment, and a general desire to not see animals suffer, influences the decision as to how, and when, to treat. The prognosis may have a large bearing on this decision. Some owners desire treatment for their animal even if the outlook is bleak. Other owners may favour euthanasia for their pet if long-term management is required, even if a successful outcome is likely.

The prognosis is usually categorised as good, fair, guarded, poor or grave. A good prognosis indicates that the animal has a good chance of making a full recovery, or having its condition successfully managed. A fair prognosis indicates that the animal has a reasonable chance of making a full recovery, or having its condition successfully managed. A guarded prognosis means that it is uncertain whether or not the animal will make a recovery. A poor prognosis means that the animal has little chance of making a full recovery, and a grave prognosis means that the animal is likely to die in the near future.

The prognosis is essentially determined by the diagnosis, but will be influenced by other factors such as the owner's commitment (both practical and financial) to the treatment regimes. The earlier a diagnosis is made, the earlier the owner can be informed about the prognosis. The majority of animals entering veterinary practices suffer from minor illnesses that have a good prognosis. In seriously ill animals, the prognosis should be determined as rapidly as possible so that the owner can make a decision about their pet. Some serious illnesses carry a good prognosis, but when the prognosis is poor or grave, euthanasia should always be considered as a potential option.

Prescribing treatment

Treatment of small animal patients can be specific or symptomatic. Specific treatments target the actual cause of the illness and can cure or control it (e.g. antibiotics for an infection, insulin for diabetes mellitus). Symptomatic treatments target the clinical signs associated with the illness. They cannot cure the underlying condition, but they can control it whilst the body heals itself or responds to a specific treatment. Symptomatic treatments can also be used to provide long-term control of incurable conditions such as atopic dermatitis or arthritis. However, symptomatic treatments should not be given in the absence of a tentative or specific diagnosis. For example, anti-emetics would be appropriate if a tentative diagnosis of gastritis had been made, but they should not be used indiscriminately to treat every animal that presents with vomiting. At best they will delay implementation of more specific therapy and at worst, they may actually harm the patient.

When treatment is prescribed, clinicians should ask themselves 'Why am I giving this specific medication and what do I hope to achieve?' The systematic review, appraisal and use of clinical research findings to ensure the delivery of optimum care for a particular condition is known as 'evidence-based medicine.' At the moment, evidence-based veterinary medicine is still in its infancy, and many drugs are prescribed on the basis of clinical and anecdotal experience. The ultimate aim is that the efficacy of all drugs and treatment regimes will have been determined on the basis of blinded, randomised, controlled trials that definitively prove their benefit. At the opposite end of the spectrum to evidence-based medicine are some old prescribing practices that appear to have survived into the modern era. One such practice is the false belief that it is beneficial to start a course of treatment by always giving an injection of a drug or vitamin solution. There is often no rationale to this approach and it has more to do with a clinician's perceived need to be seen to be doing something technical in front of the client in order to justify their fee.

Clinicians should always balance the potency or aggressiveness of a treatment regime against the severity of the disease. This follows the principle of 'First, do no harm'. An animal should never be placed in a situation where the effects of the treatment are worse than the original disease. For example, this can happen when long-term glucocorticoids are used inappropriately to treat pruritus, resulting in iatrogenic Cushing's syndrome. In addition to potential adverse effects, clinicians need to ensure that owners are aware of the cost of medications, and any associated monitoring, especially if they are required in the long term.

In most countries, the prescribing of drugs to animals is governed by law. In Europe, the process is regulated by asking veterinarians to follow a prescribing cascade. This states that drugs should be chosen in the following order:

- The first choice of drug should be a veterinary product that is licensed to treat a specific condition in a specific species
- If a specific product in this category is not available, clinicians should choose a veterinary product that is licensed in the species to treat a similar condition (e.g. the treatment of *Cheyletiella* mite infestation with selamectin)
- If no such product exists, a product licensed for use in other veterinary species to treat similar conditions should be considered (e.g. the use of ivermectin to treat refractory canine demodicosis)
- If there are no appropriate licensed veterinary products to treat the condition, clinicians can then consider using either human drugs (e.g. the use of azathioprine to treat immune-mediated diseases) or importing a veterinary drug from another country under license (e.g. the use of milbemycin to treat refractory canine demodicosis).

The treatment of animals with generic human drugs, where equivalent licensed veterinary products exist, is illegal. It is also illegal to progress down the prescribing cascade in order to save costs.

When prescribing treatment, clinicians should also consider the complexity of the treatment regime, and how it will fit in with the owner's lifestyle. Lack of owner compliance is common, both in human and veterinary medicine. The easier the treatment is to administer, the more likely that it will be done properly. In general, drugs that can be given once daily are more likely to be administered correctly than drugs requiring three times daily dosing.

Compliance is also more likely if time is taken (by the veterinary surgeon or nurse) to ensure that the owner is able to medicate their pet in an efficient manner.

Re-check examinations

Re-check examinations are not required if the owner can adequately assess the outcome of a treatment course. This is likely to be the case when the condition has an obvious clinical sign, such as vomiting or diarrhoea. However, a re-check will be necessary if the response to treatment can only be assessed by a trained clinician. This would be the case if further physical examination were required, such as abdominal palpation or auscultation of the chest. Re-checks should not be arranged just to see how the animal is 'doing'. There must be a specific purpose for the re-check and the clinician needs to decide in advance why the animal needs to come back, what milestones it should have reached, and what decisions will be made, based on how it has responded. If the animal is on long-term treatment, periodic re-checks may be necessary for monitoring, fine-tuning and to comply with local rules or legislation requiring animals to be under the veterinarian's care before prescribing drugs.

During a re-check, the diagnostic approaches outlined above can all be used, but usually in a truncated form. The history can be brief and the physical examination can focus on the abnormality being treated. However, if the animal is not responding as expected, it may be necessary to re-evaluate the whole diagnostic approach to ensure that nothing has been missed. For example, if the animal has been treated on the basis of a pattern or probability diagnosis, it may be necessary to consider a wider problem-oriented approach which brings in some other differential diagnoses. Additional testing may then be warranted. In the absence of a definitive diagnosis, it is not appropriate to just keep changing treatments to see if another drug would work better.

In some cases, it is necessary for a different clinician to see an animal for a re-check. Although this is not ideal in terms of continuity, it is sometimes unavoidable for practical or logistical reasons. In such cases, it is essential that the first clinician provides medical records that clearly indicate to the second clinician what the owner is expecting. An example might be 'If no response to nonsteroidal anti-inflammatory drugs (NSAIDs), advise radiography.' This ensures that the owner receives consistent advice. Accurate medical records, stating clearly what was observed during the first consultation, and consistent use of terminology, are also important so that clients realise the two clinicians are talking about the same thing.

Clinicians should not deliberately book cases in to see a different veterinarian in order to avoid seeing a difficult or frustrating case. If a second opinion is required, it

should be discussed with the owner and second veterinary surgeon in advance.

Hospitalised patients

If an animal needs to be admitted into the veterinary clinic, it needs to be carefully monitored by the nursing staff and thoroughly examined on at least a daily basis so that the effects of any treatments can be assessed. One way of monitoring such patients is to use the 'SOAP' system (Subjective Objective Assessment Plan). The subjective parameters include such things as whether the dog looks brighter, has started to eat, or has stopped vomiting. The objective parameters include things such as the temperature, pulse rate, respiratory rate or volume of water drunk. Based on the subjective and objective parameters, the clinician can make an assessment. This might be something like 'The dog is brighter, the vomiting has stopped and the temperature is back to normal. Much improved from yesterday'. After the assessment, the clinician can make a plan. For example, in the above case the plan might be to 'introduce small amounts of food, monitor for vomiting and keep in until tomorrow'. The hospitalised animal is 'SOAPed' each day until the plan is to send it home.

The role of specialists

Within the first year of entering general practice, new graduates will have built up a wide portfolio of experience that covers many of the common conditions seen in small animals. By that stage, they should feel confident and competent in their abilities to handle routine cases. However, the explosion of knowledge in veterinary medicine has resulted in large numbers of rare diseases being described and the emergence of ever more advanced forms of diagnostic testing. It is no longer possible for general practitioners to be informed about all the advances in all disciplines, and to develop the technical expertise to conduct all the procedures. In addition, management of complex cases can require specialist experience and monitoring. It is no longer acceptable for a clinician to attempt to diagnose and manage a complex condition of which they have no previous experience, without having received further training in that discipline or having suggested referral to the owner. Veterinarians should, therefore, consider referral to a specialist as a normal extension of their everyday practice, as it is in the medical field. It is certainly not a sign of failure.

In general, referral should be recommended at the outset if an unfamiliar disease is encountered. It is far better for the animal and owner to see the specialist immediately than as a last resort after multiple consultations and a whole series of tests. In some cases, an initial specialist opinion can also save the owner money, because it may be possible to avoid unnecessary tests. When it is not initially obvious that the case is going to be difficult to diagnose, the 'three-consultation rule' can be used as a general guide to determine if referral should be offered. This states that when an animal is seen for the same complaint, a clinician should have made a definitive diagnosis within three consultations. If at the end of the third consultation, the clinician is no nearer to establishing a definitive diagnosis than they were at the outset, the owner should be offered a referral. Referral should also be offered when a condition that requires specialist management is diagnosed. Examples of when cases should be referred are highlighted throughout this book.

Clinicians should be selective in their choice of a specialist. To develop specialist expertise in a specific discipline requires many years of advanced training, typically acquired during a residency under the close supervision of qualified specialists. At the end of this training period, the clinician should obtain a Diploma or become Board Certified in their speciality. Some veterinary clinicians offer referral services without having received such training or qualifications. In some countries, lesser qualifications (e.g. the certificate system in the UK) might be put forward as providing eligibility to provide a referral service. These qualifications were never intended to assess a candidate's ability to practice referral medicine and in no way compare to the level of knowledge and clinical training that is required to obtain a Diploma. Therefore, when offering a referral, clients should be made fully aware of the options available so that they can make an informed choice. They may decide to consider factors such as travel distance in preference to level of expertise, but that must remain their choice, and should not be imposed on them without prior discussion.

Section 1
Health checks and vaccinations

Geoff Shawcross

A new puppy or kitten will be presented either by an existing client who has acquired another pet, or by a new client who has never been to the practice before. The purpose of this consultation is to evaluate the clinical well-being of the pet, advise on diet and discuss preventative medicine. However, during this time, the client will also be forming their opinion of the expertise, compassion and efficiency of the whole practice team.

Pre-purchase advice

Clients may occasionally ask veterinarians for advice about choosing particular breeds. However, what appears to be a simple question can have a very complicated answer. Choosing a breed of dog or cat is a very personal matter, so the final decision can rest only with the purchaser. Potential owners should be advised to do some research into the breeds they are considering, and ensure that they have the time, facilities and financial resources to own the breed that they choose. Factors that need to be considered are the size of the animal, the amount of exercise it will need and its likely temperament. In particular, veterinarians need to be aware of the many breed predispositions to disease so that they can answer specific questions when asked. For example, potential owners may want to know if the breed they would like to buy is prone to joint disease, skin problems or cancer.

If there is the opportunity to advise the client before they actually purchase their new pet, it should be suggested that finalising the purchase should be dependent on a satisfactory report from a veterinary surgeon. If the clinician subsequently finds a problem that could be detrimental, or have long-term financial implications, the animal then can be returned. The clinician should appreciate, however, that the majority of clients 'bond' very quickly with their new pet and cancelling the purchase, even after an unsatisfactory veterinary surgeon's report, is rarely an option. Indeed, many owners will feel that they have 'rescued' their new pet if they felt that the breeder/supplier would not look after it properly were it

to be returned, and are often prepared to invest the necessary care and finances to resolve the problems. If the animal is to be returned, treatment (especially surgical procedures) should not be instigated unless there are significant welfare issues.

The first consultation

The pet may be presented as soon as it has been acquired, but it is often better to see the animal after it has had the chance to settle in its new home for a few days and the owner has had the opportunity to observe its behaviour and demeanour. The owners can then describe any issues of concern and may describe signs that warrant further evaluation during the clinical examination. In most cases, puppies and kittens will be presented when they are 8–10 weeks of age, at which time they require their first vaccinations.

It is always helpful if reception or nursing staff can obtain the signalment (breed, age and sex) before the clinician sees the animal. It is permissible for them not to know that the dog is a Nova Scotia Duck-Tolling Retriever and not a mongrel but, unfortunately, not the veterinary surgeon!

Many owners are worried that their newly acquired pet will be exposed to infections at the practice and this concern should be appreciated. Practice policy may include keeping kittens and puppies contained within a pet carrier, or even waiting outside the building in the car, pending their appointment. At all times, the examination room, equipment and clinician should appear to be scrupulously clean. Owners of pedigree pets should be asked about the future use of the animal, whether it is for breeding, working or simply a family pet. Owners who wish to show their animals should be advised to seek the opinion of a recognised judge of the breed, if conformation is an absolute priority. The clinician's opinion should be confined to veterinary matters.

The clinician should check through any paperwork that the client has been given by the breeder/supplier. Often, they will have been given copies of the results of breed-related health schemes of the parents (e.g. hip scores, elbow scores, eye schemes) and this will introduce a discussion about diseases that will not be apparent at the time of the examination but may develop as that animal gets older (such as hip dysplasia, elbow dysplasia, cataracts, retinopathies, heart disease). In addition, the client

100 Top Consultations in Small Animal General Practice, First Edition
By Peter Hill, Sheena Warman and Geoff Shawcross
© 2011 Blackwell Publishing Ltd

is likely to have been given a diet sheet, together with advice about worming and vaccinations. This information should be checked, to make sure it is broadly consistent with practice policy. Any differences in advice should be explained to the client.

The clinical examination

Time taken to ensure the consultation is pleasurable for the pet will pay dividends later. Forceful restraint and painful manipulations may make the animal fearful at future visits.

The physical examination should be thorough and follow the general principles outlined in the Introduction. Particular attention should be focussed on signs of infectious and congenital disease. The limitations of the examination should be explained to the owner and the results of all parameters that have been checked (whether normal or not) must be recorded.

General findings

- Puppies and kittens should be alert, bold and inquisitive, but it should be appreciated that some individuals are naturally reserved in a strange environment. Young animals that are genuinely ill are invariably lethargic, disinterested in their surroundings and reluctant to eat
- Coughing (dogs) and sneezing (cats) initially should be considered as signs of an infectious disease
- Diarrhoea is common and often associated with a change in diet but if the animal has diarrhoea when purchased, this concern should be addressed as it could have an infectious cause. Diarrhoea in young cats can be frustrating to treat
- Neurological signs such as intention tremors, ataxia or dysmetria may or may not progress, but rarely improve
- Breeds that have extreme characteristics (e.g. dwarfism, hairlessness, excessive skin folds) have their own 'in-built' problems and these should be mentioned, so that the owner knows what to look out for/expect as the animal matures. However, it would be unwise to make disparaging remarks about the characteristics of a particular breed to the owner, because often it is the eccentricity that has attracted the owner to the breed in the first place.

The head

- The mucous membranes should be normal. Abnormalities, such as cyanosis or pallor, are serious and will be associated with other clinical signs
- The mouth should be checked for cleft palates and normal primary dentition. Acceptable dental occlusion varies with the breed standards, although in most breeds maxillary prognathism (overbite) is a fault. Although malocclusions are a serious show fault, they are rarely of clinical significance for the pet animal
- The eyes should be clear and bright, with no ocular discharges or epiphora. The eyelids should not show signs of entropion, which if present can lead to severe corneal damage. A degree of ectropion is a characteristic of certain breeds and would have to be deemed normal in such individuals. The nictitans should be in the correct position and there should be no deformity of its free edge. The globes and pupils should be of equal size, and there should be no signs of a strabismus or nystagmus. The identification of lens defects and retinopathies in very young animals requires considerable expertise, and it is often difficult to obtain the necessary restraint required for a thorough ophthalmoscopic examination. Rather than carry out a poor ophthalmoscopic examination, it may be preferable to outline the conditions that may exist (within the breed) and advise referral to a specialist at the appropriate age
- The ear canals should be clean and odour-free. Infestation with ear mites (*Otodectes cynotis*) is quite common and requires prompt treatment. The pinnae of most prick-eared dogs will not be erect until they are several months of age
- The nose should be free of discharges. The external nares are often small in brachycephalic breeds (both dogs and cats) and although this may accepted as part of the breed standard, extreme stenosis may result in respiratory problems as the animal matures.

Chest and abdomen

- Auscultation of the lungs should not reveal any abnormal sounds
- The heart should be carefully evaluated on both sides of the chest, over the entire cardiac area, listening for heart murmurs that would suggest a congenital heart defect (see Chapter 56). Some murmurs associated with congenital heart disease can be very focal. If there is any doubt about the origin or significance of a murmur, the opinion of a specialist should be sought
- The rib cage should be palpated for symmetry
- Abdominal palpation need not be exhaustive, especially if it is being resented, as it is rarely productive. In the absence of other gastro-intestinal signs, thickening of the intestines would suggest a significant worm burden

- Umbilical hernias are very common and some may warrant surgical correction. This, however, is rarely urgent and can usually be deferred until the vaccination course is complete. In bitches, it can often be corrected at the same time as neutering. Inguinal hernias are much less common and can be difficult to detect. They carry a higher risk of complications later in life and should be repaired when the animal is reasonably mature
- Cryptorchidism is common but the testicles of very small animals can be difficult to palpate. It is a serious defect in animals that are to be shown or used for breeding and the clinician must be confident before declaring both testicles are present. If there is any doubt, the clinician should defer making a decision.

Skeletal system

- Limbs of chondrodystrophic or giant breeds can be difficult to evaluate but should always appear symmetrical when viewed from the front and rear. Growth plate disorders are uncommon but can lead to limb deformity that develops at an alarming rate. If such a deformity is suspected, expert advice should be sought at an early stage.

Skin

- The coat should be clean and should not smell
- The skin should be examined carefully for evidence of parasites
- Pruritus is common and may even lead to areas of excoriation. Allergic skin disease (atopic dermatitis, dietary) is uncommon in the puppy or kitten, and pruritus is usually caused by ectoparasites (whether obvious or not).

Taking the temperature of puppies and kittens is not particularly helpful unless they appear unwell. If it is done, it should be left until the end of the clinical examination, as the procedure is often resented. Elevated temperatures are common, especially in nervous puppies, and should be interpreted with care and in the context of the animal's demeanour.

Vaccination

One of the main reasons for the puppy or kitten consultation is to start the vaccination programme. However, it is unwise to administer vaccines until the animal has had time to settle into its new environment in case it is incubating any infectious diseases. If the animal develops signs of illness shortly after being acquired, the clinician and owner will then know that it was not induced by the vaccine.

Dogs are typically vaccinated against distemper, parvovirus, infectious canine hepatitis (adenovirus-1) and leptospirosis. In some countries, rabies vaccination is also required. Protection can also be given against canine kennel cough organisms by vaccinating for canine parainfluenza and *Bordetella bronchiseptica*. The necessity for these latter vaccines should be based on a risk–benefit analysis. The clinical signs that can be seen with these diseases is summarised in Table 1.1.

Cats are typically vaccinated against feline viral rhinotracheitis (herpes virus, FHV), feline calicivirus (FCV), and feline panleukopenia (feline parvovirus). In some countries, rabies vaccination is also required. Protection against feline leukaemia virus (FeLV) should also be advised in cats that are at risk of contracting this infection (especially outdoor cats or in multi-cat households). Vaccination against feline immunodeficiency virus is

Table 1.1 Clinical signs of the infectious diseases that dogs are normally vaccinated against.

Disease	Signs and symptoms
Distemper	Oculo-nasal discharge, conjunctivitis, coughing, dyspnoea, vomiting, diarrhoea, lethargy, anorexia, fever followed by neurological signs (seizures, vestibular disease, cerebellar signs, paresis or involuntary twitching)
Parvovirus	Vomiting, diarrhoea (often haemorrhagic), lethargy, anorexia, fever, dehydration and shock
Infectious canine hepatitis	Corneal oedema (blue eye), vomiting, diarrhoea, abdominal pain, hepatomegaly, jaundice, coagulopathy, lethargy, anorexia and fever
Leptospirosis	Shivering, muscle tenderness, lumbar pain, vomiting, polydipsia, jaundice, petechial haemorrhages, lethargy, anorexia and fever
Rabies	Behaviour change, difficulty swallowing, ptyalism, bark change, dropped jaw, aggression, biting, ataxia, paralysis, seizures
'Kennel cough' Parainfluenza virus *Bordetella bronchiseptica*	'Hacking' cough, sensitive trachea, nasal discharge (see Chapter 54)

Table 1.2 Clinical signs of the infectious diseases that cats are normally vaccinated against.

Disease	Signs and symptoms
'Cat flu' Herpes virus Calicivirus (*Chlamydophila felis*) (*Bordetella bronchiseptica*)	Sneezing, nasal discharge, ocular discharge, ulcer on tongue, corneal ulcers, lethargy, anorexia, fever (see Chapter 55)
Panleukopenia	Abortion of dead kittens, 'fading kittens', sudden death, vomiting, diarrhoea, extreme lethargy, ataxia, intention tremors, seizures
FeLV	See Chapter 12
FIV	See Chapter 13
Rabies	Aggression, altered voice, biting, ptyalism, ataxia, paralysis, seizures

available in certain countries, but this can complicate subsequent diagnosis of the infection using immunological tests (see Chapter 13). The clinical signs that accompany these diseases are summarised in Table 1.2.

The recommended protocols and timing of vaccination varies between manufacturers and can change as new scientific information comes to light. Veterinarians should familiarise themselves with the type of vaccines used in their particular clinic and the requirements in specific geographic locations.

Antiparasitic treatment

The first consultation is also a good opportunity to continue deworming programmes and to initiate preventative treatment against other parasites. Puppies and kittens require continual protection against the development of intestinal roundworms (*Toxocara canis*, *Toxocara felis*, *Toxascaris leonina*). They should also be treated for tapeworms (*Dipylidium caninum*, *Taenia* spp.), hookworms (*Ancylostoma caninum*, *Uncinaria* spp.) and whipworms (*Trichuris vulpis*). In endemic areas, protection against *Angiostrongylus vasorum* is also advised. In some countries, year-round protection against heartworm (*Dirofilaria immitis*) is also required.

Many pets also require protection against ectoparasites (fleas, ticks). The nature of the control programme should be based on a risk–benefit analysis for the individual

patient, as the requirement for such prophylactic treatment varies dramatically with geographic location and even microenvironment.

There are many products available for antiparasitic treatment in dogs and cats with differing active agents, spectrum of activity and routes of administration. However, as yet, there is no single product that will effectively treat and protect against all the parasites listed above. Clinicians must determine what level of protection is required for their patient against each of the parasites, bearing in mind that this requirement can change at various stages of the animal's life. In most clinics, there will be established protocols that are based on local conditions. Despite this, there is always an element of choice when selecting antiparasitic products and factors such as cost, and the ease and frequency of administration can be taken into account.

Further advice

Diet

Discussions about diet can be fraught if the clinician disagrees with the advice that the owner has received from the breeder. On this subject, the client is likely to favour the opinions of the breeder and want to continue with their recommendations. However, dietary faults, such as over-supplementation with vitamins and minerals, are common. In addition, the palatability of some diets may not suit the individual, and the quantity of food recommended by the breeder may be too much or too little. In such cases, it can be suggested to the owner that the breeder's diet should be used as a basis for a transition to an adult diet. Many practices have nursing staff who are competent at giving dietary advice but initially the veterinarian should be responsible for advising any dietary changes.

Neutering

The practice will have established its preferred times for routine neutering. Although this operation will not be carried out imminently, the subject should be broached, if only to obtain the client's views on the procedure. Neutering is not appropriate in all cases (see Chapter 3). If the animal is to be neutered, other procedures, such as hernia repair can be carried out at the same time.

Training and socialisation

Advising on this subject can be very time consuming. Many practices have lay-staff who are competent to advise on this subject, and run (or know of) suitable classes or puppy parties.

There has been a tradition in some countries to alter the appearance of some dog breeds by docking their tails, removing their dewclaws and cropping their ears. There are legal, ethical and moral issues surrounding this practice and clinicians should be aware of the legislation that exists in their own countries. For example, ear cropping is illegal in the UK but is permissible in the USA. Tail docking is now illegal in England, Wales and Scotland, although it is permitted in certain specified breeds in England and Wales if specific written evidence is provided that the dog will be involved in fieldwork. The reader is advised to consult current guidelines (e.g. RCVS website).

Additional recommendations

Some caution should be exercised when dispensing medication to young animals and the drug manufacturer's recommendations should be followed explicitly. Also, it is generally unwise to try and treat a number of different things at the same time. Initial vaccination, treatment for ectoparasites and worm infections, together with a change in a dietary regime, may result in the animal becoming unwell, without the clinician being able to know exactly why.

It is well known that clients remember few of the facts that they are told during a consultation. As this consultation has to cover a wide range of topics, much of the advice should be presented in a practice handout, so that the client can digest the information at home. However, advice should always be given confidently and preferably with a specific recommendation. Although there is a basic tenet that owners should be given all the facts so that they can make informed decisions, the clinician is in the unique position of having received considerable training and should therefore be able to suggest the most suitable course of action; the clinician should not shy away from this responsibility.

Geoff Shawcross

Traditionally, the annual health check consultation has been associated with 'booster' vaccinations. It is often considered a 'quick' or 'catch-up' consultation during a busy session. This concept is outmoded and unfair to clients. In addition to performing the vaccination, the animal should have a thorough health check and time should be taken to discuss any problems perceived by the owners, to instigate and reinforce preventative medical treatments, and to identify clinical problems at an early stage in their development.

Problems that might be raised by owners

Some clients may use the annual health check to discuss clinical concerns. This can include non-urgent medical problems that they have noticed but 'put off' until the annual vaccinations are due. Such problems might include obesity, mild lameness (stiffness on rising or reluctance to jump associated with degenerative joint disease), intermittent diarrhoea, dental problems, non-pruritic skin conditions or behaviour problems. The annual health check is also a time when owners may seek advice about breeding or neutering. Some problems (e.g. behavioural or dietary advice) can be very time-consuming to explain but as they are not urgent and will not affect the vaccination protocol, it may be sensible to arrange another consultation later. This will allow a fuller discussion with the client and can involve other members of the practice team who are qualified to give dietary or behavioural advice.

The clinical examination

The annual health check provides an opportunity to perform a full physical examination of the patient. This is particularly important if the animal hasn't been presented to the practice for a whole year, or if on recent visits it has only received a partial examination related to a specific problem. A typical protocol for such an examination is described in the Introduction: Diagnostic and therapeutic approaches. As the clinician develops an effective examination technique, it should be possible to complete the clinical examination quickly and efficiently. During the

examination, owners should be encouraged to point out areas that concern them.

Because one of the primary reasons for the consultation is vaccination, one particular aim of the physical examination should be to identify those problems that would potentially preclude vaccination. These include:

- signs of infection
- conditions requiring treatment that would interfere with the effects of vaccination such as glucocorticoids or immunosuppressive drugs
- serious illness that would make vaccination superfluous, e.g. identifying an abdominal mass.

Young animals are likely to have fewer medical problems than older ones but clinicians should be aware of problems that are breed-related and may need to be addressed at an early stage. Clinicians should be particularly careful in assessing changes that often go unnoticed by owners (e.g. cataracts, corneal opacities, eyelid tumours, dental disease, cutaneous lumps, mammary tumours) or which cannot be detected by them (e.g. heart murmurs, abdominal masses). With advancing age there is an increase in the incidence of disease, so any signs and symptoms need to be identified and their significance quantified.

Depending on the history given by the owner, or the findings of the physical examination, some animals may require additional evaluations such as ophthalmoscopic, otoscopic, orthopaedic or rectal examinations.

Recommending treatments and procedures

Following a clinical examination, a clinician may recommend some form of treatment or procedure for an abnormality that has been detected. As this may be something that the owner was not previously aware of, the subject has to be broached with some sensitivity. Some owners will want any problem identified to be dealt with, regardless of costs. However, it is not unusual for owners to want to see a cost–benefit analysis before consenting to a procedure, especially if they themselves do not perceive the condition to be clinically significant and funds are limited. They will usually consent if a tangible welfare benefit can be demonstrated in the short or medium term. As animals get older, there is also a risk-benefit to be considered. For example, the removal of a benign growth for cosmetic reasons may be appropriate in a middle-aged animal but

100 Top Consultations in Small Animal General Practice, First Edition
By Peter Hill, Sheena Warman and Geoff Shawcross
© 2011 Blackwell Publishing Ltd

not in a geriatric patient, where anaesthesia may pose a significant risk. The following chapters are designed to help clinicians make prudent decisions and give the appropriate advice.

A recent trend is the recommendation to take blood samples from older patients that are clinically normal, with a view to detecting early degenerative changes in the major organs. This is partly due to the increased availability of in-house analysers, which have made it easier to process the blood samples. Veterinarians must be aware that the costs involved in running such tests may be beyond the means of some clients, and a refusal to accept the clinician's advice on this matter does not constitute neglect. Furthermore, if such tests are recommended, the results of these analyses (especially if they show only marginal abnormalities) should be viewed critically and with some circumspection before advising the client, and embarking on what may be a long-term treatment plan. It is common for routine haematological and biochemical analyses to reveal values that are outside the normal ranges, but this does not always mean there is a clinical problem (see the Introduction: Diagnostic and therapeutic approaches, for further details). However, clinicians need to be aware when abnormal test results need to be followed up. For example, mild azotaemia does not necessarily indicate renal failure, but it would be important to follow this up with a urine analysis to assess the renal concentrating ability.

Vaccination

Many clients will regard this as the major reason for annual attendance at a veterinary practice. Most practices send booster-reminder letters to their clients, which should not only inform the owner that the inoculations are due, but explain that a thorough clinical examination will take place and that there will be opportunities for the client to discuss any problems they feel are important. It should be pointed out to clients that the responsibility to present their pet for vaccination within the prescribed period rests entirely with them and that booster-reminders are a service provided by the practice but should not be relied upon. Failure to make this clear could make the Practice liable for any financial implications that may arise, such as restarting a lapsed vaccination programme or the need for additional laboratory tests (e.g. rabies titres for travelling pets).

Vaccination protocols will have been established by the individual practice, taking into account the vaccine manufacturer's recommendations and the level of disease risk in the animal's environment. The diseases that are typically vaccinated against are summarised in Chapter 1. As the duration of immunity varies with the individual antigens, it is unnecessary to give a full booster for every vaccine every year. Clinicians will therefore need to familiarise themselves with the protocols recommended by the manufacturer of the vaccines they use, while owners will also need to be told why the vaccine may be different in one year compared to another, as this may influence cost. It is best if the vaccines are given towards the end of the consultation, when it is clear that nothing is going to interfere with the protocol.

Other forms of preventative medicine

The annual health check also provides an opportunity to reinforce other aspects of preventative medicine in addition to vaccination. Three important issues worthy of specific mention are parasite control, dental care and obesity. The client should be reminded that parasite control is not only beneficial to the long-term welfare of their pet, but also of public health importance. Parasites that require control measures include intestinal helminths and cestodes, fleas, ticks, biting flies and heartworm, but some of these have restricted geographical distribution (see Chapter 1). In recent years, there has been a substantial increase in the number of products available to treat all types of parasites, and improvements in the mode of their administration have helped increase owner compliance with dosage regimes. All members of the practice, veterinary surgeons, nurses and receptionists, should be giving the same advice regarding parasite control; the protocols should be decided and agreed upon in the light of product efficacy, spectrum of activity and cost. Whenever possible, explanations should be kept simple so that the client can remember what they are trying to achieve and what it is they must do.

Dental care is often neglected in pet dogs and cats. The annual health check is a good time to reinforce prophylactic measures such as tooth brushing or the use of dental chews. It is also a good time to recommend routine dental work such as ultrasonic scaling that can prevent the subsequent development of more serious problems such as periodontal disease.

Obesity is a common but particularly difficult problem in small animal practice. The clinical problems caused or exacerbated by obesity (see Appendix 4) are well documented and despite widespread acceptance of these problems, owners of obese pets are often very resistant to suggestions that their pet needs to be on a weight-loss diet. It can take considerable tact and encouragement to convince them that their pet will benefit by being slim and fit. Nurse-run 'weight-watcher' clinics can be particularly helpful in motivating owners. The annual check-up is an ideal time to weigh the animal and record its condition score. Keeping a record will not only monitor changes in weight but also help if dispensing 'over-the-counter' preparations, when the pet is not presented.

Geoff Shawcross

Neutering (desexing) pets is a routine procedure in general practice but because it is so common, there is a danger that the veterinary surgeon will assume that an owner fully understands the advantages, disadvantages and risks that are associated with the procedure. It is prudent for the veterinary surgeon to discuss the procedure to ensure that it is both appropriate for the animal and will achieve the owner's aim. All animals presented for surgical neutering should have a pre-surgical physical examination, to detect any problems that may increase anaesthetic risk, and to check that both testicles have descended in males and that females are not in oestrus.

Reasons for neutering

- Prevention of unwanted puppies and kittens. This is the most common reason for neutering and is frequently promoted by animal charities in an attempt to reduce the unwanted and abandoned animal population. The charities often support neutering schemes financially
- Modification of behaviour associated with reproduction. During oestrus, vulval bleeding and the bitch's desire to escape can be problematic for some owners. The 'calling' behaviour of queens can be both persistent and recurrent, leading to a loss of bodily condition and attracting the unwanted attention of local tomcats. Neutering male cats and dogs reduces (but does not eliminate) territorial aggression, territorial marking and the desire to roam
- Modification of general behaviour. Neutering only affects those behaviour patterns associated with the sex hormones and not those that are inherited or learned. In this context, neutering will have little effect on the general behaviour of cats of either sex, or on bitches. Owners should be warned that neutering in an attempt to modify undesirable behaviour (e.g. in aggressive dogs) may be helpful but is not reliable, and invariably requires additional behaviour-modification techniques

- Prophylaxis of medical conditions. Spaying will prevent pyometra and false pregnancies, and can reduce the incidence of mammary tumours if performed before the female's second season. The overall incidence of male genital disease is lower but castration removes the risk of testicular neoplasia and reduces the incidence of prostatic disease in dogs and fight-associated diseases in the cat (e.g. cat bite abscesses, FIV). Males with one or both testicles undescended should always have both removed, as retained testicles are more likely to become neoplastic
- Treatment of medical conditions. Surgical neutering is used to treat testicular and ovarian disease and pyometra, and often as adjunctive treatment where it is thought that the sex hormones have a role in the cause or maintenance of the disease (e.g. diseases of the mammary glands, vaginal tumours, perineal hernias, prostatic disease, circum-anal adenomas and diabetes mellitus in bitches)
- Prevention of transmission of inherited diseases. Breeders will usually neuter animals that carry serious heritable defects.

Disadvantages or complications associated with surgical neutering

- It is irreversible, leaving no opportunity for future breeding
- It may have an effect on coat texture and colour. Some dogs of both sexes will develop or retain a juvenile texture or colour to their coat. Owners of colour point breeds (Siamese, Birman, etc.) should be warned that the coat colour will be darker over the surgically prepared site when it re-grows
- There are general surgical risks, such as wound infections, haemorrhage and risks associated with general anaesthesia. The risk of intra-operative haemorrhage is significantly higher if surgery is performed when the animal is in oestrus. In part, this is due to the effects of oestrogen on coagulation, but the genital tract also becomes more vascular and friable. The possibility of coagulation defects in susceptible breeds (e.g. von Willebrand's disease in the Doberman Pinscher) should also be considered

100 Top Consultations in Small Animal General Practice, First Edition
By Peter Hill, Sheena Warman and Geoff Shawcross
© 2011 Blackwell Publishing Ltd

- Urinary incontinence due to sphincter mechanism incompetence is eight times more common in spayed bitches, and is more likely if the procedure is performed before the first season. This disorder can require prolonged medication, or even corrective surgery
- Neutering may contribute to obesity. Some breeds, such as the Labrador, Golden Retriever, spaniels and collies, have a great propensity to become obese after neutering. Regular weighing and attention to diet and exercise should minimise this risk. There is also a tendency for cats, particularly those offered ad-lib food, to become obese, which carries a heightened risk of developing diabetes mellitus and hepatic lipidosis
- Persistence of infantile genitalia may occur. This would only be significant in bitches, which can subsequently develop vulval fold dermatitis. The incidence and severity of vulval fold dermatitis is exacerbated by obesity and urinary incontinence
- Some male dogs, particularly those with an inherently placid temperament, become extremely lethargic and disinterested in their surroundings after castration
- Failure to remove all ovarian tissue will result in recurrence of oestrus behaviour
- Failure to remove the entire uterus can result in the development of a stump pyometra.

Recommended age for neutering

There is general agreement that cats of both sexes can be neutered before puberty without the risk of undesirable side-effects developing. This would typically be performed around 5–6 months of age. Opinions are divided, however, on the best age to neuter dogs. The protagonists for neutering before puberty cite improved prophylaxis and the rapid recovery from a simplified surgical procedure as the main advantages. Conversely, neutering after puberty may reduce the risks of complications such as urinary incontinence developing later. There is general agreement that there is no advantage in letting bitches or queens have one litter before neutering.

If a bitch is not neutered before her first season, then the best time to neuter her is between seasons, as this is when the hormonal activity is at its lowest. As most bitches come into season every 6 months, it would normally be recommended that neutering takes place three months after the bitch has been in season.

Chemical control of breeding

Oestrus can be inhibited in both the bitch and queen by the administration of progestagens, either by injection or by tablet. These methods are used when breeding cycles need to be controlled but not eliminated, where surgical risks are high, or where the owner finds the risk of undesirable side-effects unacceptable. Return of oestrus following cessation of the drug is unpredictable and there is an increased risk of pyometra, diabetes mellitus and mammary tumours in animals treated with progestagens. For further details the reader is referred to Chapter 72 (Oestrus control, misalliance and false pregnancies).

Delmadinone acetate (Tardak, Pfizer) is a progestagen that can be used as an adjunct in the treatment of prostatic disease and for male-hormone dominated behavioural problems but it is not a sterilising agent. If treatment of a medical or behavioural problem with the drug has the desired effect then surgical castration can be carried out later, with increased certainty of achieving the desired result.

Currently, there is no satisfactory method of chemically sterilising male cats, although there have been recent advances in chemical sterilisation of the male dog. Suprelorin (Virbac), available as a subcutaneous implant containing deslorelin, reduces libido and spermatogenesis in adult dogs, effectively sterilising them and reducing the effects of testosterone on behaviour and medical conditions. Deslorelin is a gonadotropin-releasing hormone (GnRH) agonist and acts by suppressing the function of the pituitary–gonadal axis when given as a low, continuous dose. This suppression results in the failure to synthesise and/or release follicle-stimulating hormone (FSH) and luteinising hormone (LH), the hormones responsible for the maintenance of fertility. The effects of the drug are temporary and wear off after six months unless the dog is re-implanted and is, therefore, likely to be considered an option for owners who are undecided about surgical castration. Currently, treatment with deslorelin would be expensive in the long-term.

An alternative approach available in some countries is intra-testicular injection of zinc gluconate (Neutersol). Neutersol is a Food and Drug Administration (FDA)-approved injectable sterilant used for chemical castration ('sterilization') of male dogs 3–10 months of age. According to the manufacturer, Neutersol is a safe, effective, and convenient alternative to surgical castration and is 99.6% effective. Employing Neutersol for castration takes a fraction of the time of surgical castration. This drug is registered for use in dogs only. The technique involves injecting Neutersol into each testicle. The volume injected is based on the testicular width as determined by measuring each testicle at its widest point using a metric scale (millimeter) caliper. Its active ingredient, zinc gluconate, causes atrophy of the testes and the prostate, rendering male puppies sterile. Injections must be properly placed. In dogs that are likely to struggle, sedatives are generally recommended. A major drawback of this product is that testosterone levels are unaffected, so unacceptable male behaviour is likely to persist.

Overall recommendations

It is necessary to explain the pros and cons of any treatment protocol to the owner, in order to obtain their informed consent to carry out the procedure. However, the clinician should bear in mind that most owners have little or no veterinary medical knowledge and may need to be guided towards making a reasonable decision. Clinicians should be able to put the potential risks of the procedure into a proper perspective for the owner, as in most cases the benefits will out-weigh the perceived risks.

Section 2
General signs and illnesses

Sheena Warman

Inappetence is defined as a reduction in appetite, whilst anorexia is defined as a complete lack of dietary intake. They are common presenting signs but are non-specific indicators of systemic disease and may reflect underlying nausea. Inappetence should be differentiated from a fussy appetite, which is common particularly in small breed dogs.

Common differential diagnoses

- Inability to smell food, e.g. cat flu
- Pyrexia
- Pain
- Dental disease
- Gastrointestinal disease, especially foreign bodies, intestinal neoplasia, severe gastroenteritis, intussusception
- Renal failure
- Hepatic disorders
- Pancreatitis
- Heart failure
- Anaemia
- Neoplastic disease
- Metabolic abnormalities, e.g. hypokalaemia, hypercalcaemia, hypoadrenocorticism

Diagnostic approach

A detailed history should be obtained, as other clinical signs are likely to be more useful in diagnosing the underlying disease (refer to relevant chapters for further information). In order to ascertain the significance and effects of the inappetence or anorexia, the owner should be asked what percentage of its normal daily dietary intake the pet has been eating, for how long appetite has been reduced, whether any weight loss has occurred, and whether or not the pet is drinking normally. Physical examination should be thorough, with all body systems carefully evaluated. The abdomen in particular, should be palpated carefully for masses because these can be easily missed.

Attention should be paid to body condition score, hydration status, and indicators of any underlying disorders.

The diagnostic investigation will be influenced by the presence or absence of signs of a specific illness. If no specific clinical signs are apparent, and inappropriate diet has been excluded, a blood sample should be taken for haematology and biochemistry. Biochemistry should include a minimum of urea, creatinine, albumin, globulin, liver enzymes and function tests (e.g. dynamic bile acids), sodium, potassium, calcium, phosphorus and glucose. Urinalysis (specific gravity, dipstick examination ± sediment examination) can be helpful, particularly if azotaemia becomes apparent on serum biochemical testing, as this will help differentiate between pre-renal and renal azotaemia. If haematology, biochemistry and urinalysis are unremarkable, survey radiographs of the abdomen and chest are indicated.

Treatment

Identification and treatment of the specific underlying cause will allow the appetite to return. During the convalescent period, owners should be advised to offer small meals of warmed, palatable food such as boiled chicken or fish, or commercial convalescent diets. Some pets may benefit from hand-feeding, but force-feeding should be avoided as it may result in food aversion. Some pets, especially cats, refuse to eat whilst hospitalised and a decision may have to be taken to discharge the animal earlier than would have been desired.

What if it doesn't get better?

Complete anorexia for more than three days in cats, or five days in dogs, warrants urgent intervention. This is particularly important in cats due to the high risk of hepatic lipidosis. The patient should be

100 Top Consultations in Small Animal General Practice, First Edition
By Peter Hill, Sheena Warman and Geoff Shawcross
© 2011 Blackwell Publishing Ltd

hospitalised and supportive care provided, with intravenous fluids if necessary to treat dehydration and provide ongoing maintenance fluid requirements. Additional problems (e.g. hypokalaemia) should be addressed as appropriate. Nutritional support should be by the enteral route (i.e. allowing the food to be absorbed via the gastrointestinal tract) whenever possible. Resting daily caloric requirements (kcal/24 h) for hospitalised dogs and cats can be calculated as (30 × body weight in kg) + 70.

If the patient remains anorexic, tube-feeding should be instituted. Naso-oesophageal tubes are usually well-tolerated, are relatively straightforward to place, and are ideal for short-term nutrition in patients that are not vomiting and do not have oesophageal disease. Patients can still eat voluntarily with these tubes in place. Some patients will tolerate syringe feeding but this should only be carried out by competent individuals because of the risk of aspiration, and should not be continued if the patient appears to resent the procedure.

Appetite stimulants can be helpful in some cases and include intravenous diazepam (cats) or oral cyproheptadine or mirtazapine (dogs or cats). Suspected nausea can be treated with maropitant or metoclopramide. Supplementation with vitamin B12 is sometimes undertaken, but is likely to be helpful only in patients with low B12 concentrations (e.g. some patients with gastrointestinal disease). Corticosteroids should not be used empirically as appetite stimulants and should be reserved for patients in which an underlying corticosteroid-responsive disease has been identified, or for palliative treatment of very sick patients if owners will not allow any further investigations/treatment.

Parenteral nutrition (i.e. by the IV route) is only appropriate in a small proportion of patients whose intestinal function is severely compromised, and would not generally be undertaken in general practice. Note that isotonic glucose-containing intravenous fluids, and amino acid supplements, provide only a very small proportion of daily caloric requirements, and must not replace the provision of adequate enteral nutrition, as outlined above.

If the patient does not begin to eat after a specific underlying cause has been identified and treated, clinicians should look for an additional cause of the signs. The physical examination should be repeated to ensure that more specific clinical signs have not developed or been overlooked. Blood test results and radiographs should be re-evaluated to ensure that nothing has been missed.

The low-cost option

Costs can be minimised if the underlying cause can be identified using history and clinical examination alone. Performance of unnecessary tests will rapidly escalate the cost. Investigations can be prioritised and then performed sequentially rather than all at once, as long as the condition of the animal allows this. However, clients must be made aware that some of the potential diagnoses can only be made following diagnostic tests and some may require long-term treatment, both of which can lead to considerable expense.

When should I refer?

Referral should be discussed when the patient fails to improve despite attempts at encouraging them to eat, and when an underlying disease has not been identified during investigations which can be performed within the practice. Referral should also be considered if facilities/personnel are not available to provide nutritional support to patients that have been anorexic for more than a few days.

Sheena Warman

Dogs and cats in ideal body condition should have easily palpable ribs with a slight fat covering, and a visible waist behind the ribs when viewed from above. In most cases, changes in body weight are noticed in relation to deviations from this ideal body condition score. However, an owner's interpretation of changes in their pet's weight can be misleading; for example, dogs with a combination of abdominal distension (e.g. due to ascites) and muscle wastage might be thought by the owners to have gained weight, despite an actual weight loss. Weight loss rarely occurs in growing animals, but they can fail to gain weight adequately and be too thin for their age.

Weight loss can occur for a variety of reasons and should always be considered pathological unless the owner has reduced their pet's food intake or increased its exercise regime. If weight loss is gradual, it may take some time before the owner appreciates a significant change. It is therefore good practice to record the animal's weight and body condition score (see Appendix 4) at each visit to the practice, so that changes can be accurately monitored.

Common differential diagnoses

- Inadequate caloric intake, caused by:
  - Poor quality or inadequate quantity of food
  - Systemic disease, resulting in inappetence or anorexia (e.g. chronic renal failure)
  - Inability to eat, e.g. facial trauma
  - Increased exercise/work
- Inadequate absorption of food, caused by:
  - Intestinal parasitism
  - Gastrointestinal disease (particularly those causing malabsorption, maldigestion or protein-losing enteropathies)
  - Exocrine pancreatic insufficiency
- Inability to utilise calories absorbed, caused by:
  - Diabetes mellitus
  - Hepatic disease
  - Severe protein-losing nephropathy
- Excessive metabolic rate, caused by:

- Cachexia associated with neoplastic disease or cardiac failure
- Hyperthyroidism (cat)
- Chronic inflammatory or infectious diseases

Note that weight loss can be multifactorial in an individual patient, and probable differentials will be influenced by the age of the pet. For example, weight loss in an old cat would most probably be due to renal failure, hyperthyroidism, diabetes mellitus and/or neoplasia, whereas poor weight gain in a puppy would most probably be due to poor quality diet or intestinal parasitism.

Diagnostic approach

A thorough history should be obtained, especially regarding quantity and quality of diet, worming routine, changes in exercise regime, and additional clinical signs which might be helpful to establish a diagnosis. The duration and severity of the weight loss should be recorded. Physical examination must be thorough, with particular attention to body condition score and any indicators of underlying disease.

The diagnostic approach will be influenced by both the age of the animal, and the presence or absence of other specific clinical signs (see appropriate chapters). The urgency of the investigation will also be influenced by the rate at which weight loss is occurring. If inadequate intake of food has been excluded and no other clinical signs are apparent, then samples should be taken for haematology, biochemistry (including urea, creatinine, albumin, globulin, liver enzymes and bile acid stimulation test, sodium, potassium, calcium, phosphorus and glucose) and urinalysis (specific gravity and dipstick examination, with urine protein:creatinine ratio performed if there is significant proteinuria). Serum thyroxine (T4) concentration should be measured in older cats. In puppies and kittens, in the absence of specific clinical signs, a faecal sample should be submitted for parasitology and/or appropriate worming treatment prescribed, before pursuing further diagnostic testing.

100 Top Consultations in Small Animal General Practice, First Edition
By Peter Hill, Sheena Warman and Geoff Shawcross
© 2011 Blackwell Publishing Ltd

Treatment

If an inappropriate type or quantity of diet is being fed, advice should be given as necessary. If there is any concern regarding inadequate worming, particularly in young animals, appropriate treatment should be prescribed. In most cases, effective treatment relies on identification and management of the underlying disease. For advice regarding inappetent patients, refer to Chapter 4.

What if it doesn't get better?

If weight loss persists and no underlying disease is identified on initial investigations, further diagnostic procedures are appropriate. Survey thoracic and abdominal radiographs may indicate the presence of conditions which were not apparent on physical examination (e.g. neoplastic disease). Some patients with gastrointestinal disease or exocrine pancreatic insufficiency may not have significant vomiting or diarrhoea, or gastrointestinal signs may not have been noticed by the owner (e.g. outdoor cats); in these patients measurement of trypsin-like immuno-reactivity (TLI), B12 and folate may be helpful. Further investigations, including abdominal ultrasound, endoscopy and biopsies may be necessary to achieve a definitive diagnosis (Figure 5.1). Tests for infectious disease are appropriate in some cases, although most patients will exhibit additional clinical signs, e.g. FIV, FeLV or feline infectious peritonitis (FIP) infection in cats; leishmaniosis in dogs which have travelled to endemic areas.

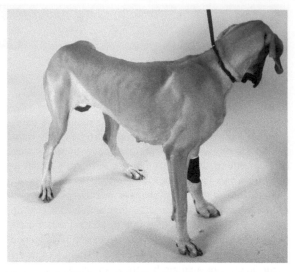

Figure 5.1   **Underweight Great Dane diagnosed with inflammatory bowel disease**

The low-cost option

It is important to confirm that an appropriate diet is being fed (and consumed) prior to embarking on expensive diagnostic tests. In puppies and kittens, it is often more economical to prescribe de-worming medications than to perform faecal parasitology in every case of suspected intestinal parasitism. Clues to an underlying condition can often be detected on a thorough physical examination, and will help prevent unnecessary tests being performed.

When should I refer?

Referral should be discussed if no underlying cause is identified during investigations which can be undertaken within the practice.

Sheena Warman

Polyuria and polydipsia (often abbreviated to PUPD) are common presenting signs in small animal practice. Polydipsia is defined as persistent water intake in excess of 100 ml/kg bodyweight per day and polyuria is the passing of unusually large volumes of urine. Accurate measurement of water intake can be difficult, particularly in multi-pet households or those with outdoor access, but for practical purposes water intake which is consistently more than 2–3 times normal for the individual pet is likely to be significant. A change of diet from wet to dry food is likely to cause an increase in thirst, although not true polydipsia. Polydipsia is most commonly a consequence of a disease or abnormality causing polyuria, typically due to osmotic diuresis or impaired response to anti-diuretic hormone (a mechanism known as secondary nephrogenic diabetes insipidus). It is important to remember that PUPD nearly always reflects a serious underlying disease.

Common differential diagnoses

- Endocrine disorders, e.g. diabetes mellitus, hyperadrenocorticism, hyperthyroidism (cats), hypoadrenocorticism
- Renal disease, e.g. chronic renal failure, pyelonephritis
- Pyometra
- Electrolyte disorders, e.g. hypokalaemia, hypercalcaemia
- Drug administration, e.g. furosemide, glucocorticoids, phenobarbitone.

Less common differentials include hepatic disease (e.g. portosystemic shunt, hepatic failure), polycythaemia, congenital renal diseases, primary diabetes insipidus and primary (psychogenic) polydipsia.

100 Top Consultations in Small Animal General Practice, First Edition
By Peter Hill, Sheena Warman and Geoff Shawcross
© 2011 Blackwell Publishing Ltd

Diagnostic approach

A logical approach is essential for investigation of cases of PUPD and the first step is to confirm the diagnosis. If practical, the owner should be asked to measure the water intake, to confirm the presence of polydipsia. Polyuria is more difficult to recognise, especially in cats, and it should be differentiated from urinary incontinence or dysuria. Dogs with urinary incontinence will often leave patches of urine on their bed, or leak urine intermittently, whereas dogs with polyuria will usually ask to be let outside, or leave large puddles of urine next to the door. However, concurrent polyuria can result in worsening of signs of incontinence. Dysuria is characterised by frequent attempts to void small volumes of urine. Other historical features that may be helpful in establishing a diagnosis are age, neuter status, appetite, changes in weight, and any recent drug administration. A full physical examination may reveal signs of the underlying cause such as a vaginal discharge in bitches with pyometra, tachycardia or goitre in hyperthyroid cats, coat changes with hyperadrenocorticism, or enlarged lymph nodes or anal sacs which could be consistent with a neoplastic cause of hypercalcaemia.

The next step is to analyse a free-catch urine sample (for specific gravity, dipstick and sediment analysis) to assess urine concentration and as a screening test for diabetes mellitus (glucosuria) or pyelonephritis (which may show evidence of inflammation on urine sediment analysis). Free-catch samples from dogs should be collected mid-stream into a clean container. Owners should be provided with containers to avoid the possible use of old jars which may contain substances that affect the test results, such as jam, resulting in artefactual glucosuria. Urine samples can be obtained from cats by providing non-absorbable litter in a litter tray. In some dogs and cats, it is more convenient to collect a sample by catheterisation or cystocentesis.

Haematology and biochemistry should be performed in all cases of PUPD, regardless of the information obtained from the history, physical examination and urinalysis, because more than one disease can occur concurrently. Useful biochemical parameters include glucose, urea, creatinine, albumin, globulin, liver enzymes and bile acid stimulation test, sodium, potassium, calcium and cholesterol. These initial blood tests allow identification of patients with diabetes mellitus, renal insufficiency, hepatic disease or electrolyte disorders. They may also give clues regarding hyperadrenocorticism (steroid leukogram, elevated alkaline phosphatase (ALKP), elevated cholesterol) or hypoadrenocorticism (hyponatraemia, hyperkalaemia), which would warrant further investigation (see below). In elderly cats, serum thyroxine should be measured.

If a diagnosis is not reached on these initial investigations, further tests should be performed. In entire bitches, evaluation for pyometra (e.g. ultrasound) should be a priority. If pyelonephritis is suspected, a cystocentesis sample should be obtained for bacterial culture. However, bacterial shedding with pyelonephritis can be intermittent, and trial treatment with antibiotics is sometimes appropriate if there is a high index of suspicion.

If hyperadrenocorticism is suspected, based on additional clinical signs or laboratory results (see Chapter 74), an adrenocorticotrophic hormone (adrenocorticotropin; ACTH) stimulation test should be performed. This test can also be used to confirm a diagnosis of hypoadrenocorticism (note that not all hypoadrenocorticoid dogs have abnormal electrolytes). If the ACTH stimulation test is normal, or equivocal, hyperadrenocorticism should be definitively excluded by performing a low-dose dexamethasone suppression test or urinary cortisol:creatinine ratio, even if there are no additional signs of hyperadrenocorticism.

Once the common conditions have been ruled out (which can be difficult to do with complete certainty in the case of hyperadrenocorticism, early renal disease, or pyelonephritis), then the remaining differentials are primary polydipsia or diabetes insipidus. Investigation of these requires either a water deprivation test or trial treatment with a vasopressin analogue (desmopressin or DDAVP). Water deprivation tests are associated with significant risks (particularly if underlying renal disease has not been detected) and are challenging and time-consuming to perform. Interpretation of water deprivation tests and trial DDAVP treatment can also be fraught with difficulty. It is often beneficial to discuss such cases with an internal medicine specialist prior to undertaking these procedures.

Treatment

There is no symptomatic treatment for PUPD, and successful management requires identification and appropriate treatment of the underlying disease (refer to specific chapters). Severe PUPD in a dog can be inconvenient for owners if it needs to urinate overnight; however, they should be warned against water restriction as this could be dangerous.

What if it doesn't get better?

Effective treatment of cases of PUPD requires identification and appropriate treatment of the underlying disease (see appropriate chapters). However, owners should be told if the condition being treated is incurable and that, in such cases, lifelong management will be required. Owners should also be warned that the polydipsia may not always resolve despite rational treatment, especially in the case of renal failure or hepatic disease. If the PUPD fails to resolve despite the clinician's expectations, the possibility of concurrent diseases or incorrect diagnosis should be considered.

The low-cost option

There are no causes of PUPD that can be managed cheaply. Costs will be minimised if the logical, step-wise approach outlined above is taken, as the most common conditions will be identified on initial laboratory testing. However, diagnosis, treatment and monitoring of many of these conditions is expensive, and in some cases financial limitations may mean that euthanasia must be discussed as an option at an early stage, particularly in patients which are showing additional signs of clinical deterioration.

When should I refer?

Most routine cases of PUPD can be diagnosed and managed in general practice. However, referral should be discussed if a diagnosis cannot be reached using investigations that can be performed within the practice, or if a condition does not respond to treatment as the clinician expects. Specialist expertise may be required for the interpretation of tests for hyperadrenocorticism, water deprivation tests, trial therapy with DDAVP, assessment of glomerular filtration rate and investigation of porto-systemic shunts. Complex management issues that may benefit from referral may be seen in some cases of diabetes mellitus, hyperadrenocorticism, hyperthyroidism, hypoadrenocorticism, pyelonephritis, hepatic disease and diabetes insipidus.

Sheena Warman

Pyrexia means an abnormal increase in body temperature. Increased body temperature can have a variety of causes, many of which are not infections (see differential list below). 'True' fever is caused by the production of endogenous pyrogens, which raise the normal set-point in the thermoregulatory centre in the anterior hypothalamus, causing the core temperature to be increased through a combination of increased heat production and conservation. This is a protective mechanism for fighting infection, for example, by slowing viral replication and increasing leukocyte function. Body temperature can also be increased as a result of inadequate dissipation of heat (heatstroke), or excessive muscular activity.

Normal rectal temperature in dogs and cats is generally between 38 and 39°C. Temperatures in excess of 41.5°C can result in permanent organ damage or even death, and are more likely to be associated with heatstroke or excessive muscular activity than with true fever.

Common differential diagnoses

- True fever
  - Infectious disease (bacterial, viral, fungal, or protozoal)
  - Non-infectious inflammatory disease (e.g. pancreatitis)
  - Immune-mediated disease
  - Neoplastic disease (particularly myeloproliferative disorders)
  - Tissue trauma/necrosis
- Inability to dissipate heat (heat stroke)
  - Excessive environmental temperature and/or humidity
  - Respiratory obstruction
- Excessive muscular activity
  - Strenuous exercise
  - Prolonged seizure activity.

Diagnostic approach

The first step is to establish if the pyrexia is significant. Veterinary attention for animals with true fever is usually sought because of other clinical signs such as lethargy or inappetence. Mild elevations in temperature (39.0–39.5°C) can be an incidental finding in an otherwise well patient and can be caused by physical factors such as high ambient temperature or excitement. These patients, and patients with heat stroke, will usually be trying to dissipate heat by panting and postural changes, in contrast to patients with true fever, where the altered thermoregulatory set-point does not provoke this mechanism.

Animals with heatstroke or excessive muscular activity are often dangerously hyperthermic (>41.0°C). A rapid history and assessment of cardiovascular and respiratory systems should be performed and emergency treatment measures instituted immediately (see below).

In patients where true fever is considered likely, a full history should be obtained, paying particular attention to any historical or clinical signs that could indicate the source of the pyrexia, e.g. coughing, sneezing, signs of lower urinary tract disease, or diarrhoea. The vaccination status of the animal should be confirmed, and any history of foreign travel noted (in case of exotic infectious diseases).

A thorough physical examination must be performed to try to find the likely cause of the pyrexia. Findings which might indicate a bacterial cause include abscesses, dental infections, purulent nasal discharge, increased chest sounds (e.g. pneumonia), reduced chest sounds (e.g. pyothorax), a newly identified heart murmur (e.g. endocarditis), focal abdominal pain (e.g. pyelonephritis), generalised abdominal pain (e.g. peritonitis), vaginal discharge (pyometra), prostatic pain (prostatitis), spinal pain (e.g. discospondylitis), joint pain/effusion (e.g. septic arthritis), bone pain (e.g. osteomyelitis), or anal sac pain (abscessation). Viral disease, including respiratory infections, FIV, FeLV or FIP, should be considered in cats (see relevant chapters). Signs suggestive of an immune-mediated disease or non-septic inflammatory disease might include swollen or painful joints

100 Top Consultations in Small Animal General Practice, First Edition
By Peter Hill, Sheena Warman and Geoff Shawcross
© 2011 Blackwell Publishing Ltd

(e.g. polyarthritis), pain on manipulation of the neck or spine (e.g. polyarthritis or meningitis), cranial abdominal pain (e.g. pancreatitis), anaemia, or serious skin abnormalities. Careful examination for tumours should include palpation of the lymph nodes and abdomen (in particular the spleen). Note that many of the above symptoms have multiple causes and will require further investigation for confirmation of the diagnosis.

It should also be noted that some patients with significant pyrexia will have no other apparent abnormalities even on thorough physical examination; these patients are classified as 'pyrexia of unknown origin' (PUO) and can represent a diagnostic challenge and therapeutic dilemma.

Treatment

In patients with a rectal temperature in excess of 41°C (usually secondary to heatstroke or seizures), urgent treatment is required. These patients often show signs of dehydration and/or hypovolaemic shock. Patients should be cooled using cool water fans, and by application of surgical spirit to paws. Cold water and ice should be avoided as they result in vasoconstriction and impaired heat loss. Cooling measures should stop when the temperature is 39.5–40°C to prevent the development of rebound hypothermia. Cooled or room-temperature intravenous isotonic crystalloids should be administered as required to help support the cardiovascular system, and oxygen supplementation should be provided by flow-by, face-mask or nasal catheter techniques to optimise oxygen delivery to tissues.

In patients with true fever, any specific cause of pyrexia identified on physical examination should be treated or investigated further, as appropriate. If a bacterial cause is identified, appropriate antibiotic therapy should be initiated. Intravenous fluids are not necessary unless the patient is dehydrated, hypovolaemic, or has a rectal temperature >41°C. Active cooling techniques as described above can be counter-productive as they will have no effect on the animal's altered thermoregulatory set-point, and the patient will expend further energy trying to maintain its elevated body temperature.

In pets with PUO, the approach will depend on the severity of other signs. If the patient is severely unwell (e.g. several days of inappetence or clinical signs of dehydration), further investigations (initially haematology, biochemistry and urinalysis) should be considered. If a pet with PUO has been unwell for no more than 24–48 hours and seems reasonably bright, empirical therapy can be justified. It is possible that many of these patients would recover without drug treatment, but owners are usually keen for treatment that will improve their animal's demeanour as quickly as possible. Good client communication is essential, with explanations of the reasoning behind the choice of treatment and the need to re-examine the patient being emphasised.

It is important to note (and explain to owners) that not every animal with pyrexia has a bacterial infection. Antibiotics should be used in patients where a bacterial cause seems particularly likely, e.g. cats which are known to spend time outdoors and are likely to be involved in fights, or in patients with a previous history of urinary or respiratory tract bacterial infections. A short course of antibiotics may also be considered in other cases of PUO, as some of the bacterial infections listed above can be difficult to detect in the early stages.

A single dose of an NSAID can be considered, either as sole therapy or in conjunction with antibiotics, in order to improve the patient's demeanour and appetite by lowering the body temperature for 24–48 hours. This may give the patient time for its underlying problem to resolve spontaneously, whilst being unlikely to mask the signs of serious underlying disease. Although pyrexia may be a protective mechanism in patients with infectious disease, there is little evidence that a single dose of NSAIDs will cause problems in a dog or cat in which a thorough physical examination has not yielded any clues as to the cause.

The specific approach taken can only be decided upon by the attending clinician, taking into account all the relevant factors about the case. However, a short course (5–7 days) of oral antibiotics such as ampicillin or amoxicillin, and/or a single subcutaneous injection of a NSAID to lower the animal's thermoregulatory set-point, are possible starting points. Irrespective of the treatment given, the patient should be re-examined if there is no improvement or if signs relapse within 24–48 hours.

What if it doesn't get better?

Appropriate treatment of specifically identified bacterial infections usually leads to rapid improvement with a good prognosis, unless there is an underlying severe systemic disease. The practice of changing antibiotics every few days to assess response is inappropriate; if there is no response to initial antibiotic treatment, a straightforward bacterial infection is unlikely. Some of the other causes of pyrexia carry a poorer prognosis despite appropriate treatment, such as FeLV, FIP, fungal or protozoal infections, lymphoproliferative neoplasia and some immune-mediated diseases.

If the animal has been initially treated for PUO with antibiotics, with or without NSAIDs, and has relapsed or failed to respond, further diagnostic tests should be performed. In many cases, additional clinical signs will have become evident allowing more specific treatment and/or investigations. A thorough physical examination should be repeated and haematology, biochemistry and urinalysis (including culture) should be performed. In cats, FIV and FeLV testing should be undertaken, and FIP considered. Fine needle aspiration should be performed on any suspicious swellings or abnormal masses.

If the cause is still elusive, an underlying infectious, immune-mediated or neoplastic process should be investigated using survey thoracic and abdominal radiographs and abdominal ultrasound when available. In some cases, more specialised tests will be required, e.g. biopsy of abnormal masses, echocardiography, blood cultures, joint taps, CSF taps or bone marrow biopsies.

The low-cost option

The majority of patients with pyrexia will improve within 24–48 hours. In most cases it is not clear whether this is because of, or in spite of, empirical therapy. If empirical antibiotic therapy is given, then costs can be minimised by using antibiotics such as ampicillin or amoxicillin.

Patients with persistent PUO can be expensive and frustrating to investigate, and even in specialist centres a diagnosis may not be reached in 10–15% of cases. If owners will not permit further investigations, trial therapy with a prolonged course of broad-spectrum antibiotics may be necessary. If there is no response to antibiotics, trial treatment with immunosuppressive doses of corticosteroids is occasionally recommended in case of undiagnosed immune-mediated disease. However, if corticosteroids are used, the owner must be made aware that death may result if dissemination of an unidentified infectious process occurred.

When should I refer?

Referral should be discussed if the animal does not respond to initial treatment or relapses frequently, and an underlying disease is not identified using facilities available within the practice. Further investigation of cases of pyrexia using advanced procedures such as echocardiography, blood cultures, joint taps, CSF taps or bone marrow biopsies should only be undertaken by clinicians with expertise in these techniques. Cases should be discussed with the specialist prior to referral, as it is often more economical for the patient to be examined when it is symptomatic and has not received any treatment for at least a few days. Medical management of some of the causes of pyrexia can also benefit from specialist input.

Sheena Warman

Anaemia means reduced numbers of circulating red blood cells (RBCs) and is a common finding in dogs and cats. Owners are generally unaware that their pet is anaemic, but will seek veterinary attention for the resulting clinical signs, such as lethargy or collapse, or because of clinical signs associated with an underlying disease. Anaemia occurs as a result of one of three mechanisms:

- Haemorrhage (loss of RBCs)
- Haemolysis (destruction of RBCs)
- Inadequate RBC production.

Haematological analysis allows anaemias to be classified as regenerative (with evidence of ongoing RBC production) or non-regenerative (when the bone marrow is unable to respond adequately to the increased need for RBCs). This differentiation provides clues to the underlying cause, and also offers prognostic information, as persistent lack of regeneration is often a poor prognostic sign.

Common differential diagnoses

- Haemorrhage (regenerative although maximum response may take 3–5 days)
  - Trauma (e.g. road traffic accident, arterial bleed)
  - Bleeding tumour (e.g. splenic haemangiosarcoma)
  - Surgical haemorrhage
  - Gastrointestinal ulceration
  - Severe ectoparasite (or rarely endoparasite) burden
  - Disorders of haemostasis (e.g. warfarin toxicity, von Willebrand's disease, thrombocytopenia, disseminated intravascular coagulation)
- Haemolysis (regenerative although maximum response may take 3–5 days)
  - Immune-mediated haemolytic anaemia (IMHA) may be primary or secondary to underlying disease; a small proportion are non-regenerative due to destruction of RBC precursors in the bone marrow
  - Infectious diseases (babesiosis, ehrlichiosis, *Mycoplasma haemofelis* in cats)
  - Toxins (zinc, paracetamol, onions)

- Inadequate RBC production (non-regenerative)
  - Bone marrow disorders (including FeLV and FIV infection in cats, oestrogen toxicity, administration of myelosuppressive drugs, and primary bone marrow disorders)
  - Anaemia of chronic disease (many chronic inflammatory or neoplastic diseases cause mild anaemia due to an inability of the bone marrow to utilise iron as a consequence of abnormal cytokine production)
  - Iron deficiency (usually due to chronic blood loss in animals, especially from the gastrointestinal tract; can be mildly regenerative, initially)
  - Anaemia of renal disease.

Diagnostic approach

The main aims when presented with anaemia are to assess its severity and determine its cause so as to allow appropriate treatment. Anaemia may be apparent from the history and physical examination, especially when there has been obvious haemorrhage, or it may be detected on blood tests that are performed to investigate other clinical signs such as lethargy, anorexia or polydipsia.

Clues from the physical examination

Patients with anaemia vary in their clinical signs depending on the severity, duration, speed of onset and underlying cause. Mild anaemia does not cause obvious clinical signs or pallor. Moderate to severe anaemia that has developed over a period of weeks to months may cause only mild lethargy or exercise intolerance, but mucous membrane pallor will usually be evident on physical examination.

With increasing severity, or sudden development of moderate/severe anaemia, animals show pronounced lethargy, exercise intolerance or even collapse. Tachypnoea and tachycardia may occur due to lack of oxygen-carrying capacity. Haemic heart murmurs may be detected which are usually soft with a maximum grade 2/6, located at the left heart base.

100 Top Consultations in Small Animal General Practice, First Edition
By Peter Hill, Sheena Warman and Geoff Shawcross
© 2011 Blackwell Publishing Ltd

Severe haemorrhage will cause signs of hypovolaemic shock, initially with a bounding pulse, progressing to a weak and thready pulse as compensation fails. The animal's packed cell volume (PCV) may be normal, initially. Evidence of external haemorrhage may be apparent from an arterial bleed or haemorrhage around fracture sites (Figure 8.1). Internal haemorrhage should be suspected in any case of unexplained anaemia, and becomes more obvious if there is melaena or haematemesis (gastrointestinal bleeding), a fluid thrill on abdominal percussion (haemoabdomen), tachypnoea with ventral dullness on thoracic auscultation and percussion (haemothorax), or tachypnoea with audible crackles (pulmonary contusions).

Haemolytic anaemias and non-regenerative anaemias do not cause a reduction in circulating blood volume. Severe or acute-onset haemolytic anaemias result in a bounding pulse and there may be other signs such as jaundice. Non-regenerative anaemias generally develop over a period of several weeks to months, and in many cases the only clinical sign will be mucous membrane pallor.

Haematological tests

Confirmation of anaemia and its severity are achieved by routine haematological testing. Values for PCV, haematocrit, haemoglobin concentration and RBC count will be below the reference range for the species (see Appendix 5). In general, a PCV of less than about 20% in a dog or 15% in a cat would be considered severe. Clinicians should be aware that patients with acute, severe haemorrhage may have normal PCVs initially, but have clinical signs due to a sudden reduction in circulating blood volume. Once anaemia is confirmed, further history should be obtained if necessary to exclude trauma, exposure to toxins, or foreign travel.

If the anaemia is considered significant, but the patient is stable, the first step is to submit an EDTA blood sample and fresh blood smears to an external laboratory where the necessary expertise is available to evaluate and interpret haematological changes. A reticulocyte count should be requested as the presence of these red cell precursors indicates regeneration, along with other abnormalities such as increased mean corpuscular volume (MCV) and evidence of anisocytosis and polychromasia. If regeneration initially appears to be inadequate in a case with haemorrhagic or haemolytic anaemia, then full haematology and reticulocyte count should be repeated 3–5 days later, by which time regeneration would be expected

to be maximal. Full haematological analysis can also provide evidence of immune-mediated haemolysis: spherocytes, autoagglutination (Figures 8.2 and 8.3); iron deficiency: reduced mean corpuscular haemoglobin (MCH), mean corpuscular haemoglobin concentration (MCHC), and morphological abnormalities; or bone marrow disease: concurrent neutropenia and thrombocytopenia. Serum biochemistry may also provide clues to the cause of the anaemia or any underlying disease (e.g. hyperbilirubinaemia with haemolytic anaemia; azotaemia with renal failure). FeLV and FIV testing should be performed in cats if another cause of the anaemia is not apparent. Mild anaemia which is detected incidentally and not causing any clinical signs (e.g. in a patient with renal failure) does not usually need to be investigated further.

In an emergency situation, with severe or acute anaemia, there may not be time to wait for results of external laboratory tests. Rapid determination of PCV and total solids (measured on a plasma sample using a refractometer) can help to differentiate between haemorrhage and haemolysis, the most likely causes. Haemorrhage often leads to a reduction in total protein and total solids, whereas haemolysis should be suspected if there is evidence of jaundice (yellow discolouration) or haemoglobinaemia (red discolouration) in the plasma overlying a spun blood sample. If there is no obvious source of haemorrhage, abdominocentesis, thoracic/abdominal ultrasonography or radiography may detect internal bleeding. Unless there is a known cause of haemorrhage, an in-house blood smear should be examined to assess adequacy of platelet numbers (normal 10–15 per high power field), as in-house haematology analysers can sometimes provide inaccurate assessments of platelet numbers. The smear can also be used to assess for evidence of regeneration (anisocytosis, polychromasia), and other red cell changes such as spherocytosis. Further evidence of immune-mediated haemolysis can be obtained by performing an in-saline agglutination test, performed by adding a drop of saline (2 drops in cats) to a drop of EDTA blood on a glass slide, and assessing for macroscopic and microscopic agglutination (Figure 8.3). It is recommended that an EDTA blood sample and fresh smears be submitted to an external laboratory as soon as possible.

In cases where a cause for the anaemia is still not apparent, the following investigations should be considered, based on the clinician's index of suspicion for the various conditions (referral might be required for some of these procedures):

- Suspected occult haemorrhage: urinalysis, faecal occult blood testing (following 3 days of a meat-free diet) and survey imaging
- Suspected haemolytic disease: IMHA is likely if there is significant bilirubinuria, bilirubinaemia, auto-agglutination and/or spherocytosis. The diagnosis can be confirmed with a positive Coombs' test. Survey imaging should be performed to investigate any underlying diseases. Other causes of haemolysis are less common, but include access to toxins such as zinc (e.g. American pennies), paracetamol, or onions (which cause oxidative damage, especially to feline RBCs)
- Suspected *Mycoplasma haemofelis* infection: polymerase chain reaction (PCR) test
- Suspected exotic disease with history of travel abroad: PCR tests for ehrlichiosis, leishmaniosis and babesiosis
- Suspected bone marrow disorder: bone marrow biopsy
- Suspected disorders of haemostasis: useful tests include platelet count, buccal mucosal bleeding time (if platelets are adequate), and assays of clotting times such as prothrombin time (PT) and activated partial thromboplastin time (APTT). The laboratory should be contacted in advance for advice regarding sample submission
- Suspected inherited disorders: e.g. genetic tests for pyruvate kinase deficiency in Basenjis, phosphofructokinase deficiency in Springer Spaniels, or measurement of vitamin B12 for cobalamin deficiency in Border Collies and Giant Schnauzers.

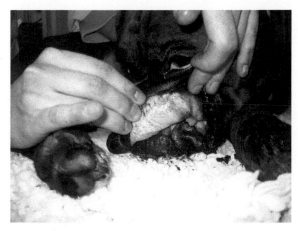

Figure 8.1 Boxer with pale mucous membranes caused by gastric haemorrhage

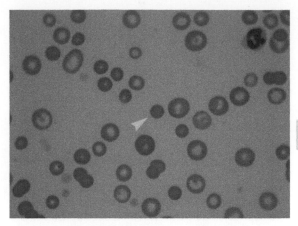

Figure 8.2 Blood smear from a dog with IMHA. Arrow points to a spherocyte

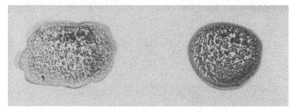

Figure 8.3 A positive in-saline agglutination test; microscopic agglutination should be confirmed under the microscope

Treatment

If the animal is reasonably bright, with normal heart rate, respiratory rate and pulse quality, then initial management is focussed on identifying the cause of the anaemia, in order to initiate appropriate treatment. In more severe, but not life-threatening cases, stress and exercise should be avoided until the investigations are complete.

If the animal is showing clinical signs of hypovolaemia due to acute haemorrhage, it should be treated initially with intravenous crystalloids ± colloids, with attempts made to control haemorrhage. Pressure bandages should be applied to areas of external haemorrhage. An abdominal bandage can be placed on patients with abdominal bleeding whilst the patient is stabilised prior to surgery. If bleeding cannot be controlled, then blood transfusion may become necessary. Patients with pulmonary contusions require cautious fluid therapy as it is very easy to cause worsening of pulmonary haemorrhage and irreversible respiratory failure.

Patients with haemolytic or chronic non-regenerative anaemia are generally euvolaemic and will not benefit from treatment with crystalloids or colloids. However, they may show signs of lack of oxygen-carrying capacity such as weakness, tachycardia, tachypnoea and bounding pulses. If this is the case, the animal is likely to benefit from a transfusion of whole blood, packed red blood cells or a haemo-globin-based oxygen carrying solution.

Patients with suspected gastrointestinal bleeding should be treated with gastroprotectants such as omeprazole and sucralfate. If rodenticide toxicity is suspected, vitamin K treatment should be administered. Administration of iron or vitamin B12 is not indicated unless a specific deficiency has been demonstrated. Further treatment will depend on the cause of the anaemia (such as erythropoietin in renal failure) and specialist advice should be sought, if necessary.

What if it doesn't get better?

Successful treatment of anaemic patients requires identification and treatment of the underlying disease. If bleeding patients do not respond to initial treatment, a search for an ongoing source of haemorrhage should be made. Iron deficiency should be considered if there has been chronic external blood loss. Therapy of patients with haemolytic anaemia will depend on the underlying cause and if there has been no response within a few days to specific treatment, the diagnosis should be re-evaluated. If haematological analysis reveals persistent non-regenerative anaemia, it is important to identify the precise cause in order to determine if treatment could reverse the condition. For example, some cases of primary bone marrow disease can be successfully treated, but many will require specialist input and/or have a poor prognosis.

The low-cost option

Costs can be minimised by paying meticulous attention to the historical and physical findings and taking a logical approach to identifying the underlying cause. Initial in-house tests including PCV, total solids, examination of a blood smear and, if necessary, an in-saline agglutination test, can be performed quickly and cheaply, although more reliable information is likely to be obtained from an external laboratory. In cats, infectious disease testing (FeLV, FIV, *Mycoplasma haemofelis*) should be performed early in the course of investigations. Complicated cases requiring extensive investigations, and emergency cases requiring blood transfusions or surgery, are likely to incur substantial costs of which the owner must be made aware.

When should I refer?

General practices should be well equipped to deal with anaemia due to acute haemorrhage or chronic disease. Referral should be recommended for patients in which the diagnosis remains elusive following investigations performed within the practice, and for patients requiring treatment with blood products and/or intensive care, if the practice cannot provide these facilities. Conditions which may benefit from specialist input include disorders of haemostasis, IMHA, bone marrow disorders and inherited causes of anaemia.

Sheena Warman

Jaundice is the term used to describe the yellow discolouration of skin, mucous membranes and sclera due to the accumulation of bilirubin (Figure 9.1). Bilirubin is a natural by-product of RBC breakdown. Normally, it is metabolised by the liver and excreted in bile but it will accumulate if the extent of breakdown exceeds the capacity of the liver to metabolise it, if there is hepatic dysfunction, or if there is biliary obstruction/leakage. These three mechanisms are classified as pre-hepatic, hepatic and post-hepatic, respectively. Usually, jaundice is not clinically evident until serum bilirubin exceeds about 25 µmol/l (typical reference interval 0–10 µmol/l).

Common differential diagnoses

Pre-hepatic disease

- Haemolysis, e.g. immune-mediated haemolytic anaemia, *M. haemofelis* infection in cats.

Hepatic disease (see Chapter 42 for full details)

- Acute hepatitis (drugs, toxins, leptospirosis, infectious canine hepatitis [CAV-1])
- Chronic hepatitis (immune-mediated, drugs, e.g. phenobarbitone, inherited disease, e.g. copper-associated hepatopathy)
- Cholangitis
- Neoplasia (primary or metastatic)
- Hepatic lipidosis (cats)
- FIP (cats)
- Cirrhosis
- Sepsis.

Post-hepatic disease

- Pancreatitis or pancreatic tumour
- Biliary duct neoplasia
- Biliary rupture (bile peritonitis).

100 Top Consultations in Small Animal General Practice, First Edition
By Peter Hill, Sheena Warman and Geoff Shawcross
© 2011 Blackwell Publishing Ltd

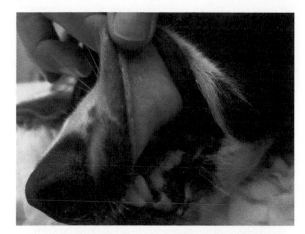

Figure 9.1   Springer Spaniel with severe jaundice

Diagnostic approach

A detailed history should be obtained from the owner, paying particular attention to vaccination status, clinical signs such as inappetence, altered thirst, vomiting or diarrhoea, and exposure to drugs or toxins. A complete physical examination should be performed, although it is not possible to differentiate the underlying causes of jaundice on physical examination alone. The presence of obvious pallor makes haemolytic disease more likely. The presence of an enlarged liver or cranial abdominal mass may suggest neoplasia but hepatomegaly can also be associated with non-hepatic causes, such as haemolytic anaemias. Large pancreatic masses may also be palpable, but can be difficult to distinguish from hepatic tumours or other masses in the cranial abdomen.

Further investigation of jaundice requires diagnostic tests. The first step is to perform haematological and biochemical analysis. It can be difficult to detect pallor in severely jaundiced mucous membranes, but normal PCV (or RBC, haemoglobin or haematocrit) would allow haemolytic disease to be excluded. Haemolysis usually causes a strongly regenerative anaemia. Spherocytosis, agglutination and/or a positive Coombs' test are likely in the case of immune-mediated haemolysis.

Serum biochemistry is usually performed to aid diagnosis and assess the general health of the patient, although it cannot be relied upon to identify the cause of the jaundice. Biochemical analysis should include alanine transferase (ALT), ALKP, total bilirubin, urea, creatinine, albumin, globulin, glucose, sodium, potassium, calcium and cholesterol; plus γ-glutamyl transferase (GGT) in cats. Of these parameters, liver enzymes can be useful in helping to determine the cause of jaundice, but it is important to note that all causes of jaundice can cause some elevation in liver enzymes. ALT is a marker of hepatocellular damage, whereas ALKP, GGT and cholesterol are markers of cholestasis; the relative degree of increase may help determine the underlying disease. Haemolysis can cause hypoxic damage to the liver, resulting in mild (2–3 fold) elevations in liver enzymes. In hepatic disease, all liver enzymes are likely to be markedly elevated (>4–5 fold increase), but in some conditions where the liver mass is markedly reduced (e.g. terminal cirrhosis) they can be normal. In cases of biliary obstruction, ALKP, GGT and cholesterol are likely to be more markedly elevated than ALT; however ALT is often moderately to markedly elevated due to the toxic effects of bile acids on hepatocytes. Measurement of GGT in cats is particularly useful as it is usually elevated with cholangiohepatitis, but not with hepatic lipidosis. There is little value in performing bile acid assays in jaundiced patients, as the jaundice is likely to interfere with the assay. Measurement of bilirubin will confirm jaundice if there is any doubt clinically, and provides a baseline for monitoring response to treatment; it will not help identify the cause of the jaundice. Assays of conjugated and unconjugated bilirubin are unreliable and are no longer recommended.

Other biochemical parameters are not useful to help determine the cause of the jaundice but are measured to assess other aspects of the patient's health. Severe jaundice is likely to interfere with measurement of creatinine and phosphorus, depending on the technique used by the laboratory. Measurement of serum amylase and lipase might be useful in some cases of acute pancreatitis; a 4–5 fold increase in a patient with appropriate clinical signs is consistent with acute pancreatitis. However, they are neither particularly sensitive nor specific, and measurement of species-specific pancreatic lipase immunoreactivity (cPLI or fPLI) is preferred (see Chapter 43).

Abdominal ultrasound by a competent ultrasonographer is the most useful investigation to differentiate hepatic from post-hepatic causes. Hepatic size and architecture can be assessed, and may suggest abnormalities such as neoplasia. If there is complete post-hepatic biliary obstruction, gall bladder and common bile duct distension will become apparent within 24 hours, and intrahepatic bile duct distension within 7 days. The pancreas should also be assessed and canine or feline pancreatic lipase (PLI) measured, if pancreatitis is suspected. Ultrasound will also identify any fluid accumulation, which could be caused by portal hypertension associated with end-stage liver disease, or could suggest bile peritonitis. Radiography can be useful to evaluate hepatic size, to help identify mass lesions, or to suggest the presence of free abdominal fluid, but it is inferior to ultrasonography for identification of the cause of jaundice.

Other tests that may need to be considered (depending on the case) include *Leptospira* serology, further investigation of suspected FIP in cats (see Chapter 14), abdominocentesis, hepatic aspirates, or liver biopsies (following assessment of clotting profiles). If haemolysis and infectious/toxic causes of hepatitis have been excluded, and ultrasound is not available (or is not diagnostic), there are three options. The patient can be provided with supportive care for a few days (see below) and carefully monitored; exploratory surgery can be considered to identify the cause; or the patient can be referred to a specialist for ultrasonographic assessment and further investigation/treatment, as appropriate. It should be noted that surgical investigation and treatment of post-hepatic causes of jaundice is challenging and is best carried out by a specialist.

Treatment

The treatment of jaundice requires identification of the underlying cause. In cases with primary immune-mediated haemolytic anaemia, treatment should be started with immunosuppressive doses of corticosteroids and supportive care with blood products as required.

Further details of the management of hepatic causes can be found in Chapter 42. Many patients will be dehydrated due to reduced voluntary water intake and inappetence, and will benefit from intravenous fluid therapy and encouragement to eat whilst results of investigations are awaited (see Chapter 4). Anti-emetics are indicated in vomiting patients. Patients with bile peritonitis or complete biliary obstruction require urgent surgery, and are best referred to a specialist as soon as possible.

When leptospirosis is considered likely (e.g. unvaccinated dogs with a history of swimming or contact with rats), patients should be barrier-nursed and treated with IV fluids and ampicillin. Ampicillin should be continued for at least 2 weeks and followed by a 2-week course of doxycycline, to aid clearance of the organism from the kidneys. CAV-1 is now rare in the UK, but should be considered a possibility in unvaccinated pets.

The low-cost option

When finances are limited, the most important objective is to determine a prognosis as soon as possible. However, as prognosis is essentially related to diagnosis, this may not be possible without performing the diagnostic sequence outlined above. Measurement of PCV can be used to rapidly eliminate haemolysis as a cause. Once this is done, clinicians may be forced into basing a prognosis on the likelihood of the various conditions being present. Development of jaundice in an elderly dog or cat is most likely to be due to end-stage liver disease or neoplasia and euthanasia should be considered.

Antibiotics can be considered as a trial treatment for patients in which haemolysis has been excluded but further investigation has been declined. In dogs this is rarely effective, as bacterial causes of jaundice (other than leptospirosis) are uncommon. In cats (in which suppurative cholangitis is more common), initial treatment with broad-spectrum antibiotics might be beneficial, adding anti-inflammatory doses of prednisolone if there is no improvement. Owners should be made aware of the potential risks associated with giving prednisolone, both in terms of side-effects and if there is undiagnosed infectious disease (see Chapter 42).

What if it doesn't get better?

Successful treatment of jaundiced patients requires identification and treatment of the underlying disease. Conditions such as immune-mediated haemolytic anaemia, toxin-induced hepatopathy, hepatitis, leptospirosis, hepatic lipidosis and pancreatitis carry a fair prognosis and appropriate treatment may allow a full recovery. However, in cases of cirrhosis or neoplasia, the prognosis is poor and euthanasia may have to be considered as an option.

When should I refer?

Referral should be discussed if the diagnosis is not apparent following investigations within the practice. In particular, a thorough ultrasonographic assessment by a specialist can be invaluable. Surgical treatment for post-hepatic causes of jaundice can be fraught with complications and is best performed by a specialist.

Sheena Warman

'Collapse' can be caused by loss of consciousness or the inability to support normal posture. Additionally, owners will often use the term to describe any pet which is recumbent and will not rise with gentle encouragement. Possible causes for collapse can be loosely described in three different categories. *Sudden collapse* refers to patients in which an acute pathophysiological insult results in collapse. *Episodic collapse* describes patients who suffer recurrent collapsing episodes, which may be due to an intermittent problem, or a chronic problem with acute exacerbations (e.g. cardiac disease exacerbated by exercise). These episodes are often very short in duration and the patient often appears normal on arrival at the veterinary practice. *Apparent collapse* describes recumbent patients who have the ability to move, but would prefer not to.

Common differential diagnoses

Causes of sudden collapse

- Hypovolaemic shock, e.g. bleeding due to trauma or splenic tumour rupture, septic shock, gastric dilation and volvulus (GDV)
- Cardiac disease, e.g. severe congestive heart failure, pericardial effusion, aortic thromboemboli in cats
- Respiratory disease, e.g. airway obstruction, pneumonia, pleural space disease
- Orthopaedic disease, e.g. limb fractures
- Metabolic disorders, e.g. hypoglycaemia, hypoadrenocorticism, severe electrolyte disturbances, hepatic encephalopathy, diabetic ketoacidosis, blocked bladder
- Neurologic/neuromuscular diseases, e.g. head trauma, brain tumours, toxin ingestion, vestibular disease, central nervous system (CNS) inflammatory diseases, botulism
- Spinal disease, e.g. fractures, disc disease, fibrocartilaginous embolism, infarction, atlanto-axial subluxation (some of which suffer recurring collapsing episodes)
- Severe anaemia.

Causes of episodic collapse

- Seizures due to intracranial disease, extracranial disease (such as hepatic encephalopathy or episodic hypoglycaemia), or idiopathic epilepsy (see Chapter 84)
- Syncopal episodes
  - Cardiac disease, e.g. sub-aortic stenosis, pulmonic stenosis, intermittent dysrhythmias (bradydysrhythmias or sustained tachyarrhythmias), dilated cardiomyopathy, hypertrophic cardiomyopathy (cats)
  - Metabolic abnormalities, e.g. intermittent hypoglycaemia in patients with insulinoma
  - Hyperviscosity, e.g. polycythaemia
  - Orthostatic hypotension, vasomotor instability (poorly defined in dogs and cats)
- Neuromuscular disorders, e.g. myasthenia gravis, narcolepsy/cataplexy, inherited myopathies
- Collapsing episodes precipitated by exercise in patients with chronic cardiac, respiratory or neuromuscular disease.

Causes of apparent collapse

- Orthopaedic disease, e.g. osteoarthritis, polyarthritis, bilateral cruciate ligament disease
- Severe pain, e.g post-surgery or trauma
- Neuropathies and myopathies, e.g. corticosteroid-induced myopathy
- Some patients with sudden collapse can be persuaded to stand and sometimes walk, depending on the severity of the disease.

Diagnostic approach

On arrival at the practice, the collapsed pet should have a rapid triage assessment (initial evaluation of respiratory and circulatory systems), to identify any immediately life-threatening problems. This involves assessment of the respiratory system (respiratory rate, effort and pattern), cardiovascular system (pulse rate and quality, mucous membrane colour, heart rate and rhythm), neurological system (mentation, any evidence of seizure activity, spinal reflexes),

100 Top Consultations in Small Animal General Practice, First Edition
By Peter Hill, Sheena Warman and Geoff Shawcross
© 2011 Blackwell Publishing Ltd

a brief assessment of whether the patient is capable of standing or walking, and whether there is evidence of a blocked bladder (cats). Rectal temperature should be obtained if there is any suspicion of hypo- or hyperthermia.

Patients with life-threatening abnormalities detected during this period should be stabilised before a full clinical examination is carried out and a detailed history obtained. Samples should be taken for an emergency database, to include a minimum of PCV, total solids, urea, glucose, sodium and potassium. A blood smear should be made for later examination, and samples stored for further haematological and biochemical assessment if necessary. Imaging techniques (radiography and/or ultrasound) can be used to investigate further when appropriate. Sedation is rarely required in the collapsed patient. Ultrasound is particularly useful for rapid identification of intracavity fluid accumulations, e.g. haemorrhage. Further investigations will depend on the abnormalities detected on physical examination.

Patients with episodic collapse may be clinically normal at the time of examination. Owners should be questioned regarding the nature, duration and frequency of the episodes, whether they occur at rest or on exercise, any abnormalities or changes in the environment prior to collapse, any change in consciousness or respiratory pattern, and whether there are any autonomic signs such as urination, defecation or salivation during episodes. It is helpful to establish whether the collapsing episodes are more consistent with syncope or seizure. Syncope usually occurs during excitement or exercise, and lasts for a few seconds during which the animal may appear 'floppy'; recovery is usually rapid and complete. Seizures are more likely to occur at rest and last for seconds to minutes; they are often associated with tonic–clonic muscle activity with autonomic signs, and post-ictal signs may be apparent.

Initial investigation of episodic collapse should include full physical and neurological examination, haematology and biochemistry (including electrolytes and fasted glucose), and urinalysis. In some cases it is helpful to ask the owners to record an episode with a video camera. Further testing will vary depending on the case, but may require electrocardiogram (ECG) analysis (including 24 hour Holter monitoring, particularly important in breeds at risk of intermittent ventricular dysrhythmias such as Boxers and Dobermanns), blood pressure assessment, radiography, echocardiography, arterial blood gas analysis, ACTH-stimulation test, exercise testing, acetylcholine receptor antibody testing (for myasthenia gravis), magnetic resonance imaging (MRI), CSF analysis, or electrophysiological testing of muscle and nerves. Referral is likely to be required for many of these procedures.

Treatment

These initial investigations should identify any immediately life-threatening problems which can then be managed appropriately. For example, animals with hypovolaemic shock should receive boluses of intravenous fluids (take care in patients with suspected pulmonary contusions or underlying heart disease); those with respiratory distress should be provided with supplemental oxygen whilst the cause of the problem is established and treated; and patients with seizure activity should receive urgent treatment with anti-seizure medication, e.g. diazepam. Further management will depend on the nature of the underlying disease.

What if it doesn't get better?

Successful treatment relies on the accurate identification of the underlying cause of the collapse, using a logical, efficient approach. Some collapsed patients have terminal disease and euthanasia may be appropriate.

Investigation of episodic collapse can be expensive and frustrating, and owners should be warned of this at the outset. In patients with infrequent episodic collapse in which no abnormality is detected following initial investigations, it is often appropriate to take a 'wait and see' approach. The exception to this is breeds such as Boxers and Dobermanns which are at increased risk of intermittent, potentially life-threatening ventricular dysrhythmias, and should have Holter monitoring and echocardiography performed as a priority.

The low-cost option

An efficient triage assessment, followed by a thorough history and physical examination, is the most important aspect of assessment of the collapsed patient, and in many cases will allow a provisional diagnosis to be made. A limited emergency laboratory database is relatively cheap to perform and can quickly identify life-threatening problems. At the point of admitting the animal, and before performing further expensive tests, it is important to establish the owners' expectations. Basic first aid treatment such as oxygen supplementation or analgesia should not be withheld, but further investigations and treatment, if necessary, may need to be delayed while the financial implications are discussed. A step-wise approach should be used, and the owner informed of likely diagnosis, treatment options and prognosis as soon as possible.

When should I refer?

Referral should be considered when a diagnosis is not reached following tests performed within the practice, or if the practice does not have the facilities required to treat a particular condition (e.g. spinal surgery). Finding the cause of episodic collapse can be particularly challenging, and early referral is recommended.

Sheena Warman

Abdominal distension may be noticed by owners and be the reason for seeking veterinary attention, or may be noticed by the clinician during observation and physical examination of the patient. Distension can be caused by gas, fluid, organ enlargement, or a combination of these. Some owners may be under the impression that their pets are gaining weight, without appreciating that gradual abdominal distension can be associated with loss of body condition and muscle mass, which is usually noticeable over the spine and rump.

Common differential diagnoses

- Gastric dilatation and volvulus (GDV)
- Pregnancy or pyometra
- Blocked bladder (especially cats)
- Fluid accumulation (ascites, Figure 11.1)
  - transudate – hypoproteinaemia, prehepatic portal hypertension
  - modified transudate – liver disease, neoplasia, pericardial disease, right-sided congestive heart failure, FIP (cats)
  - exudate – peritonitis, FIP (cats)
  - other fluids – bile, blood, urine, chyle

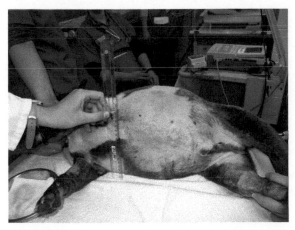

Figure 11.1 A dog with severe abdominal distension due to ascites. (Photo courtesy of Angie Hibbert)

100 Top Consultations in Small Animal General Practice, First Edition
By Peter Hill, Sheena Warman and Geoff Shawcross
© 2011 Blackwell Publishing Ltd

- Organomegaly: especially infiltrative or neoplastic disorder of liver or spleen
- Hyperadrenocorticism: due to a combination of hepatomegaly, fat redistribution and muscle weakness.

Diagnostic approach

If the problem is acute, the patient should undergo a triage assessment in order to establish whether emergency treatment is required. Patients with GDV or a blocked bladder are likely to require urgent intervention (see Chapters 44 and 66).

If the problem is chronic, a full history should be obtained from the owner, paying particular attention to reproductive and oestrus history in entire bitches. A full physical examination should be performed. Organomegaly may be palpable, although it is often difficult to identify the organ involved with certainty. Abdominal fluid may be suggested by the presence of a fluid thrill on ballottement of the abdomen. If abdominal fluid is present, the patient can be tested for hepatojugular reflux. This is performed by checking for jugular distension whilst an assistant applies consistent firm pressure over the liver, causing increased venous return to the right side of the heart; if right atrial pressures are elevated due to pericardial disease or right-sided heart failure, the right atrium may be unable to cope with the increased venous return and jugular distension may be observed. Whilst this test will not identify every such case, it is easy to perform. It is important not to overlook pericardial or right-sided heart diseases as potential causes of ascites.

If there is a high index of suspicion of fluid within the abdomen, abdominocentesis should be performed and fluid submitted for cytology, biochemistry (including total protein, albumin, and other parameters as suggested below), and possibly culture and sensitivity. Concurrent serum biochemistry is useful for comparative purposes, as well as for the identification of severe hypoalbuminaemia (generally ≤15 g/L), which could result in the formation of a transudate. The presence of toxic neutrophils with intracellular bacteria in the fluid, together with low glucose and high lactate concentrations, is indicative of septic peritonitis requiring urgent surgical investigation. In uroperitoneum, concentrations of creatinine will be higher in the fluid than in serum. In pancreatitis, amylase and lipase concentrations will be higher than in serum, and in biliary peritonitis, bilirubin concentration will be higher in the fluid. In patients with haemoabdomen, PCV and total solids may help indicate severity and chronicity of haemorrhage. Most in-house biochemistry analysers can be used for analysis of effusions.

Ultrasound can be used to confirm the presence of fluid. It can also allow identification of specific organomegaly, pyometra, or pregnancy. If organomegaly is identified, biopsy should be considered. Ultrasound is also useful for evaluating the presence of any concurrent pleural fluid; bicavitary effusions are most commonly associated with neoplasia, right-sided heart disease, hypoproteinaemia, or FIP (cats). It is also used to diagnose pericardial disease or right-sided heart failure.

Radiography may help identify mass lesions, but will be of limited use if fluid is present due to the poor detail which results. Pleural effusion and cardiomegaly can be identified using radiography.

Treatment

Initial management depends on the cause of the abdominal distension. Patients with GDV, a blocked bladder, uroabdomen, septic peritonitis, or pyometra require urgent intervention (see Chapters 44, 66 and 70). Patients with acute abdominal haemorrhage may also require urgent stabilisation with fluid therapy, an abdominal pressure bandage, and possibly surgery. Patients with pericardial effusion may require urgent pericardiocentesis, depending on the severity of the cardiac tamponade.

Other causes of abdominal distension tend to be more gradual in onset. Initial management is focussed on achieving a diagnosis and treating the underlying disease appropriately. Occasionally, severe ascites can cause the patient noticeable discomfort and therapeutic drainage of enough fluid to improve patient comfort can be helpful whilst waiting for tests to be performed. This is not recommended in cases of haemoabdomen; it may make bleeding worse, and it prevents reabsorption of haemoglobin and proteins. Repeated drainage is not usually recommended as it can deplete the animal of proteins.

What if it doesn't get better?

Successful treatment requires correct identification of the underlying disease. If the diagnosis is uncertain, physical examination should be repeated, test results reviewed, and further investigations performed as appropriate. There are certain conditions that inherently carry a poor/grave prognosis.

The low-cost option

Apart from a normal pregnancy, there are no causes of abdominal distension that can be managed at low cost. All are likely to involve either emergency medical or surgical treatment, or protracted medical management. The owner should be given an indication of the likely prognosis before embarking on extensive investigations or surgery. In chronic cases, a step-wise approach to investigation, starting with a thorough ultrasound evaluation (or abdominocentesis and fluid analysis, if fluid is present) will often lead to a tentative diagnosis. Whilst radiography may give useful information, it usually requires the additional cost of sedation, and ultrasound is more likely to be diagnostic.

When should I refer?

Most emergencies causing abdominal distension can be treated successfully within primary care facilities. Referral should be considered if appropriate facilities and expertise are unavailable for cases requiring surgical intervention, if it is thought that the patient would benefit from specialist ultrasound examination, or if unfamiliar techniques such as pericardiocentesis are necessary. Long-term management of some of the causes of abdominal distension may benefit from the input of a specialist.

Andrea Harvey

Aetiology and pathogenesis

Feline leukaemia virus (FeLV) is a retrovirus in the lentivirus genus. The virus is shed in all bodily secretions but the main route of infection is via oronasal exposure to infected saliva. Transmission of infection usually requires prolonged contact with infected secretions (e.g. mutual grooming, sharing food bowls). Transplacental infection may occur but is uncommon.

Once a cat is infected with FeLV there are three possible outcomes:

- the cat becomes persistently infected
- the cat becomes transiently infected but then eliminates the virus (can take up to 3 months)
- the cat develops a latent/focal infection whereby the virus persists in some tissues but is not detectable in the blood.

History and clinical signs

FeLV infection is most common in young cats, with FeLV-associated disease usually occurring within 3–5 years of the cat becoming infected. Because the virus is transmitted by close prolonged contact, the disease is most common in cats that have lived closely with other cats.

FeLV can be associated with a wide range of disorders that are not specific to FeLV infection. A large proportion of FeLV-positive cats will develop lymphoma (most commonly mediastinal, multicentric, renal or spinal) leading to clinical signs such as dyspnoea, lymphadenopathy, renomegaly, ataxia/paresis or other neurological signs. Anaemia is also a very common consequence of FeLV infection. This can be caused by a variety of mechanisms including immune-mediated haemolytic anaemia and bone marrow disorders. In some cases, multiple cell lines are involved, resulting in pancytopenia. Cats may, therefore, present with anything from acute regenerative anaemia to chronic non-regenerative anaemia with vague signs such as inappetence, weight loss, pyrexia, pallor, weakness or pica. FeLV may also cause immunosuppression and disease related to secondary infections, similar to those that occur with FIV (see Chapter 13).

100 Top Consultations in Small Animal General Practice, First Edition
By Peter Hill, Sheena Warman and Geoff Shawcross
© 2011 Blackwell Publishing Ltd

Specific diagnostic techniques

The aims of diagnostic testing for FeLV are to identify FeLV-associated disease in cats presenting with clinical illness, and to identify healthy cats with persistent FeLV infection that will pose a risk to other cats and have a poor medium to long-term prognosis themselves.

Diagnosis is generally based on detecting p27 antigen using an enzyme-linked immunosorbent assay (ELISA) or immunochromatographic assay (ICA). p27 is a major core protein in the virus, usually present in large amounts in the plasma of persistently infected cats. These tests can be done in-house (e.g. IDEXX SNAP®, Rhone-Merieux Witness® and Bio Veto Test Laboratories Speed-duo®) or in a commercial laboratory. If an in-house test kit is used, it is extremely important to follow the manufacturer's instructions closely, otherwise false results can occur. Even though some test kits allow the use of whole blood, it is not recommended because false-positive results are more likely than with serum or plasma. Saliva tests are also available but are not recommended because they are associated with a high number of false-positive results.

It is essential to remember that antigen detection tests for FeLV are not 100% sensitive and specific, so false-positive and false-negative results can occur. Several points therefore need to be considered when interpreting the results.

A *positive* antigen result can mean:

- The cat is persistently infected with FeLV
- The cat is transiently infected with FeLV (can last 3–16 weeks)
- A false-positive result.

A *negative* antigen result can mean:

- The cat has not been exposed to FeLV
- The cat has been transiently infected and has successfully eliminated the virus
- The cat has recently been infected and p27 antigen is not yet detectable (can take a few weeks post infection)

- The cat has a latent or focal infection and is not viraemic
- A false-negative result (this is unlikely as the antigen tests are considered reliable in this respect).

Whenever a positive FeLV antigen test is obtained, it is important to consider the health status of the cat and the prevalence of FeLV in the population being tested. For example, a false-positive result will be much more likely in a clinically healthy cat when the prevalence of FeLV infection is low, while a false-positive result would be unlikely in a clinically sick cat. A large proportion of FeLV antigen tests will be false-positives, so it is essential that a positive result is always confirmed with another test, particularly in a clinically healthy cat. Also, as it can take 3–16 weeks to clear a transient infection, repeating the test up to 16 weeks later is required to confirm persistent FeLV infection.

If a negative antigen test result is obtained, the cat is most likely free of FeLV, but this result can occur in recently infected cats, or cats with latent or focal infections (i.e. they are non-viraemic). If contact with a known infected cat had occurred, it would be advisable to re-test 9–16 weeks later to detect an early infection. If latent or localised infection was suspected (e.g. the cat had a disease known to be commonly FeLV related), performing an alternative test (see below) would be indicated.

Two other types of FeLV test are currently available at some commercial laboratories, both of which can be useful as confirmatory tests:

Immunofluorescence antibody test (IFA)

This detects neutrophil- and platelet-associated FeLV p27 antigen, indicating that bone marrow infection had occurred. The test can be performed on a fresh blood smear, a bone marrow smear or a blood sample collected into EDTA or heparin. Usually, if a cat is IFA positive it will be persistently infected. Transient viraemia is still possible, however, and interpretation should take into consideration the health status of the cat. In a clinically healthy cat, repeat testing 12–16 weeks later is indicated to confirm the FeLV status.

PCR (polymerase chain reaction)

This detects FeLV proviral DNA in a sample of blood or bone marrow (collected into EDTA). As with antigen tests, a positive PCR result can occur with transient or persistent viraemia, but it can also detect latent and recovered infections. With latent and recovered infections, ELISA/ICA and IFA tests will be negative. Quantitative PCR is a more sophisticated version of the technique which provides a measure of the total viral load: large amounts of provirus are more likely to indicate persistent viraemia whilst lower amounts of provirus may be more likely to indicate latent or recovered infections.

A summary of the ways in which the various diagnostic tests can be used is shown in Figure 12.1.

Discordant results

A discordant result is when different findings are obtained from the same cat using different FeLV tests. A commonly encountered discordant result is ELISA/ICA positive but IFA negative. The majority of these discordant results remain discordant on repeat testing, and probably represent false-positive antigen test results. However, the true significance of such a result is difficult to interpret because a number of these cats will subsequently become ELISA/ICA negative, whereas a minority will become IFA positive. Hence, continued monitoring and repetition of tests is advisable where discordancy is encountered in a clinically healthy cat.

Another type of discordant result is a positive PCR result when all other FeLV tests are negative. This most probably represents cats that have been transiently infected and have recovered, but the possibility of latent FeLV infection in these cats cannot be excluded. The clinical significance of a positive PCR result with negative ELISA/ICA or IFA results is currently unknown.

If FeLV infection has been confirmed, further investigations for evidence of FeLV-related disease and concurrent infectious diseases may be indicated, e.g. routine haematology, biochemistry, urinalysis, faecal analysis, imaging, FIV testing and *Haemoplasma* species PCR.

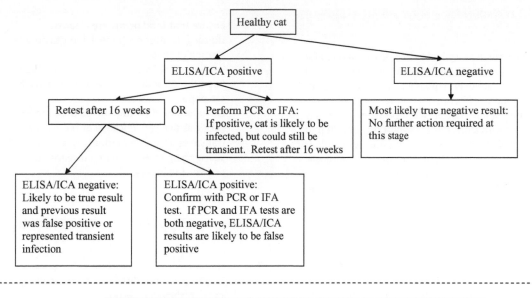

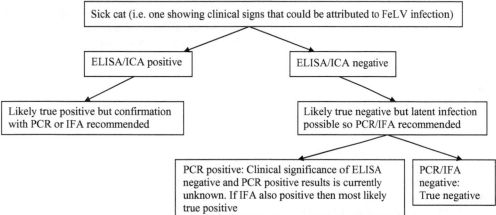

Figure 12.1 **Diagnostic algorithms illustrating the use of FeLV detection tests. In healthy cats, the route taken when positive results are obtained will have to take into account the specific circumstances and wishes of the owner**

Treatment

Routine vaccination against FeLV is recommended for all cats with access to the outdoors or in a household with an identified FeLV-positive cat. FeLV vaccines are extremely effective at preventing infection. Vaccination should not be withheld from a clinically healthy cat with a positive ELISA/ICA test or PCR (but negative IFA), as this may be a false-positive result or previous exposure, in which case not vaccinating will leave the cat susceptible to infection.

In infected cats, there is currently no specific treatment that has been proven to eliminate the virus but some treatments, such as azidothymidine (AZT) and feline recombinant interferon, have been used to try to reduce the effects of the virus. The efficacy of these treatments is controversial. For the treatment of FeLV-associated diseases, additional treatment can be beneficial. For example, for lymphoma, chemotherapy will be required, if the client chooses to pursue treatment.

Other important aspects of management to consider are similar to those used with FIV infection (see Chapter 13):

- Preventing secondary infections
    - Avoid feeding raw meat and discourage from hunting (to reduce risk of toxoplasma infection)
    - Regular flea treatment (to reduce risk of *Haemoplasma* infection)
    - Regular de-worming
    - Good diet
    - Keep indoors to reduce exposure to other infectious agents
    - Regular vaccination against herpesvirus, calicivirus and panleukopenia using killed vaccines if the cat is housed with other cats. If the cat has no contact with other cats, vaccination may not be necessary.
- Identifying and promptly treating secondary infections appropriately, e.g. bacterial infections, protozoal infections such as giardiasis, toxoplasmosis
- Reducing the risk of infection to other cats
    - If the cat is housed with other cats, maintain a stable group, and don't introduce any new cats

- Ensure that food bowls are cleaned thoroughly after each meal and discourage sharing of food bowls
- Vaccinate any in-contact cats against FeLV
- Keep the cat indoors, especially in densely cat populated areas
- Owners should be told not to breed from FeLV-positive cats because of the risk of transmission to their kittens, and the risk of succumbing to FeLV-related disease during or after pregnancy.

What if it doesn't get better?

The prognosis for FeLV-infected cats, once they succumb to FeLV-related disease is poor. However, in the short term they can respond well to treatment for specific diseases, such as lymphoma. If a FeLV-related disease is not responding to the treatment being used, consultation with a specialist or referral is worthwhile to investigate if any alternative treatments may be beneficial.

The low-cost option

Once FeLV infection has been diagnosed, further options will depend on the clinical status of the cat. If the cat is clinically healthy, the lowest-cost option will be to prevent secondary infections and transmission to other cats, and wait until the cat develops FeLV-related disease. Once this happens, the prognosis is poor and euthanasia is an appropriate option. Some owners may elect for euthanasia at the time of diagnosis.

When should I refer?

Referral may be a consideration in any FeLV-positive cat that is clinically unwell if the clinician is not confident with the management options, and the owner is keen to pursue further treatment.

Andrea Harvey

Aetiology and pathogenesis

Feline immunodeficiency virus (FIV) is a retrovirus in the lentivirus genus. The virus is shed in saliva and transmitted mainly through bite wounds. High levels of virus are present in saliva so a single bite can be sufficient. Cats that fight, especially free-roaming entire male cats and feral cats, are most at risk. Other modes of transmission are much less common but include grooming, sharing food bowls and transmission from queen to kittens, either transplacentally or via milk.

Once infected, a cat remains infected for life. However, there is a prolonged asymptomatic period, usually lasting several years, during which the cat appears clinically normal. During this time, there is progressive targeting of immune cells leading to a gradual decline in immune function. Development of FIV-related disease, therefore, does not usually occur until several years after infection, most commonly in middle aged to older cats.

History and clinical signs

FIV infection is more common in rescue cats, cats which have been strays, and those known to fight with other cats. There may be a transient period of pyrexia, malaise and possibly lymphadenopathy during the first 3 months following infection, but this often goes unnoticed.

FIV can be associated with a wide range of disorders that are not specific to FIV infection. Clinical signs may be a primary result of the FIV infection itself, including lymphadenopathy, haematological abnormalities, pyrexia, diarrhoea, uveitis, chorioretinitis, neurological disease or neoplasia. However, more typically, clinical signs are a result of immunosupression and secondary infections with bacteria (e.g. *Haemoplasma, Chlamydophila*), protozoa (e.g. *Toxoplasma, Giardia*), fungi (e.g. dermatophytes), yeast (e.g. *Malassezia*), viruses (e.g. FIP, FeLV, herpesvirus (FHV), calicivirus (FCV)), or parasites. FIV infection should be considered as a potential underlying cause of many illnesses, especially if they are recurrent or resistant to treatment. Some of the many syndromes associated with FIV include gingivitis/stomatitis, respiratory tract infec-

tions, conjunctivitis/ keratitis, anaemia, meningitis/ encephalitis and skin infections.

Differential diagnoses depend on the specific clinical signs of the individual case (refer to other relevant chapters for differential diagnoses).

Specific diagnostic techniques

Diagnosis is generally based on detecting serum antibodies to FIV viral proteins using an ELISA or ICA. These tests can be done in-house (e.g. IDEXX SNAP®, Rhone-Merieux Witness® and Bio Veto Test Laboratories Speed-duo®) or by a commercial laboratory. If an in-house test kit is used, it is extremely important to follow the manufacturer's instructions closely, otherwise erroneous results can occur.

It is essential to remember that no test for FIV is 100% sensitive or specific, so false-negative and false-positive results can occur and several points need to be considered when interpreting results.

A *positive* antibody result can mean:

- The cat is infected with FIV
- Maternally derived antibodies are present – Kittens born to FIV-positive queens can test positive due to these antibodies, but less than 25% of these kittens will develop FIV, so they should be re-tested when over 6 months old
- The cat is vaccinated against FIV – There is a vaccine available for FIV (not yet available in the UK, but likely to be in the near future). This will make diagnosis of FIV much more difficult as any vaccinated cat will be positive on an antibody test
- False-positive result – Whenever an FIV test is performed, it is important to consider the health status of the cat and the prevalence of FIV in the population being tested. For example, a false-positive result will be much more likely in a clinically healthy cat in an area in which the prevalence of FIV infection is low, while a false-positive result would be unlikely in a clinically sick cat. A positive result should, therefore, always be confirmed with an alternative test.

100 Top Consultations in Small Animal General Practice, First Edition
By Peter Hill, Sheena Warman and Geoff Shawcross
© 2011 Blackwell Publishing Ltd

A *negative* antibody result can mean:

- The cat has not been exposed to FIV
- The cat has been infected recently and has not yet developed antibodies (seroconversion). Typically, this can take up to 12 weeks after infection
- The cat is infected but has not produced antibodies, or has produced antibodies that are not detectable with the tests used (e.g. possible with ELISA/ICA)
- The cat has terminal FIV infection and antibody levels are no longer detectable
- False-negative result. Since there is a possibility in some FIV-infected cats that antibodies will not be detectable, another type of test (see below) should be performed in any cat where FIV infection is strongly suspected (e.g. presence of multiple or recurrent infections) despite a negative antibody test.

Several other types of FIV test are available at some commercial laboratories which are useful as confirmatory tests:

PCR (polymerase chain reaction)

This detects FIV proviral DNA in the blood. A positive test should be reliable provided a validated PCR test is used (reliability data should be obtained from the laboratory performing the test). PCR is useful as a confirmatory test in cats with a positive ELISA/ICA, and also in kittens (as it is not affected by maternally derived antibodies), vaccinated cats, cats that have been recently exposed to FIV which may not yet have produced antibodies, and in cats where FIV infection is strongly suspected (e.g. presence of multiple or recurrent infections) despite a negative antibody test. However, it is important in all these situations to realize that PCR may not detect all the different FIV subtypes and false-negative results can occur. A positive PCR is usually reliable, but any discordant results between PCR and an antibody test should be discussed with the laboratory running the tests. In a healthy cat, a positive result should be obtained with two different tests before concluding that it is infected with FIV.

IFA (immunofluorescence antibody test)

This detects antibodies to numerous FIV viral proteins in the blood, as opposed to just the one or two viral proteins present in an ELISA or ICA test kit. It also detects antibodies actually bound to FIV-infected cells. These features make it a much more reliable antibody test, and therefore it is useful as a confirmatory test in an ELISA-positive cat, and as an additional test in a cat where FIV is strongly suspected despite a negative ELISA/ICA. It is also valuable where there is discordance between ELISA/ICA and PCR. A positive result still needs to be interpreted carefully as described for ELISA tests, but false-positive results are less likely.

Western blotting

This also detects antibodies to a variety of FIV proteins making it more sensitive than an ELISA or ICA test, so it is another alternative to IFA. However, although it is widely used in the USA, it is not currently widely available in the UK.

Virus isolation

This detects whole virus in the blood and is, therefore, very specific (i.e. a positive result is reliable), but the test has limited availability as it is time-consuming and technically difficult to perform.

If FIV infection is confirmed, further investigations to look for evidence of FIV-related disease and concurrent infectious diseases may be indicated, e.g. routine haematology, biochemistry, urinalysis, faecal analysis, imaging, FeLV testing and *Haemoplasma* species PCR.

Treatment

Unlike FeLV, effective vaccines against FIV are not widely available. A FIV vaccine licensed in the USA is likely to become available in the UK in the near future, but its efficacy is controversial.

Once a cat is infected with FIV, the infection cannot be eliminated. There are currently no specific treatments that have been proven to inhibit FIV replication, but some treatments (e.g. AZT, feline recombinant interferon) have been used to try to reduce the effects of the virus. The efficacy of these treatments is also considered controversial. However, many affected cats can be effectively managed for long periods. Important aspects of management to consider are:

- Prevention of secondary infections:
  - Avoid feeding raw meat and discourage from hunting (to reduce risk of Toxoplasma infection)

- Regular flea treatment (to reduce risk of *Haemoplasma* infection)
- Regular worming
- Good diet
- Keep indoors to reduce exposure to other infectious agents
- Regular vaccination against herpesvirus, calicivirus and panleukopenia using a killed vaccine if the cat is housed with other cats. If the cat has no contact with other cats vaccination may not be necessary.
- Identifying and promptly treating secondary infections appropriately, e.g. bacterial infections, protozoal infections such as giardiasis, toxoplasmosis
- Reducing the risk of infection to other cats
  - Neuter entire cats
  - Keeping the cat indoors is strongly advisable, but if owners refuse, keeping the cat indoors just at night will significantly reduce the risk of transmitting infection as most cat fights occur at dawn and dusk.

The low-cost option

Once FIV infection has been diagnosed, the treatment options depend on the clinical status of the cat. The lowest cost option will be to prevent secondary infections and transmission to other cats. Euthanasia should be offered when the cat succumbs to a FIV-related disease that is affecting the cat's quality of life significantly and cannot be treated within the owner's financial limitations.

When should I refer?

Referral may be a consideration in any FIV-positive cat that is clinically unwell if the clinician is not confident with the options for management. If a FIV-related disease is not responding to the treatment as expected, consultation with a specialist, or referral, may be worthwhile to investigate whether any alternative treatments may be beneficial.

What if it doesn't get better?

Once a cat is infected with FIV it will eventually succumb to FIV-related disease. However, there is a long asymptomatic period, usually many years, before this occurs. Treatment depends on the clinical signs that arise, but most secondary infections are treatable. It should also be borne in mind that cats may also develop disorders that are unrelated to the FIV, so clinical illness should not automatically be considered terminal in a cat known to have FIV.

Aetiology and pathogenesis

Feline infectious peritonitis (FIP) is caused by a coronavirus (FCoV). FCoV is a ubiquitous RNA virus infecting large numbers of cats, particularly in multicat households. The virus is shed in the faeces and transmitted faeco-orally, with litter boxes representing the main source of infection. The virus can survive in a dry environment for 7 weeks. Indirect transmission (via litter trays, hands, clothes, etc.) can also occur. Although direct transmission from FIP cases may occur, this does not usually lead to disease. Cats are most likely to be infected following contact with FCoV in faeces from asymptomatic cats. In breeding households, kittens are usually infected with FCoV at around 5–6 weeks of age. Once a cat becomes infected with FCoV, most cats remain clinically healthy or show only a mild transient enteritis. Only a small proportion of FCoV infected cats will go on to develop FIP. Virus is shed in the faeces within 1 week of infection. The duration of shedding varies widely from weeks to months, with some cats remaining lifelong carriers.

FIP is a pyogranulomatous vasculitis. It is thought to arise through mutation of FCoV within the individual cat followed by rapid replication of the mutant virus and infection of monocytes and macrophages. Whether or not FIP develops, and the type of lesions that develop, is thought to be influenced by viral load and the cat's immune response. Cats infected with FCoV are predisposed to developing FIP if they experience stressors such as surgery, re-homing, a visit to a cattery, etc. Some breeds (e.g. Bengal, Orientals, Birman) and individual lines within breeds appear more likely to develop FIP.

History and clinical signs

The majority of cases of FIP occur in cats less than one year of age, although it can affect cats of any age. It most commonly arises in multicat households, and particularly in purebred cats.

FIP can present with variable clinical signs, depending on the distribution of pathology. FIP has been broadly classified into two forms: effusive (wet) and non-effusive

(dry), but these two forms just reflect different extremes of a continuum of clinical signs, being partly dependent on the cat's immune response to the virus.

Initial clinical signs may be non-specific, such as pyrexia, lethargy, anorexia, weight loss or failure to thrive. Pyogranulomatous and vasculitis/perivasculitis lesions may develop in any organs such as the kidneys, mesenteric lymph nodes, liver, spleen, omentum and brain. The organs affected determine the clinical signs that develop. Ascites is the most common clinical sign. Other clinical findings may include dyspnoea (most commonly due to pleural effusion, rarely due to pyogranulomatous pneumonia), palpably enlarged mesenteric lymph nodes, renomegaly, ileocaecocolic/colonic lesions, ocular lesions (uveitis, iritis, hyphaema, keratic precipitates, chorioretinitis, retinal perivascular cuffing) and neurological signs (focal, multifocal or diffuse signs involving the brain, spinal cord and/or meninges). The most common neurological signs include ataxia, hyperaesthesia, nystagmus and seizures.

Specific diagnostic techniques

There is no definitive non-invasive ante-mortem diagnostic test for FIP. Currently, definitive diagnosis can only be made on histopathology of affected tissues demonstrating pyogranulomatous inflammation. Immunohistochemistry can confirm the presence of FCoV antigen in macrophages.

There are various clinical features and laboratory abnormalities that can arise with FIP, and the more that are present, the more likely that FIP is the diagnosis. A tentative diagnosis of FIP is therefore often made by first excluding other differential diagnoses, followed by searching for abnormalities that would be indicative of FIP.

Diagnostic investigations that can be of value include:

- Ophthalmic examination: assessing for abnormalities as described above. Differential diagnoses include toxoplasmosis, FeLV/FIV, Bartonella, neoplasia, idiopathic immune-mediated uveitis

100 Top Consultations in Small Animal General Practice, First Edition
By Peter Hill, Sheena Warman and Geoff Shawcross
© 2011 Blackwell Publishing Ltd

- Complete haematology
  - Lymphopenia is common; a normal lymphocyte count makes FIP less likely
  - Mild, non-regenerative anaemia is common in FIP but is also a common finding with any chronic illness.
- Serum biochemistry
  - Hyperglobulinaemia is common, and often marked. The albumin:globulin ratio is usually <0.8. Differential diagnoses include multiple myeloma (if monoclonal gammopathy demonstrated on serum protein electrophoresis), lymphoma and other inflammatory diseases, particularly lymphocytic cholangitis if liver parameters are also elevated
  - Hyperbilirubinaemia (mild to moderate) is common and usually occurs in the absence of elevated liver enzymes
  - Liver enzymes, urea and creatinine can be elevated, depending on degree of organ involvement.
- Thoracic radiographs: mainly to detect pleural fluid. If present, the fluid should be sampled, if possible
- Abdominal ultrasound: to detect free abdominal fluid. If present, the fluid should be sampled. Other abnormalities may include mesenteric lymphadenopathy, hyperechoic mesenteric fat, irregular edges to the kidney/liver/spleen
- Abdominal/pleural fluid analysis
  - If any effusions are present, analysis of the effusion(s) is one of the most diagnostically useful assessments
  - Usually, the fluid is either an aseptic exudate or a modified transudate, being highly proteinaceous with a relatively low cellularity, usually comprising neutrophils and macrophages. Albumin:globulin ratio is usually <0.4. If it is above 0.8, then FIP is unlikely. Differential diagnoses include lymphocytic cholangitis, congestive heart failure, lymphoma, septic peritonitis
  - Immunofluoresence can be performed on the fluid to identify the virus within macrophages, which if present is considered to provide a definitive diagnosis of FIP.
- Alpha-1 acid glycoprotein (AGP). A concentration above 1500 μg/ml is supportive of FIP, but it can be elevated in other inflammatory conditions, and can be high in healthy cats infected with FCoV

- Coronavirus antibodies. Coronavirus titres do not distinguish between 'normal' coronavirus infection and FIP, but simply indicate exposure to coronavirus and are frequently positive in healthy cats. If the titres are very high (>1:16 000) this can be more suggestive of FIP. However, coronavirus antibodies are generally of limited diagnostic value since low or negative titres do not rule out FIP, and healthy cats that never go on to develop FIP can also have very high titres, particularly if they are living in multicat households. Caution must be taken to ensure that high coronavirus titres are not over-interpreted
- Neurological assessment/MRI/CSF if neurological signs are present. Such cases are best referred to specialists. Important differential diagnoses to consider in a young cat with neurological signs include metabolic disorders (e.g. portosystemic shunt), congenital neurological abnormalities (e.g. hydrocephalus), lymphoma (potentially FeLV-associated), other infectious aetiologies (e.g. Toxoplasmosis), idiopathic epilepsy, trauma, toxins, and nutritional abnormalities (e.g. thiamine deficiency).

Treatment

Sadly, FIP is still considered a fatal disease. Most cats with FIP (particularly if they are effusive) will deteriorate rapidly and should be euthanised as soon as their quality of life is reduced. A minority of cats with FIP will have a much more chronic course of disease with only mild clinical signs. In these cases, it is reasonable to treat palliatively with corticosteroids, and supportive treatments such as appetite stimulants (e.g. mirtazapine, cyproheptadine). Interferon is a controversial treatment that is recommended by some clinicians, although there is a lack of good evidence for any benefit. It is reasonable to try interferon in cases with a more chronic course of disease, if there are no financial limitations. Euthanasia should be considered once further clinical signs develop and/or the cat's quality of life is significantly compromised.

The risk of FIP is always greater in multicat households, mainly due to increased stressors and higher viral burdens. General measures for controlling infectious diseases should be employed, such as only keeping small stable groups of cats (maximum 4–5 cats) housed together. Routine hygiene measures should always be taken with all cats to reduce the risk of FCoV infection. FCoV is readily inactivated by most household detergents and bleach. There is no value in isolating a cat with suspected FIP that lives in a multicat household, as the other cats will probably be infected with FCoV and are unlikely to have any higher risk of developing FIP than any other cat in a multicat household. It is recommended to wait 2 months before bringing any new cats into a household that has had a cat with FIP.

Breeding households are the highest risk environments for FIP. Owners of kittens obtained from a breeder should be encouraged to inform the breeder if their kitten has developed FIP so that the breeder can monitor the situation. If a breeder is having multiple kittens going on to develop FIP then consideration should be given to:

- Identifying high FCoV shedders in the household, using reverse transcriptase (RT)-PCR screening of faeces. However, the value of this is controversial
- Early weaning and strict isolation and hygiene measures to prevent FCoV infection of the kittens. Again, effectiveness is controversial and the negative effects on socialisation need to be considered
- Evaluation for genetic involvement. Some individual tom cats and/or queens may produce higher proportions of kittens that go on to develop FIP and if this is identified, consideration should be given to stopping breeding with those individuals.

Currently the only guaranteed protection against FIP is preventing infection with FCoV. Being a ubiquitous virus, this is extremely difficult to achieve unless a cat is bred in a FCoV-free household and is kept indoors with no other cats, or only other FCoV-free cats. At present, there is a vaccine available for FCoV in the USA and some European countries, but not the UK. The efficacy of this vaccine is very controversial and most cats will already have been infected with FCoV prior to vaccination, in which case it is unlikely to be of value.

What if it doesn't get better?

Sadly the prognosis for cats with FIP is very poor and most cats will need to be euthanised fairly soon after diagnosis.

The low-cost option

If there is enough clinical evidence to justify a diagnosis of FIP, then given the grave prognosis, euthanasia should be considered early on in the course of the disease. In cases where there is not enough evidence to diagnose FIP, or if there are financial limitations on performing further investigations, then supportive treatment and monitoring is usually a reasonable choice. In most cases of FIP, there will be progression of clinical signs in a relatively short space of time, and the diagnosis may become more certain as further clinical features develop.

When should I refer?

Referral to a feline medicine specialist may be a consideration in any cat where FIP is a differential diagnosis but where the practitioner is unable to find enough evidence to be certain about the diagnosis, or when advanced diagnostic techniques (e.g. MRI, CSF analysis) are required. Referral is also indicated if an owner wants a specialist opinion prior to making further decisions (e.g. regarding further investigations or euthanasia) or breeders want to discuss any implications on their breeding programmes.

Section 3
Skin problems

Peter Hill

Pruritus is a sensation in the skin that leads to a desire to scratch. It is caused by stimulation of cutaneous nerve endings by inflammatory mediators and cytokines released from eosinophils, neutrophils, mast cells or lymphocytes. In dogs, signs other than scratching may be seen, including chewing, nibbling, licking, rubbing, rolling and head shaking. The skin lesions found in a pruritic dog will depend on the cause, severity and chronicity. Initially, there may be no visible lesions but most of the underlying conditions cause erythema or rashes (macular, papular or pustular eruptions). Licking and self trauma can lead to salivary staining, excoriations, self-induced alopecia or hot spots. Chronic cases may develop hyperpigmentation and lichenification. The severity of pruritus will increase if a dog has more than one pruritic skin condition at the same time, a concept known as summation.

Common differential diagnoses

In the majority of cases, pruritus in dogs is caused by ectoparasites, infectious agents or allergies. Specific details about the diagnosis and treatment of the conditions listed below can be found in subsequent chapters.

Ectoparasites

- Flea allergy dermatitis
- Lice infestation
- *Sarcoptes scabiei* infestation (sarcoptic mange, scabies)
- *Cheyletiella* infestation
- *Trombicula autumnalis* larvae infestation
- Insect bite hypersensitivity
- Demodicosis.

Infectious agents

- Staphylococcal pyoderma
- *Malassezia* dermatitis.

Allergies

- Contact dermatitis
- Adverse food reactions
- Atopic dermatitis.

---

100 Top Consultations in Small Animal General Practice, First Edition
By Peter Hill, Sheena Warman and Geoff Shawcross
© 2011 Blackwell Publishing Ltd

Diagnostic approach

The first step with any itchy dog is to consider ectoparasites or infectious agents as likely causes. Clinicians should never diagnose allergic skin problems unless they are certain that parasitic and infectious causes have been ruled out.

Fleas, flea dirt, lice and *Trombicula* larvae can be seen with the naked eye, so they should always be looked for when examining the skin of pruritic dogs. When dealing with microscopic parasites or microorganisms, the ideal approach is to try and establish a definitive diagnosis by identifying the specific agent on skin scrapings or cytology. However, for some of the parasitic and infectious conditions listed above, it is appropriate to adopt a 'pattern recognition' approach and decide if the history, lesion type and distribution provide sufficient information to make a tentative diagnosis. Flea allergy, sarcoptic mange, *Cheyletiella* infestation, *Trombicula* infestation, insect bite hypersensitivity and superficial pyoderma usually produce characteristic lesions and a therapeutic trial is an entirely appropriate and cost-effective approach, especially when time and resources are limited. If the condition responds completely to treatment, no further action is necessary. This 'pattern recognition' approach is not appropriate when dealing with demodicosis or *Malassezia* dermatitis because neither condition produces pathognomonic signs. If suspected, both these conditions require diagnostic investigation and monitoring to ensure effective treatment. Due to the prolonged treatment courses required to resolve demodicosis, skin scrapings and/ or hair pluckings must *always* be performed to confirm the diagnosis and trial therapy must *never* be prescribed. Likewise, it is not possible to diagnose *Malassezia* overgrowth on clinical signs alone and cytological examination of stained tape strips should always be performed if this condition is suspected.

If parasites or infectious agents are not involved, or if treatment of these conditions does not lead to complete resolution, allergic skin conditions should be suspected. Clinicians should remember that allergic skin diseases have specific historical and clinical features that should be used to support the diagnosis. Although rare, contact dermatitis usually causes a very typical lesion distribution pattern that allows a tentative diagnosis to be made (e.g. collar dermatitis, scrotal dermatitis). If the condition is more generalised, it is most appropriate in general practice to first rule out adverse reactions to food, even though this is much less common than atopic dermatitis. This is done by instituting a strict trial with a diet containing novel or hydrolysed ingredients. Laboratory testing for dietary allergies is currently unreliable and there is no evidence that it provides meaningful results. Commercially available limited ingredient or hydrolysed diets are the most convenient option and they should be fed for up to 6 weeks to see if there is any reduction in pruritus. If the condition improves, the diet should be continued to see if there is complete or only partial resolution. Dietary involvement is confirmed if there is a relapse when the original diet is re-introduced. Clinicians should be aware that there are many pitfalls when performing and interpreting the response to dietary changes, and failures due to poor owner compliance are not uncommon.

If dietary manipulation does not lead to complete resolution, atopic dermatitis may be suspected (see Chapter 20). A clinical diagnosis of atopic dermatitis can be made if there is a typical history, characteristic lesions with an appropriate distribution, and when parasites, infectious agents and adverse food reactions have been ruled out. In such cases, there are two main options: long-term symptomatic treatment, or allergy testing in order to identify the precise cause. Which option is taken will depend on the severity of the condition and the wishes of the client.

Clinicians should note that skin biopsies are rarely beneficial in the investigation of itchy dogs and should not be performed routinely.

symptomatic treatments merely suppress the inflammation resulting from that cause. In most cases, symptomatic treatment involves the use of glucocorticoids. These drugs can be extremely valuable for treating pruritic dogs, providing short-term relief whilst the specific treatment is taking effect, but they can also be abused and should never be prescribed in the absence of a diagnosis. It is appropriate to use concurrent glucocorticoid therapy for all the diseases in the above differential diagnosis list with three exceptions. Glucocorticoids should *never* be given to dogs with demodicosis because, although they may relieve the itching, they make the condition worse. Glucocorticoids should also be avoided when treating superficial pyoderma or *Malassezia* dermatitis. The pruritus associated with these two conditions responds reliably to antimicrobial therapy and the degree of response allows clinicians to determine if there is an underlying cause of the infections. For the remaining conditions, glucocorticoids are very useful for providing immediate control of the pruritus associated with superficial ectoparasites and they may also be needed both in the short- and long-term for the management of allergic skin conditions. The type of glucocorticoid used depends on the duration of effect that is required. For very short-term effects (up to 3 days), an injectable glucocorticoid such as dexamethasone would be acceptable. For longer term effects, oral therapy with prednisolone or methylprednisolone at daily or alternate day doses of 0.4–1.0 mg/kg are the most appropriate options. Long-acting injectable glucocorticoid preparations do not allow daily dosage control and should be avoided. Specific glucocorticoid treatment regimes can be found in the chapters on parasitic or allergic diseases.

Treatment

When dealing with pruritus, clinicians should always try to prescribe specific treatments for specific diagnoses (see relevant chapters). Prescribing a combination of ectoparasiticides, antibiotics and glucocorticoids to every itchy dog is neither cost-effective nor good medicine. Management of pruritus in dogs can involve both specific and symptomatic treatments. Specific treatments can be curative because they target the actual cause of the pruritus, whereas

What if it doesn't get better?

In most cases, failure of the pruritus to resolve indicates failure to make a correct diagnosis. Clinicians should re-evaluate the diagnostic approach to see if any of the differentials listed above have been missed, bearing in mind that more than one condition can be present in the same patient at the same time. In non-responding or complex cases, or if multiple or allergic aetiologies are suspected, a more complete diagnostic investigation is indicated, involving coat brushings, skin scrapings, hair plucks and cytological examination. This may require the dog to be hospitalised to allow time for the procedures to be performed. In the case of confirmed allergic skin conditions, clients must be made aware that lifelong treatment is required in order to control the pruritus. If the dog does not respond to apparently rational therapy, clinicians should consider poor owner compliance, resistance to specific treatments (antiparasitics, antibiotics) or uncommon diseases (e.g. cutaneous lymphoma) as possible explanations.

The low-cost option

Costs can be minimised by making a precise diagnosis as soon as possible based on relevant historical and clinical findings. Diagnostic testing can be avoided in many cases (as described above), leaving more funds available for treatment. Drug costs can be minimised but false economies (such as recommending poor flea control products) should be avoided. Clients must be made aware that ownership of an allergic dog will incur a degree of lifelong expense.

When should I refer?

Referral of itchy dogs to a dermatologist should be recommended if a diagnosis or satisfactory outcome hasn't been achieved after three consultations. Investigation and management of complex cases by a dermatologist may save the owner time and money, and shorten the time to satisfactory resolution or control. Despite the routine availability of serum-based allergy tests, investigation of allergies is best undertaken by dermatologists, who have the necessary experience to fully evaluate the case and recommend long-term treatment options.

Peter Hill

The presenting signs seen in itchy cats are significantly different from those seen in dogs. Cats are more secretive than dogs and may suffer from pruritus without their owners being aware of it. Cats also use their tongue to 'scratch' themselves whenever they can and this can be misinterpreted as normal grooming behaviour. They tend to use their claws only in areas they cannot lick, such as around the head and neck. These methods of alleviating pruritus explain some of the presenting signs seen in cats with pruritus, such as extensive areas of alopecia over the trunk or severe excoriations around the head. In many cases, it is only when such skin lesions become apparent that owners present their cat for veterinary attention. Lesions seen in itchy cats can be divided into four distinctive syndromes. These are:

- miliary dermatitis
- symmetrical alopecia
- the eosinophilic granuloma complex
- head and neck pruritus.

Miliary dermatitis is characterised by small, crusted papules (the lesions look and feel like small scabs) most commonly over the dorsum and around the neck. Self-induced alopecia is often seen (Figure 16.1).

Symmetrical alopecia is characterised by bilaterally symmetrical alopecia most commonly over the ventral abdomen, medial hindlimbs and lateral abdomen. The dorsum is not usually affected. The hair loss is self-induced and any remaining or surrounding hair may appear stubbly. The skin is not usually grossly inflamed (Figure 16.2).

The eosinophilic granuloma complex comprises three distinctive lesions: indolent ulcers (formerly known as rodent ulcers), eosinophilic plaques and eosinophilic granulomas. These lesions occur at sites where cats can lick and may be present separately, in combination with each other, or with other pruritic syndromes. Indolent ulcers are well demarcated ulcers that occur unilaterally or bilaterally on the upper lips (Figure 16.3).

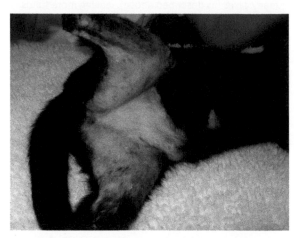

Figure 16.2 Self-induced symmetrical alopecia in a cat

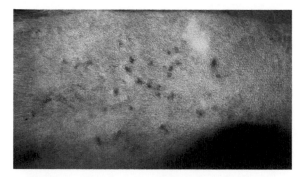

Figure 16.1 Miliary dermatitis in a cat. The area has been clipped to aid visualization of the lesions

100 Top Consultations in Small Animal General Practice, First Edition
By Peter Hill, Sheena Warman and Geoff Shawcross
© 2011 Blackwell Publishing Ltd

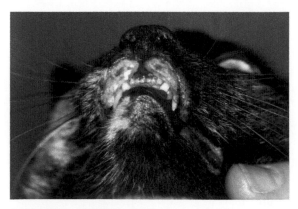

Figure 16.3 Indolent ulcers on the lips of a cat

Eosinophilic plaques are well demarcated, alopecic, raised plaques with a moist, red surface which may be eroded or ulcerated. They are usually located on the ventral abdomen, thorax and medial aspect of the hind legs (Figure 16.4). Eosinophilic granulomas are well-defined, firm, raised, yellow to pink lesions that typically occur on the caudal aspect of the hindlimbs or in the oral cavity (Figure 16.5).

Head and neck pruritus is characterised by excoriations and self-induced ulceration around the head and neck (Figure 16.6). Some cats focus the self-trauma on the cheeks.

Common differential diagnoses

Despite the specific appearances of the above syndromes, they can all be caused by a number of underlying pruritic diseases. Some of the common causes are shown below, and as with dogs, ectoparasites or allergies are frequently involved. However, unlike dogs, pruritic superficial staphylococcal pyoderma or *Malassezia* dermatitis are rare in cats.

Ectoparasites
- Flea allergy dermatitis
- Lice infestation
- *Cheyletiella* infestation
- *Otodectes cynotis* infestation
- *Trombicula autumnalis* (harvest mite) larvae infestation
- Insect bite hypersensitivity
- *Notoedres cati* infestation (notoedric mange, feline scabies); common in some countries but not seen in the UK
- Demodicosis: seen in some countries but extremely rare in cats in the UK.

Infections
- Dermatophytosis.

Allergies
- Adverse food reactions
- Atopic dermatitis.

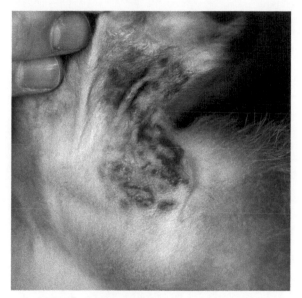

Figure 16.4 Eosinophilic plaques in the axilla of a cat

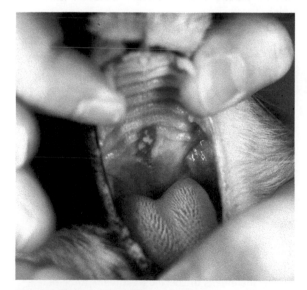

Figure 16.5 Eosinophilic granuloma on the hard palate of a cat

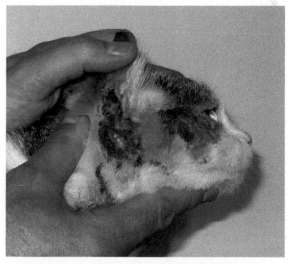

Figure 16.6 Severe facial pruritus and self trauma in a cat

Diagnostic approach

The first step is to confirm that the cat has one of the four pruritic syndromes. With miliary dermatitis and head/neck pruritus, this can be done on clinical signs alone. For symmetrical alopecia, it is worth confirming that the hair loss is self-induced by performing a trichogram (examining plucked hairs under the microscope). This will reveal that the ends of the hairs have been broken off (Figure 16.7). Although the lesions of the eosinophilic granuloma complex are distinctive, cytological examination of an impression smear is helpful in confirming the cellular component and to determine the degree of secondary bacterial infection that may be present (Figure 16.8).

Once the condition has been characterised, it is necessary to find an underlying cause. Some diagnoses may be suspected immediately on clinical examination, such as infestations with fleas, lice, *Cheyletiella*, *Otodectes* or *Trombicula*. If there is no obvious evidence of these parasites, flea allergy dermatitis is still the most likely cause and a thorough flea control programme is indicated as part of the diagnostic plan. If flea control does not resolve the problem, skin scrapings should be performed to check that other ectoparasites have not been missed. If there is a prominent alopecic component to the condition, dermatophytosis should be considered as a differential diagnosis and a Wood's lamp examination and fungal culture are indicated.

If the lesions persist after ruling out ectoparasites and dermatophytosis, allergic skin conditions should be considered. In general practice, it is most appropriate to first rule out adverse food reactions by instituting a strict dietary trial (as described in the previous chapter). This can be very difficult in cats that have free access to the outside because they can obtain food from other sources. This may be a major reason for the failure of many cats to respond to dietary manipulation.

In refractory cases, atopic dermatitis should be considered, but investigation of this disease is best undertaken by dermatologists. Identification of relevant allergens in cats by intradermal testing or IgE serology is fraught with difficulties and there is ample scope for misdiagnosis.

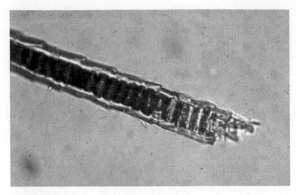

Figure 16.7   Fractured hair tip due to excessive licking

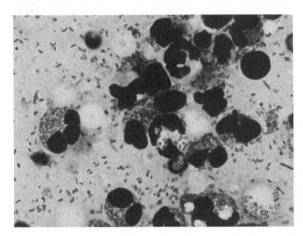

Figure 16.8 **Cytological appearance of an eosinophilic plaque with secondary infection (Diff-Quik stain)**

Treatment

Although it is critical to investigate these syndromes thoroughly, to allow identification and treatment of an underlying cause, it is often necessary to provide symptomatic treatment to ameliorate the pruritus whilst tests and specific treatments are being performed. However, symptomatic treatment should not be used instead of a diagnostic evaluation. For the more severe lesions of miliary dermatitis, head and neck pruritus, or lesions of the eosinophilic granuloma complex, an initial course of glucocorticoids is indicated. Prednisolone at 1–2 mg/kg daily for 5–14 days, followed by tapering of the dose, is most appropriate. The glucocorticoids should be discontinued to allow the effects of specific treatments to be determined, such as the response to flea control or food trials. Long-term depot injections of glucocorticoids should be avoided because they may prevent evaluation of the response to specific treatments and interfere with future testing (especially intradermal testing). If dermatophytosis is suspected, glucocorticoids should not be used until it has been ruled out by negative culture.

If ulcers or excoriations are present and there is evidence of secondary bacterial infection on cytology (especially with the eosinophilic granuloma complex or head/neck pruritus), systemic antibiotics should be prescribed for 2–3 weeks, in conjunction with glucocorticoids if necessary. Appropriate choices would be amoxicillin/clavulanic acid, cefalexin or cefovecin.

Symptomatic treatment of feline symmetrical alopecia is not usually necessary because the skin is not inflamed and the severity of the condition is less than with the other syndromes. In such cases, the best approach is to monitor the response to the specific treatments alone, but hair growth is slow so the response time will be much longer.

facial pain syndrome (head and neck pruritus). For refractory indolent ulcers, surgical resection can be curative in some cases.

Some pruritic cats defy a diagnosis and remain idiopathic, or cannot be controlled with specific treatments due to poor owner compliance. These may require long-term symptomatic therapy with glucocorticoids, ciclosporin, antihistamines, essential fatty acids or some combination thereof. In these circumstances, owners should be made aware of the possible adverse effects associated with long-term use of these drugs. Despite a labelled indication for the treatment of miliary dermatitis and the eosinophilic granuloma complex, the progestagen megestrol acetate (Ovarid; Virbac Limited) should not be routinely used for control of pruritus in the cat, due to the risk of development of diabetes mellitus and mammary hyperplasia.

What if it doesn't get better?

As with dogs, failure of the pruritus to resolve may represent a misdiagnosis. The case should be reviewed to ensure that all diagnostic steps have been performed correctly and that the client has adhered to the treatment protocol. Clinicians should then consider other less likely differential diagnoses for lesions which may look similar to those described above. These might include cowpox infection (miliary dermatitis); feline paraneoplastic alopecia or hyperadrenocorticism (feline symmetrical alopecia); squamous cell carcinoma (indolent ulcers); mast cell tumours or cutaneous lymphoma (eosinophilic plaques); and feline herpes virus infection or oro-

The low-cost option

Costs can be minimised by making a diagnosis as quickly and efficiently as possible. Most of the initial diagnostic tests are relatively cheap to perform. Short- and long-term symptomatic treatment with glucocorticoids is inexpensive in cats.

When should I refer?

Referral to a dermatologist should be recommended if a diagnosis or satisfactory progress hasn't been achieved after three consultations. Investigation of cats for possible atopic dermatitis is best undertaken by a dermatologist.

Peter Hill

Aetiology and pathogenesis

Superficial ectoparasites are a common cause of pruritic skin disease in dogs and cats. Pruritus may be caused both by physical irritation and the development of hypersensitivity reactions to the parasite's saliva.

History and clinical signs

The typical clinical signs seen with parasite infestations are variable degrees of pruritus and skin lesions that occur at specific sites. Figure 17.1 summarises the lesions and distribution patterns for the most common superficial ectoparasites. Figures 17.2 to 17.5 illustrate some of the clinical features of these conditions.

Figure 17.1 **Summary of lesions and typical distribution patterns for superficial ectoparasites that cause pruritus in dogs and cats (Photo of** *Notoedres cati* **courtesy of Francesco Albanese)**

Ectoparasite	Associated lesions	Distribution
Fleas 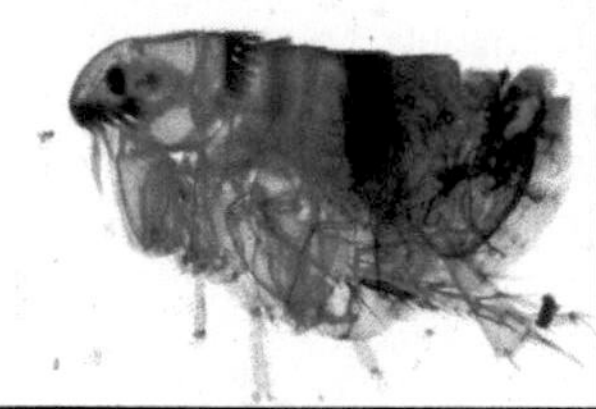	Papules Self-induced alopecia Hot spots Lichenification Hyperpigmentation	Dorsal lumbo-sacral *Affects dogs and cats* 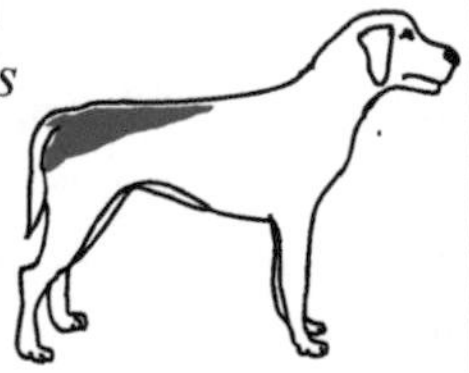
Lice 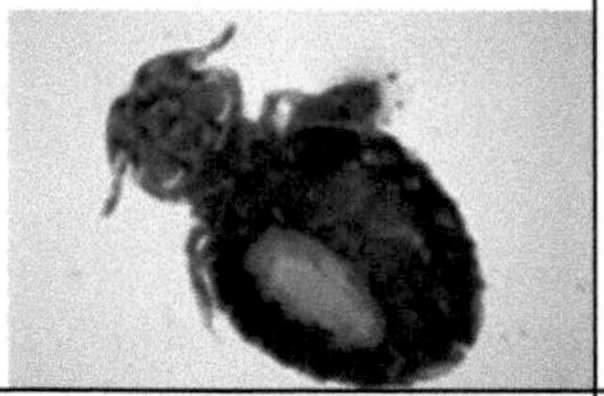	Mild scaling	Trunk Head *Affects dogs and cats* 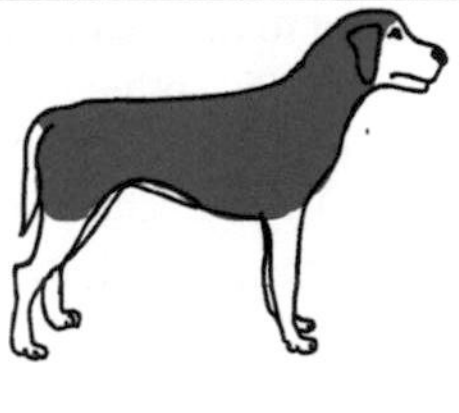
Sarcoptes scabiei 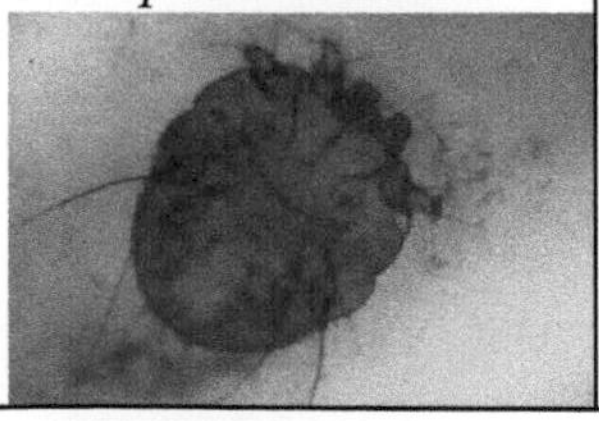	Papules Erythema Scaling Crusting	Ear margins Lateral pinnae Elbows Hocks Ventrum *Affects dogs only* 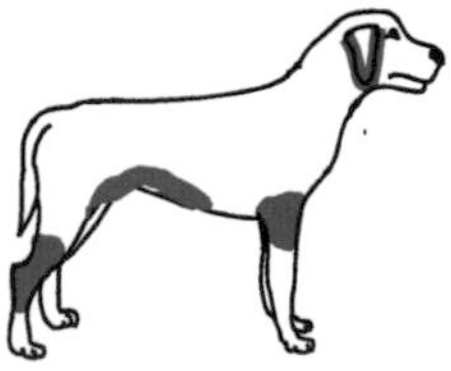

100 Top Consultations in Small Animal General Practice, First Edition
By Peter Hill, Sheena Warman and Geoff Shawcross
© 2011 Blackwell Publishing Ltd

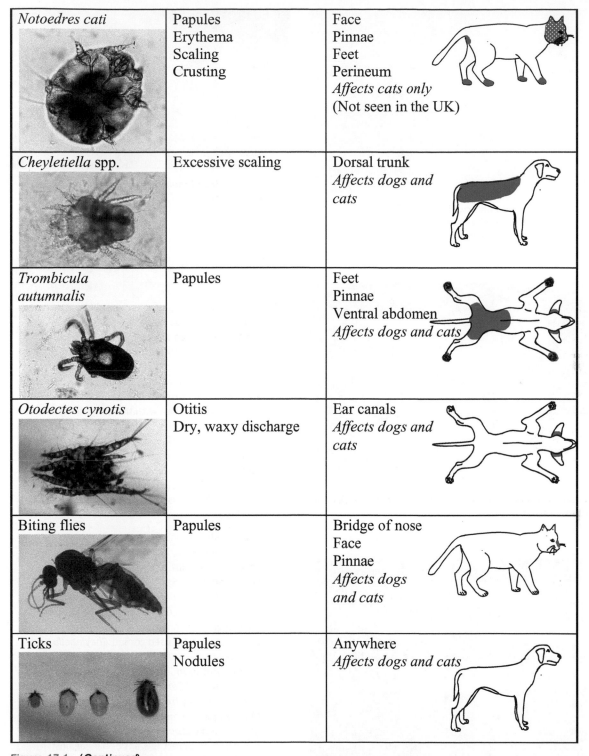

Notoedres cati	Papules Erythema Scaling Crusting	Face Pinnae Feet Perineum *Affects cats only* (Not seen in the UK)
Cheyletiella spp.	Excessive scaling	Dorsal trunk *Affects dogs and cats*
Trombicula autumnalis	Papules	Feet Pinnae Ventral abdomen *Affects dogs and cats*
Otodectes cynotis	Otitis Dry, waxy discharge	Ear canals *Affects dogs and cats*
Biting flies	Papules	Bridge of nose Face Pinnae *Affects dogs and cats*
Ticks	Papules Nodules	Anywhere *Affects dogs and cats*

Figure 17.1 (*Continued*)

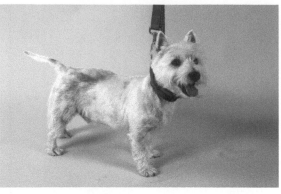

Figure 17.2 **Flea allergy dermatitis in a West Highland White Terrier. Note self-induced alopecia over the caudal dorsum and hindlimbs**

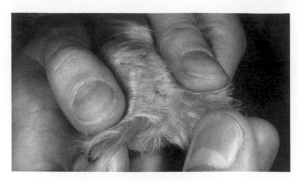

Figure 17.5 ***Trombicula* larvae in the interdigital space of a dog**

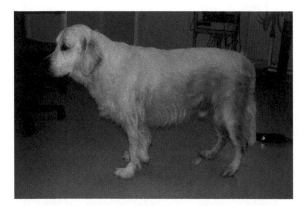

Figure 17.3 **Sarcoptic mange in a Golden Retriever. Lesions are present on the pinnal margins, hocks and elbow region**

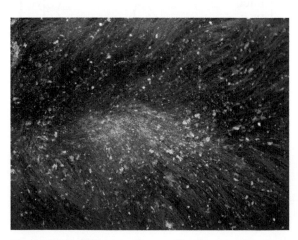

Figure 17.4 **Diffuse scaling on the dorsum of a dog with cheyletiellosis**

Specific diagnostic techniques

A definitive diagnosis of a superficial ectoparasite infestation can only be made by identifying the parasite on the skin of an affected animal. The parasites that may be seen with the naked eye are fleas, lice, *Trombicula* larvae and ticks. *Sarcoptes*, *Notoedres* (not seen in the UK) and *Cheyletiella* mites can only be seen with a microscope. Otodectes is also microscopic but it can be seen with the magnifying lens on an otoscope. Biting flies such as *Culicoides* midges, mosquitoes and blackflies are only transient visitors to the skin and won't be found on the animal. Their involvement can only be suspected based on the season and clinical lesions seen.

Tests that can be used to detect cutaneous parasites include:

- Gross examination of coat brushings: can be used to find fleas, flea dirt (reddish brown specks of dirt that turn red on moist cotton wool) and lice
- Microscopic examination of coat brushings: can be used to find lice and *Cheyletiella*
- Microscopic examination of 'sticky tape' strippings: can be used to find *Cheyletiella* and *Trombicula*
- Microscopic examination of skin scrapings: can be used to find *Sarcoptes*, *Notoedres*, *Cheyletiella* and *Trombicula*
- Microscopic examination of ear wax: can be used to find *Otodectes*
- Blood test to detect IgG antibodies against *Sarcoptes*: can be used to detect exposure to the mite but a positive result does not definitively confirm current infestation. The test

can also be negative in the early stages of infestation. Taking into account the cost of the test, it is not recommended for routine diagnostic use.

Which test (or tests) is performed will depend on the index of suspicion for a particular condition. It is important to remember that these tests can be negative, even if the animal has the disease. Hence, a presumptive diagnosis may have to be made based on history and clinical signs, and a therapeutic trial may be needed to rule the condition out. This 'pattern recognition' approach is particularly appropriate if time and resources are limited, but it is important to confirm complete resolution following successful treatment.

Treatment

Successful resolution of skin diseases associated with ectoparasites requires elimination of the parasite and prevention of reinfestation. This may entail treating the environment and 'in-contact' animals as well as the affected pet. When choosing an ectoparasiticide, it is important to follow the prescribing cascade (or local rules governing the use of such products). Table 17.1 summarises the products currently licensed in the UK and their indications.

Most modern ectoparasiticides are highly effective and competing products are rarely superior to each other. When different products are available to treat the same parasite, clinicians should take into account other factors that may be relevant to the case such as spectrum of activity, the requirement for prevention as well as treatment, ease of application, the pet's and owner's lifestyle, and cost. Clinicians and owners should follow the manufacturer's recommendations regarding the use, contraindications and safety precautions to be taken for each product. Particular care should be taken to ensure that owners do not apply permethrin-based products to cats as they are extremely toxic and can result in fatalities.

For the elimination of fleas, attention needs to be paid to the environmental stages of the life-cycle in addition to the adults that are on the host. These stages can persist for prolonged periods after the affected animal has been treated, providing a source of future reinfestation. Some 'spot-on' products provide environmental control because they contain either insect growth regulators (e.g. methoprene) or agents that pass into the environment in the flea faeces. Alternative products are also available to specifically deal with the environmental stages, such as environmental sprays or systemic agents containing lufenuron. When deciding on a flea control programme, clinicians should assess the severity of a particular case in order to decide what level of intervention would be appropriate.

Treatment of lice and mite infestations is usually easier than flea eradication because there are no environmental life-cycle stages. A product should be given that will provide therapeutic cover just throughout the duration of the parasite's life cycle. As 'spot-ons' are typically administered once a month, a course of two doses is usually sufficient.

For prevention of *Trombicula* or tick infestations, appropriate products need to be used throughout the relevant season, usually the summer and autumn in the UK. Removal of small numbers of attached ticks can be achieved using mosquito forceps or tick removal tools, but care should be taken to avoid leaving the mouthparts in the skin.

If a superficial parasite is causing severe pruritus, symptomatic treatment with a short course of glucocorticoids at anti-inflammatory doses may be indicated to provide relief whilst the specific agents are taking effect. If complete parasite elimination is not possible, such as with *Trombicula* or biting flies, longer term glucocorticoid therapy may be required.

Table 17.1 Licensed products (UK) for the treatment or prevention of parasitic skin disease in dogs and cats (2010).

Trade name	Active agents	Licensed species	Licensed indications	Unlicensed uses	Application intervals	Recommendations, contraindications and adverse effects
Acclaim (VetKem)	Methoprene Permethrin	Household spray	Environmental flea control	None	6 months	Harmful to fish
Advantage (Bayer)	Imidacloprid	Dogs Cats Rabbits	Fleas	Lice	4 weeks	Do not treat puppies and kittens less than 8 weeks of age and rabbits less than 10 weeks of age Can occasionally cause topical irritation Do not get into eyes or mouth
Advantix (Bayer)	Imidacloprid Permethrin	Dogs	Fleas Ticks Sandflies Mosquitoes	Lice Other biting flies? *Trombicula*	3–4 weeks (2 weeks for sandflies)	**Extremely toxic to cats – can be fatal** Do not treat puppies less than 7 weeks of age Dangerous to fish – do not allow dogs to swim for 48 hours Can occasionally cause topical irritation Do not get into eyes or mouth
Advocate (Bayer)	Imidacloprid Moxidectin	Dogs Cats	Fleas Ear mites Sarcoptes Demodex Heartworm Roundworms	*Cheyletiella*	4 weeks	Author's experience has not confirmed efficacy for demodicosis Do not use in puppies under 7 weeks Do not use in kittens under 9 weeks Oral ingestion may lead to neurological signs, especially in Collies and related breeds Can occasionally cause topical irritation Do not get into eyes or mouth
Aludex (Intervet)	Amitraz	Dogs	Demodex Sarcoptes	*Cheyletiella*	7 days	Do not use on Chihuahuas or dogs under 5 kg or 3 months old Not recommended on cats; toxic for horses and fish Do not use on dogs suffering from heat stress, in pregnant or lactating bitches or by owners suffering from diabetes. Can cause skin irritation, sedation, lethargy, CNS depression, bradycardia and shallow breathing. These effects normally subside within 24 hours. If the symptoms are severe and persistent, the dog should be washed in warm water and dried. The symptoms can be reversed by administering atipamazole hydrochloride (Antisedan; Janssen Animal Health) at a dose of 0.2 mg/kg IM
Capstar (Novartis)	Nitenpyram	Dogs Cats	Fleas	None	One-off or occasional use	Do not use on animals less than 4 weeks old or 1 kg in weight

Product	Active ingredient	Species	Parasites		Duration	Notes
Frontline (Merial)	Fipronil	Dogs Cats	Fleas Ticks Lice	*Cheyletiella Trombicula*	Ticks: 4 weeks Fleas: 8 weeks (dogs) or 5 weeks (cats)	**Do not use on rabbits – can be fatal** The spray can be used in puppies and kittens from 2 days of age The spot-on can be used in puppies or kittens from 8 weeks of age Harmful to fish – do not allow dogs to swim for 2 days after application Rarely causes cutaneous reactions at the site of application Do not get into eyes or mouth Severe and persistent flea infestations will require monthly treatment
Frontline combo (Merial)	Fipronil Methoprene	Dogs Cats	Fleas Ticks Lice (also provides environmental flea control)	*Cheyletiella Trombicula*	Dogs Ticks: 4 weeks Fleas: 8 weeks Cats Ticks: 2 weeks Fleas: 4 weeks	**Do not use on rabbits – can be fatal** Do not treat puppies or kittens less than 8 weeks of age Harmful to fish: do not allow dogs to swim for 2 days after application Rarely causes cutaneous reactions at the site of application Do not get into eyes or mouth Severe and persistent flea infestations will require monthly treatment
Indorex (Virbac)	Pyriproxyfen Permethrin	Household spray	Environmental flea control	Dustmites	6 months	Harmful to fish
Prac-Tic (Novartis)	Pyriprole	Dogs	Fleas Ticks	None	4 weeks	Do not use on cats or rabbits Do not use on dogs less than 8 weeks of age or 2 kg in weight Can occasionally cause local reactions at the site of application Do not get into eyes or mouth Do not bathe for 48 hours before or 24 hours after application May be harmful to aquatic organisms
Program tablets and suspension (Novartis)	Lufenuron	Dogs Cats	Immature fleas (environmental flea control)	None	4 weeks	None

(Continued)

Table 17.1 (*Continued*)

Trade name	Active agents	Licensed species	Licensed indications	Unlicensed uses	Application intervals	Recommendations, contraindications and adverse effects
Program Plus (Novartis)	Lufenuron Milbemycin	Dogs	Immature fleas (environmental flea control) Roundworms Hookworms Whipworms Heartworm	None	4 weeks	None
Program injectable (Novartis)	Lufenuron	Cats	Immature fleas (environmental flea control)	None	6 months	Injection site reactions may occur in some cats
Promeris (Fort Dodge)	Metaflumizone	Cats	Fleas	None	4–6 weeks	Do not use in kittens under 8 weeks of age Do not get into eyes or mouth
Promeris Duo (Fort Dodge)	Metaflumizone Amitraz	Dogs	Fleas Ticks	None	4 weeks	Do not use in cats Do not use in puppies under 8 weeks of age Do not get into eyes or mouth Do not allow into streams for 24 hours after treatment Avoid intense exposure to water Amitraz side-effects may occur such as sedation, lethargy, CNS depression, hyperglycaemia, bradycardia and shallow breathing. These effects normally subside within 24 hours. If the symptoms are severe or persistent, the symptoms can be reversed by administering atipamazole hydrochloride (Antisedan; Janssen Animal Health) at a dose of 0.2 mg/kg intramuscularly
Scalibor collar (Intervet)	Deltamethrin	Dogs	Ticks Sandflies	Other biting flies	6 months	
Stronghold (Pfizer)	Selamectin	Dog Cats	Fleas Ear mites Sarcoptes Lice Roundworms Heartworm	*Cheyletiella*	4 weeks	Do not use in animals under 6 weeks of age Keep out of water for 2 hours after application Rarely causes topical irritation Do not get into eyes or mouth

What if it doesn't get better?

If the treatment fails, clinicians should first establish that the products have been applied correctly. If they have, and the diagnosis is certain, another product licensed to treat the parasite should be prescribed. If the diagnosis is not certain, clinicians should make attempts to confirm it, or consider other differential diagnoses that may be causing the problem.

The low-cost option

It is rarely cost-effective to use ectoparasiticides that are not listed in Table 17.1. Products such as flea collars and shampoos containing pyrethroids may be cheaper but they are not 100% effective and have poor residual activity. Prompt treatment with an effective product is likely to minimise the expense associated with the problem becoming more chronic. However, the costs associated with prophylactic use of ectoparasiticides may not be necessary if the location or lifestyle of the individual animal suggests it is at low risk.

When should I refer?

Referral of pets suffering from superficial parasite infestation is not required.

Peter Hill

Aetiology and pathogenesis

Demodicosis is a skin disease associated with excessive proliferation of the mites *Demodex canis*, *Demodex injai* or an un-named short-bodied *Demodex* mite. Small numbers of demodex mites are part of the commensal fauna in all domestic animals, and in man where they inhabit the hair follicles around the face and eyelids. In animals, the mites are acquired during the first few days of life during suckling. The dog is the only species that is commonly affected by demodicosis. In dogs under 18 months of age, demodicosis is thought to arise because of a specific defect that prevents the host's immune system from keeping the mites under control. In adult dogs, the development of demodicosis may be associated with glucocorticoid therapy, cytotoxic drug therapy, hyperadrenocorticism, hypothyroidism, neoplasia or it may be idiopathic.

History and clinical signs

Demodicosis typically presents as a visible skin disease characterised by hair loss (Figure 18.1). About 30% of cases are also pruritic. Demodicosis may have a localised, generalised or pedal distribution (Figure 18.2). In some dogs, the skin is erythematous (Figure 18.3), whereas in

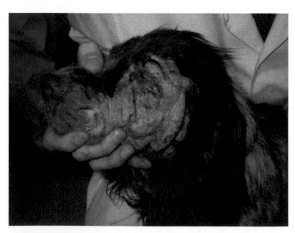

Figure 18.1 Hair loss on the face of a dog with demodicosis

100 Top Consultations in Small Animal General Practice, First Edition
By Peter Hill, Sheena Warman and Geoff Shawcross
© 2011 Blackwell Publishing Ltd

others it may be of normal colour or hyperpigmented (Figure 18.4). Close examination of the skin often reveals comedones or follicular casts, indicating the presence of follicular hyperkeratosis (Figure 18.5). In some cases, secondary bacterial infection may be present resulting in the presence of pustules, nodules or draining tracts.

Specific diagnostic techniques

Demodicosis should be considered as a differential diagnosis in any dog that presents with focal, multifocal or generalised alopecia (whether pruritic or not), or in pruritic dogs in which there is no other obvious diagnosis. A diagnosis of demodicosis can only be made by finding demodex mites on samples taken from the skin. Clinicians should never make a diagnosis of demodicosis based on clinical signs alone because the treatment course is a lengthy commitment, and continuous monitoring of mite numbers is required to achieve a successful outcome.

Tests that can be used to detect demodex mites include:

- Deep skin scrapings – the skin should be scraped until there is mild capillary oozing. The sample is best placed in mineral oil on a glass slide and scanned under the ×4 lens on the microscope. In dogs with demodicosis, mites should easily be demonstrated (Figure 18.6). A common misconception is that a few demodex mites can be found on skin scrapings from normal dogs. *This is not true: demodex mites are only found on skin scrapings when clinical demodicosis is present*. The population of commensal mites is too low to detect by this method
- Hair pluckings (trichogram) – these are easier to perform than skin scrapings, especially around the head or on the feet. Mites are found around the hair bulbs and shafts
- Skin biopsy – this test should not be necessary to diagnose demodicosis. When a diagnosis is obtained by this route, it usually means that the clinician has not evaluated the clinical aspects of the case appropriately.

Localised demodicosis
Usually juvenile onset and non-pruritic or mildly pruritic.

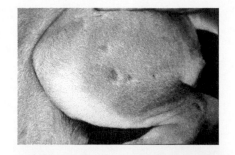
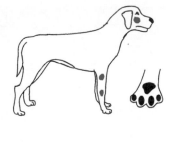

Generalised demodicosis
May be juvenile or adult-onset, and pruritic or non-pruritic. The skin may be very erythematous, scaly or in chronic cases, a slate grey colour.

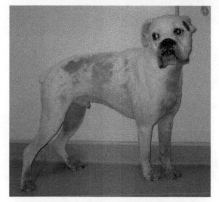
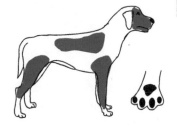

Demodectic pododermatitis
Affects the feet, often with secondary infection.

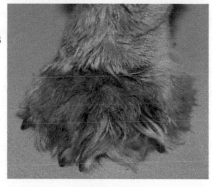
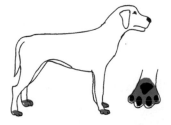

Figure 18.2   The three major presentations of demodicosis

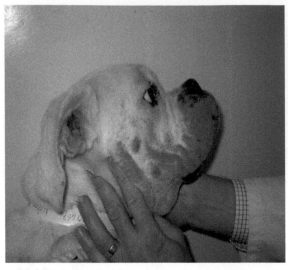

Figure 18.3 **Diffuse erythema on the face of a dog with demodicosis**

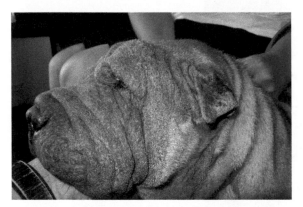

Figure 18.4 **Blue–grey hyperpigmentation on the face of a dog with demodicosis**

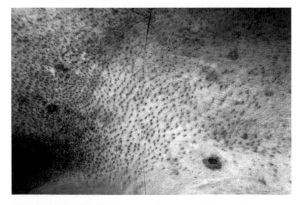

Figure 18.5 **Multiple comedones on the ventral abdomen of a dog with demodicosis**

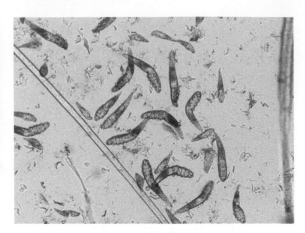

Figure 18.6 **Multiple demodex mites in a skin scraping. Larvae and eggs can also be seen**

Treatment

Successful resolution of demodicosis requires both 'clinical cure' (i.e. the animal looks normal) and 'parasitological cure' (i.e. it is no longer possible to detect demodex mites on samples taken from the skin). This is a major difference compared with the treatment of other ectoparasitic diseases. The rationale for this recommendation is that mites can still be present after the skin appears to have resolved, resulting in a subsequent relapse. For this reason, cases of demodicosis must be monitored throughout treatment by taking skin scrapings and/or hair pluckings.

In young dogs with mild, localised demodicosis, 90% of cases will resolve spontaneously as the immune system gains control over the mite population. In such cases, the most appropriate course of action is to discuss the condition with the owner, delay treatment and arrange a revisit four weeks later to check that the condition is resolving. This approach will help to determine if a dog is likely to have problems with demodicosis in the future, especially if immunosuppressive drugs were to be prescribed for treatment of other diseases. If treatment of localised demodicosis were considered necessary at the outset, especially due to client pressure, it would be appropriate to use relatively mild treatments such as spot-on moxidectin (Advocate, Bayer) or localised topical application of amitraz (Aludex, Intervet).

With more severe and widespread lesions, spontaneous resolution is not likely and treatment is necessary. Currently, only topical amitraz and 'spot-on' moxidectin are licensed for the treatment of demodicosis and clinicians should use one of these products first. However, in the author's experience, 'spot-on' moxidectin is not a reliable treatment for generalised disease and should either be avoided, or used as a preliminary treatment with the intention of changing to amitraz if it is not working.

A typical treatment protocol involves weekly amitraz washes and monthly rechecks. In long-coated dogs, it is advisable to clip the coat to aid penetration to the skin surface. Prior washing with a benzoyl peroxide shampoo can be beneficial if the skin is covered in scale or crust. If performed by the owner, they should be instructed to wear gloves and a protective apron, and carry out the bath in a well-ventilated area. The amitraz solution should be prepared according to the manufacturer's recommendations, applied over the whole body with a sponge and left on to dry. Cotton wool or cotton buds can be used to apply the solution to difficult areas such as around the face. Treatment of the feet is best achieved by standing the dog in the solution as the rest of the body is being covered. Licking should be prevented as the dog is drying. Potential adverse effects and contraindications of amitraz can be found in Table 17.1 in the previous chapter.

Skin scrapings should be performed at monthly intervals to determine the therapeutic endpoint. Treatment can be stopped when the lesions have resolved and two sets of completely negative scrapings have been obtained one month apart. This means that in most cases, treatment is likely to be necessary for at least two months but in severe cases, it may take three to six months.

Some important points to remember to ensure satisfactory resolution are:

- Never administer glucocorticoids to a dog with demodicosis, even if it is highly pruritic. It will prolong the course of treatment and prevent resolution.
- If there is secondary bacterial infection, the dog should be treated concurrently with systemic antibiotics until the pyoderma has resolved
- Entire bitches should be spayed when the disease has been brought under control but before treatment is stopped. The hormonal changes occurring around oestrus can destabilise the interaction between the bitch's immune system and the mite population, resulting in potential relapses

- If the disease develops when the dog is an adult, check for systemic disease, perform routine haematology, biochemistry and urine analysis, and rule out hyperadrenocorticism.

What if it doesn't get better?

Most cases of demodicosis will resolve if the above guidelines are followed carefully and for long enough. However, in some cases, the mites persist despite improvement in the lesions. If the dog has already been treated with 'spot-on' moxidectin, it should be treated with amitraz. If the dog has been treated appropriately with amitraz and the mites are still present after three to six months of treatment, a non-licensed treatment can be considered. The most commonly used options are oral administration of ivermectin (Panomec, Merial) or milbemycin (Interceptor, Novartis). Clinicians should only use these drugs if they are fully familiar with the dosage schedules and risk of adverse effects. In some dogs, the mites cannot be completely eradicated with any of the available treatments and a lifelong maintenance regime is required.

The low-cost option

A prompt diagnosis at the first visit will allow available funds to be targeted correctly and not wasted on ineffective symptomatic treatments. Demodicosis can still be an expensive disease to treat because of the long treatment courses and the requirement for monitoring. Costs can be minimised by teaching the owners how to conduct the washes at home.

When should I refer?

Referral should be offered if the case has not responded to a licensed treatment protocol and the clinician is not experienced in the use of non-licensed alternatives. Clinicians who are not able to perform the necessary monitoring of microscopic samples should also refer cases for effective management. Cases of demodicosis that occur concurrently with allergic skin disease are very challenging to manage and would benefit from the expertise of a dermatologist.

Peter Hill

Aetiology and pathogenesis

Both of these conditions are caused by commensal organisms that can colonise and infect the skin when conditions become favourable. Pyoderma is virtually always caused by *Staphylococcus pseudintermedius*, a bacterium that normally resides in the nasal passages, oral cavity and around the anus. *Malassezia* dermatitis is caused by an overgrowth of *Malassezia pachydermatis*, a yeast that normally resides around the mouth, anus and in the ears. Cutaneous infection with either organism can occur when the microclimate or resistance of the skin is changed by some underlying factor. Common underlying conditions include allergic skin diseases, endocrine diseases, ectoparasite infestation, seborrhoeic skin disease, immunodeficiency (e.g. chronic glucocorticoid therapy) and breed-related susceptibility (a genetic tendency to develop primary dermatological infections).

History and clinical signs

Both staphylococcal pyoderma and *Malassezia* dermatitis are usually pruritic conditions but lesions seen with the conditions differ substantially. Staphylococcal pyoderma can produce superficial or deep lesions. Superficial pyoderma will be described by the owner as a rash and can present as a papular eruption (Figure 19.1), pustular erup-

tion (Figure 19.2) or with staphylococcal rings or epidermal collarettes (Figure 19.3). Staphylococcal rings are circular areas of erythematous alopecia which are sometimes lightly pigmented in the centre. They are often surrounded by an epidermal collarette which is a circular rim of peripheral scaling. These lesions are virtually pathog-

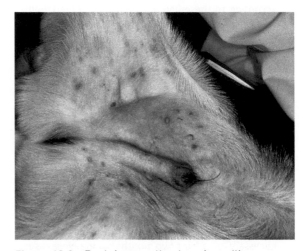

Figure 19.2 Pustular eruption in a dog with staphylococcal pyoderma

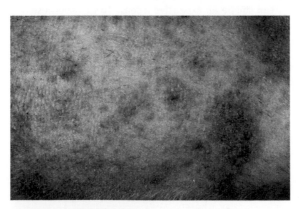

Figure 19.1 Papular eruption in a dog with staphylococcal pyoderma

100 Top Consultations in Small Animal General Practice, First Edition
By Peter Hill, Sheena Warman and Geoff Shawcross
© 2011 Blackwell Publishing Ltd

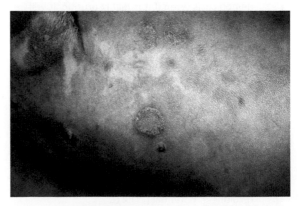

Figure 19.3 Staphylococcal rings and epidermal collarettes in a dog with pyoderma

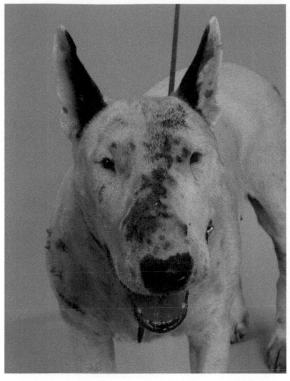

Figure 19.4 Nodules, draining tracts and ulcers in a dog with deep pyoderma

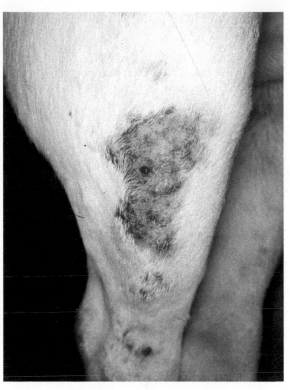

Figure 19.5 Nodules and draining tracts on the leg of a dog with deep pyoderma

nomonic for superficial pyoderma because they are rarely seen with any other condition. Superficial pyoderma typically affects the ventral abdomen and trunk and usually spares the head and distal limbs. Deep pyoderma is characterised by nodules and draining tracts which occur as a result of furunculosis (rupture of hair follicles). The draining exudate is usually purulent or blood-tinged. Lesions may occur on the chin (acne), head (Figure 19.4), limbs (Figure 19.5) or be more generalised.

Malassezia dermatitis is characterised by a more diffuse erythema that typically affects the interdigital skin (Figure 19.6), axillae (Figure 19.7), ventral neck, perineum, lips and skin folds. The skin may feel moist and be covered in a yellowish, greasy material. Chronic lesions may become lichenified and hyperpigmented. *Malassezia* overgrowth can also lead to a ceruminous otitis externa. Any breed may be affected by *Malassezia* dermatitis but Basset Hounds and West Highland White Terriers appear particularly predisposed.

Specific diagnostic techniques

The lesions of superficial pyoderma are often distinctive enough to make a clinical diagnosis on gross appearance alone. In such cases, the diagnosis can be definitively confirmed if the lesions respond completely to appropriate antibacterial therapy. If there is any doubt, initial confirmation of the diagnosis can be attempted by examining cytological samples taken from the skin by impression smear or clear sticky tape. This test is most likely to yield definitive results if pustules are pricked with a needle and then sampled (Figure 19.8). Obtaining samples from papules and epidermal collarettes is often unrewarding. Bacterial culture and sensitivity testing is not indicated at the first presentation of superficial pyoderma, but should be performed if there is not a good response to initial treatment. With deeper lesions, cytological examination and bacterial culture/sensitivity testing is recommended from the outset, to ensure that other types of organisms are not present.

Malassezia dermatitis can only be diagnosed by examining stained sticky tape preparations. This test is performed by repeatedly sticking a piece of tape onto an area of skin until it has lost its adhesiveness (usually after 10–20 applications). The tape is then stained with Diff-Quik and examined under the oil immersion lens on the microscope. *Malassezia pachydermatis* has a characteristic oval, peanut or 'Russian doll' shape, allowing easy identification (Figure 19.9). Observation of one or more organisms per field is consistent with cutaneous overgrowth, but this number can be considered normal in samples obtained from the ear canal and higher numbers are seen in otitis.

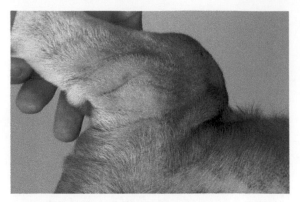

Figure 19.7 **Diffuse axillary erythema and scaling in a dog with *Malassezia* dermatitis**

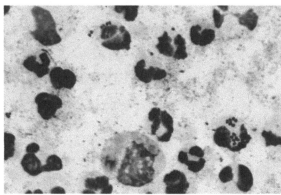

Figure 19.8 **Cytological appearance of staphylococcal pyoderma**

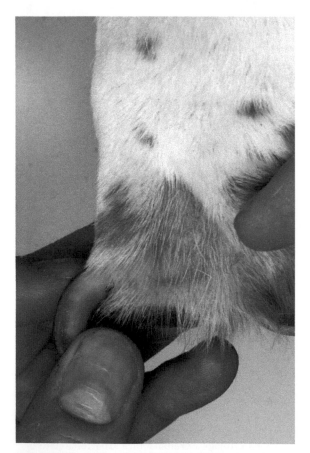

Figure 19.6 **Diffuse interdigital erythema in a dog with *Malassezia* dermatitis**

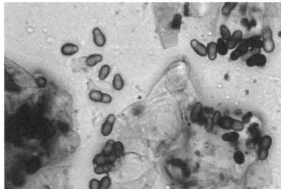

Figure 19.9 **Cytological appearance of *Malassezia pachydermatis* overgrowth**

Treatment

On diagnosing a case of pyoderma or *Malassezia* dermatitis, the clinician should always check the animal for clinical signs that might support an underlying condition, thus prompting further investigation. If no apparent condition is obvious on the first visit, it is appropriate to treat the infections and monitor the response. If the lesions resolve and do not relapse, no further investigation is required.

Staphylococcal pyoderma is treated using antibiotics that are effective against gram-positive, beta-lactamase-producing cocci. Appropriate choices include cefalexin, amoxicillin/clavulanic acid, clindamycin, potentiated sulphonamides or cefovecin. Although effective, fluoroquinolones should be reserved for confirmed infections involving gram-negative organisms, which are extremely rare in the skin. For superficial infections, a three-week course is usually required. For deep infections, longer courses are necessary and the clinician should judge the endpoint based on clinical resolution, stopping treatment two weeks after all signs have resolved. Topical therapy with an antibacterial shampoo can be a useful adjunctive treatment for both superficial or deep infections, as long as the owner is able to perform baths 2–3 times weekly. Suitable choices include benzoyl peroxide, ethyl lactate or chlorhexidine.

Malassezia dermatitis is usually treated using topical miconazole/chlorhexidine shampoo (Malaseb, VetXX). Initially, the dog should be bathed three times weekly for three weeks, as long as the owner is capable of doing this. Follow-up cytological samples should be obtained at this stage to ensure microscopic as well as clinical resolution. Systemic therapy with ketoconazole or itraconazole should be reserved for very severe cases, if the owner is unable to bathe their dog, or if topical therapy has been unsuccessful, because these treatments are unlicensed.

Glucocorticoids should be avoided when treating pyoderma or *Malassezia* dermatitis unless the condition has occurred secondarily to a confirmed underlying allergic dermatitis for which glucocorticoids are required as part of the ongoing management plan.

- If the initial lesions resolve, but the dog is still pruritic, it is likely that another pruritic disease is underlying the infection, especially ectoparasites, atopic dermatitis or adverse food reactions
- If the initial lesions resolve and the dog is no longer pruritic, but the infection relapses some time later, it is possible that a non-pruritic underlying condition is present. The most likely possibilities would be early stage atopic dermatitis, demodicosis, hypothyroidism, hyperadrenocorticism, systemic disease, neoplasia, immunodeficiency, or breed-related susceptibility
- If the initial lesions of infection do not appear to resolve following appropriate treatment, clinicians should consider staphylococcal resistance, uncommon organisms, poor owner compliance or other differential diagnoses. In such cases, culture of suspected bacteria is indicated as emergence of meticillin resistant staphylococci is becoming a major problem in some countries. Clinicians should also remember that glucocorticoids may inhibit host defences against the above organisms and, in some cases, may delay or prevent complete resolution of the infection.

The low-cost option

When treating pyoderma, costs can be greatly minimised by using potentiated sulphonamides. However, there is a greater risk of adverse effects with these drugs compared with penicillin derivatives or macrolides (see Appendix 1). The treatment of *Malassezia* dermatitis with miconazole/chlorhexidine shampoo should not result in high costs. Microscopic monitoring will add to the cost of treatment but should be considered essential for optimal management. Chlorhexidine surgical hand-wash can be used as a low cost (but less effective) alternative to antibacterial and anti-fungal shampoos.

What if it doesn't get better?

In most cases, failure of either of these infections to resolve completely indicates failure to identify an underlying condition.

When should I refer?

Referral should be offered if a dog suffers from recalcitrant or recurrent pyoderma or *Malassezia* dermatitis and an underlying cause cannot be found.

Peter Hill

Aetiology and pathogenesis

In humans, the term 'atopic' refers to a triad of allergic conditions comprising rhinitis, asthma and atopic dermatitis. In dogs, only atopic dermatitis is recognised. A form of atopic dermatitis is thought to occur in cats but the disease has not been well characterised (see Chapter 16). Atopic dogs inherit genes that result in excessive IgE synthesis and impaired epidermal barrier function. IgE antibodies are produced to environmental proteins that are absorbed through the epidermis, most commonly to house dust mite antigens (*Dermatophagoides farinae*, *Dermatophagoides pteronyssinus*) but also to pollens (from trees, weeds and grasses), human and animal danders, moulds (household or from crops) or to allergens from staphylococci and *Malassezia* organisms. The allergen-specific IgEs bind to mast cells in the dermis; on further exposure, the mast cells degranulate and release histamine, leukotrienes, prostaglandins, proteases and cytokines into the dermis. These potent inflammatory mediators cause vasodilation, inflammatory cell infiltration and pruritus. Further release of cytokines by lymphocytes leads to chronic cutaneous inflammation.

History and clinical signs

Atopic dermatitis is most common in West Highland White and Cairn Terriers, Golden and Labrador Retrievers, Boxers, Bulldogs, Irish and English Setters, Shar Peis, Dalmations, Lhasa Apsos, and German Shepherd dogs. Most cases become symptomatic between 6 months and 3 years of age, but occasionally dogs develop clinical signs after this. The most prominent clinical sign is pruritus, which may be seasonal but is more commonly continuous. Initially, affected areas may look grossly normal but they typically become erythematous with time. In the majority of cases, the face, ears and feet are affected but the ventral abdomen, axillae and perineum can be involved, especially when there is secondary infection (Figure 20.1). In an individual case, there can be considerable variation from this classic pattern and some dogs may present solely as 'foot chewers', 'face rubbers' or 'ear scratchers'.

Specific diagnostic techniques

A diagnosis of atopic dermatitis can only be made if there is a typical history, typical clinical signs (lesions and distribution) and when other pruritic dermatoses caused by ectoparasites, infections and adverse food reactions have been ruled out (the approaches described in Chapters 15, 17 and 19 should be followed meticulously). In such a case, the clinician has two options:

- Long-term symptomatic management
- Allergy testing to confirm IgE hypersensitivity and identify allergens for immunotherapy.

Which route is taken depends on a number of factors, including the severity of the pruritus, age of the dog, financial considerations and what the owner wishes for their pet. In some cases, symptomatic treatment may be recommended initially and allergy testing performed at a later date if the condition worsens.

Two methods of allergy testing are currently available: intradermal skin testing and serological measurement of allergen-specific IgE. Many practitioners wrongly believe that a positive result in either of these tests is diagnostic for canine atopic dermatitis. Positive results can be obtained with either test in clinically normal dogs and dogs with other skin diseases. The test result is only meaningful if the dog has clinical signs consistent with atopic dermatitis and all other potential causes of the pruritus have been ruled out. Most dermatologists believe that intradermal testing is superior to the measurement of IgE in the blood because it evaluates the hypersensitivity reaction in the target organ. However, if the case has been meticulously evaluated, either test can be used successfully to identify allergens for inclusion in immunotherapy vaccines.

100 Top Consultations in Small Animal General Practice, First Edition
By Peter Hill, Sheena Warman and Geoff Shawcross
© 2011 Blackwell Publishing Ltd

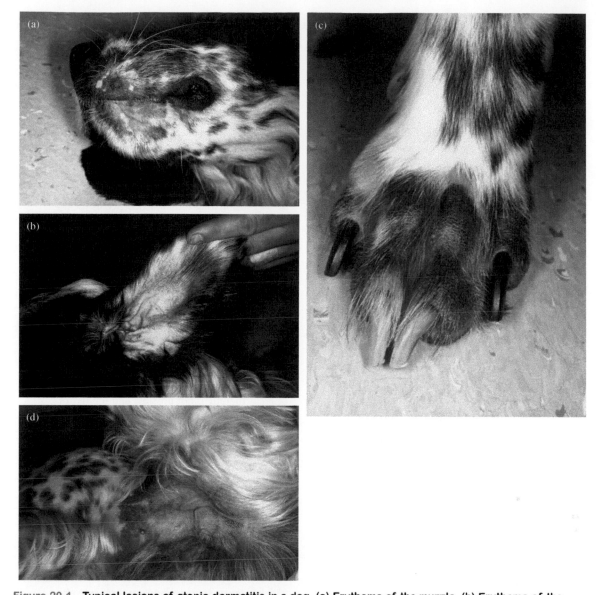

Figure 20.1 **Typical lesions of atopic dermatitis in a dog. (a) Erythema of the muzzle, (b) Erythema of the medial pinna, (c) Pedal erythema and self-induced alopecia, (d) Erythema of the ventral abdomen**

It is important to note that atopic dermatitis is an incurable disease and clients must be informed of this at the outset so that they don't have unrealistic expectations. Treatment is therefore life-long, and based on management rather than cure. This makes it especially important that other potential skin problems have been ruled out, or controlled, prior to starting therapy. The treatment of atopic dermatitis may involve the following modalities: allergen avoidance, allergen-specific immunotherapy, glucocorticoids, ciclosporin, antihistamines, essential fatty acids, Chinese herbs, topical therapy, and control of secondary skin and ear infections. In a typical case, up to three of the above treatments may be needed at the same time, especially if an attempt is made to avoid, or minimise the use of, glucocorticoids. Very severe cases may require four or five treatments, all given concurrently. The clinician's job is to find the right combination of treatments that control the clinical signs without inducing severe adverse effects, all at an appropriate cost for the owner.

Allergen avoidance would be the ideal method of controlling atopic dermatitis but, in reality, it is difficult to achieve. Attempts to control dust mite populations or avoid pollens rarely have significant effects.

Allergen-specific immunotherapy can only be undertaken if the dog has previously had an allergy test. Immunotherapy is beneficial in 50–75% of cases but it takes 2–9 months to take effect. During the early stages, it is often necessary to use concurrent symptomatic therapy to control the clinical signs. The risk of adverse effects is very low and serious complications such as anaphylaxis are extremely rare.

Glucocorticoids are probably the most commonly used drugs in the management of atopic dermatitis. They are effective in virtually 100% of cases and are very cheap. However, compared to other treatment modalities, they cause the most adverse effects, especially when given in the long term (see Appendix 2). They are best used in the following circumstances:

- as a short-term treatment for the initial management of severe pruritus or flare-ups (as long as infections have been controlled)
- as a long-term treatment for cases in which financial limitations do not permit other forms of treatment, or owners are not prepared to pursue other forms of treatment
- as an adjunctive treatment in cases that respond inadequately to other treatment modalities
- in cases of seasonal atopic dermatitis lasting 3 months or less
- in the early phases of immunotherapy if the pruritus is severe.

There are two main objectives when using long-term glucocorticoids for the management of atopic dermatitis: to ascertain the minimal effective dose and to achieve alternate day therapy. Initial doses of prednisolone of 0.5–1.0 mg/kg/day should be given for 5–10 days. After that, the daily dose can be given every 48 hours. For long-term use, the alternate day therapy should be gradually reduced to the lowest dose that is capable of controlling the pruritus. Long-acting injectable glucocorticoids are not recommended because precise dosage control cannot be achieved, alternate day therapy is not possible and the risk of adverse effects is therefore higher.

Ciclosporin (Atopica, Novartis) is a licensed treatment for canine atopic dermatitis and is highly effective in about 80% of cases. The main disadvantage of the drug is cost. It is given at a dose of 5 mg/kg, once daily. The capsules should be given on an empty stomach as food reduces bioavailability. It may take 4–6 weeks before maximum efficacy is reached. If a good response is seen, it may be possible to give the drug on alternate days, or even twice weekly. Ciclosporin has fewer short-to-medium term side effects than prednisolone, although the incidence and nature of long-term adverse effects is currently not known. The most common side effect is vomiting when the drug is first introduced. This is usually a transient effect and can be overcome by temporarily reducing or stopping the dose, or giving it initially with food. Less common adverse effects include gingival hyperplasia, hypertrichosis and papillomatosis.

Antihistamines are weak anti-pruritic drugs that are rarely effective on their own but may be helpful as adjunctive treatments. They are not licensed for use in dogs, but can be beneficial in up to 20% of cases, especially if mild or in the early stages. When prescribing antihistamines, it is important to try at least three different drugs for a week each before determining the overall efficacy and selecting the most appropriate drug for that patient for longer term use. Appropriate choices include chlorpheniramine (Piriton, 0.4 mg/kg TID), diphenhydramine (Nytol, 2.2 mg/kg TID), hydroxyzine (Atarax, 2.2 mg/kg TID) and clemastine (Tavegil, 0.05 mg/kg BID). The main adverse effect of antihistamines is drowsiness. If this occurs, the drug should be discontinued.

Essential fatty acids (EFAs) may also be beneficial in up to 20% of cases, and there can be a synergistic effect if combined with antihistamines. They need to be given for 6–8 weeks for maximum effect. Antihistamines and EFAs only work in a few cases because they are more specific than steroids or ciclosporin, and are unable to control the more widespread inflammation that is mediated by T cells and cytokines.

Phytopica (Schering Plough) is a food supplement containing three different Chinese herbs, used as an aid in the management of atopic dermatitis. It is beneficial in approximately 20% of cases.

Topical therapy may take the form of shampoos or ointments. Shampoo therapy is valuable when treating atopic dermatitis because it can help to manage secondary bacterial or yeast infections, remove surface antigens and scale, and provide soothing effects (although these only last for 24–48 hours). Topical glucocorticoids may also be very helpful, especially if inflammation of a particular body area is proving difficult to control (e.g. the perineum, a foot, the medial pinna).

What if it doesn't get better?

The dog will only be perceived to have got better by the owner if long-term maintenance treatment is prescribed that provides continuous control, rather than intermittent 'stop–start' therapy prescribed at multiple visits. However, the treatment options for atopic dermatitis are not universally effective and if a case is not responding, it is necessary to try other options until adequate control is achieved. Common causes of a poor outcome are misdiagnosis, failure to control secondary infections before assessing the efficacy of anti-pruritic drugs, and instituting immunotherapy on the basis of a serum-based allergy test without undertaking a full diagnostic and therapeutic evaluation. Flare-ups in a previously well-controlled case should be carefully evaluated because they may be due to another skin disease rather than worsening of the atopic dermatitis.

The low-cost option

Atopic dermatitis is a life-long disease and requires life-long treatment. Inevitably, this will involve a degree of life-long expense. The cheapest option for long-term management is to use glucocorticoids, but owners must be made aware of the potential for adverse effects (see Appendix 2).

When should I refer?

The diagnosis and management of some cases of atopic dermatitis requires considerable dermatological expertise and referral to a specialist dermatologist may be advisable if the owner seeks optimal management. Cases may also need to be referred if intradermal skin testing is desired.

Peter Hill

Aetiology and pathogenesis

Hot spots (acute moist dermatitis, pyotraumatic dermatitis, acute exudative dermatitis, wet eczema) are highly pruritic, focal lesions. They occur due to self-trauma, and are often secondary to the pruritus associated with flea bite hypersensitivity, anal sacculitis, otitis externa, atopic dermatitis, adverse food reactions or staphylococcal pyoderma. However, some cases appear to occur without any association with another skin disease. Once the self-trauma commences, an 'itch–scratch' cycle develops resulting in maceration of the epidermis and secondary colonisation by bacteria. Hot spots are not seen in cats.

History and clinical signs

Hot spots appear suddenly, often without the owner being aware of an existing skin problem. They are usually seen on the rump, neck or face. Without effective treatment, dogs will lick, nibble or scratch at hot spots incessantly. On examination, they appear as well circumscribed, exudative, eroded lesions, often covered by matted hair. They can be painful, fairly extensive and may be malodorous.

Specific examination techniques

The clinical appearance of a hot spot is very characteristic, allowing them to be easily recognised. To allow closer scrutiny and effective treatment, the matted hair over the lesion and surrounding skin should be gently clipped off. As the lesions can be painful and clipping is often resented, the dog should be adequately restrained and the clippers used as carefully as possible. In some cases, sedation may be necessary. The lesion should then be examined carefully to determine the extent of bacterial involvement. If it is just a well demarcated erosion and the surrounding skin appears normal, it is known as a superficial hot spot (Figure 21.1). If the lesion is a

thickened, oozing, purulent plaque and the surrounding skin contains what are known as satellite lesions (papules, pustules, nodules), it is known as a deep hot spot (Figure 21.2). This distinction is important when it comes to treatment.

In addition to characterising the lesion correctly, clinicians should check the rest of the skin for evidence of underlying causes (as outlined above) that will also need to be treated.

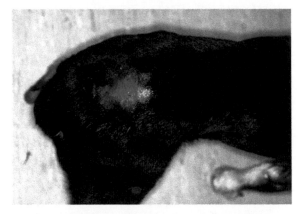

Figure 21.1 **Appearance of a superficial hot spot**

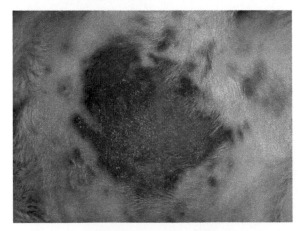

Figure 21.2 **Appearance of a deep hot spot, with thickened skin, oozing and satellite lesions**

100 Top Consultations in Small Animal General Practice, First Edition
By Peter Hill, Sheena Warman and Geoff Shawcross
© 2011 Blackwell Publishing Ltd

Treatment

After removal of the matted fur, hot spots should be cleaned with a dilute solution of chlorhexidene or povidone–iodine to remove exudate and crusts. Due to the severe pruritus associated with both superficial and deep hot spots, treatment with glucocorticoids is indicated to break the itch–scratch cycle. A short-acting injection of dexamethasone or a 3–5 day course of oral prednisolone at anti-inflammatory doses is usually sufficient. Once or twice daily topical application of an antibiotic/glucocorticoid cream is also beneficial to provide further localised anti-pruritic effects and to treat the surface bacterial colonisation. The lesion should be treated until the pruritus has subsided and the skin surface has healed.

If the lesion is a deep hot spot, a 2–3 week course of systemic antibiotics is also required. Appropriate choices would be amoxicillin/clavulanic acid, cefalexin, clindamycin, potentiated sulphonamides or cefovecin.

Some clinicians use an Elizabethan collar to prevent further self-trauma to hot spots. Whilst this is undoubtedly an effective strategy, the collars can be poorly tolerated and, in larger dogs, can be difficult to manage within a furnished house. Collars also have no direct therapeutic effect and should not be used as an alternative to anti-pruritic treatment. In the author's opinion, the compromise in the dog's welfare rarely justifies their use in this condition.

Appropriate treatment for any underlying causes is also required. This might entail flea control, expression of the anal sacs, treatment of otitis externa or management of underlying allergies.

What if it doesn't get better?

Hot spots usually respond rapidly to treatment. If the lesion persists, clinicians should make sure that they haven't treated a deep hot spot as a superficial one. Systemic antibiotic therapy would be indicated in such cases. If the lesion still fails to improve, further investigations such as cytology and biopsy are indicated to check for unusual infections or neoplasia.

If the lesion responds completely to appropriate treatment, but relapses subsequently, further attempts should be made to identify an underlying cause. If a cause cannot be found, the lesions will need to be treated symptomatically whenever they occur. In such cases, it is useful for owners to have a tube of antibiotic or glucocorticoid cream at home for use in emergencies. Prompt treatment can prevent the lesion from rapidly worsening.

The low-cost option

Treatment of superficial hot spots should not incur high costs. The costs associated with systemic antibiotic therapy for deep hot spots can be minimised by using potentiated sulphonamides.

When should I refer?

Hot spots are manageable in general practice and referral is not usually indicated, unless they are recurrent and a manifestation of an underlying allergic skin disease that is proving difficult to manage.

Peter Hill

Aetiology and pathogenesis

Acral lick dermatitis is caused by persistent licking at a distal extremity. The precise reason for this behaviour can be difficult to determine in an individual case but three main possibilities need to be considered:

1. The licking is due to pruritus, either focally at the site, or as a manifestation of a more widespread pruritic skin disease. Possible causes include staphylococcal folliculitis or furunculosis, demodicosis, a foreign body, fungal infection, atopic dermatitis, adverse reactions to food, or neoplasia.
2. The licking is due to pain or discomfort, typically as a manifestation of a neuromuscular or skeletal disorder. Possible causes include underlying joint disease, nerve dysfunction, brachial plexus or pelvic nerve tumours, or the presence of surgical implants.
3. The licking may have a behavioural or psychological component, although this is usually seen in association with the former aetiological categories. Possible contributing factors include anxiety, boredom, separation, or obsessive compulsive disorders.

History and clinical signs

Acral lick dermatitis appears as a well-circumscribed, alopecic, ulcerated plaque, usually seen on the distal limbs (Figure. 22.1). The most commonly affected site is over the carpus but lesions can also be seen in the tarsal area. Owners typically report that the dog persistently licks or nibbles at the affected area. Occasionally, owners may mention that the dog is pruritic, albeit less severely, at other sites.

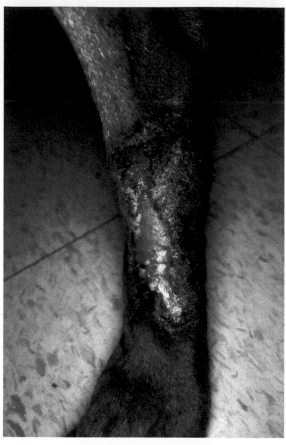

Figure 22.1 **Acral lick dermatitis on the metatarsal region of a dog**

100 Top Consultations in Small Animal General Practice, First Edition
By Peter Hill, Sheena Warman and Geoff Shawcross
© 2011 Blackwell Publishing Ltd

Specific diagnostic techniques

The lesion should be carefully examined, palpated and squeezed to check for signs of deep infection or foreign bodies. Cytological examination of an impression smear and a deep skin scraping can quickly determine if bacterial infection or demodicosis is involved. A good history and general physical examination is essential to determine if there is evidence of other underlying causes. Any historical or physical signs of pruritus elsewhere may point to a more widespread problem. The affected limb should be carefully examined for signs of pain or lameness, and the axillae and inguinal regions should be carefully palpated for the presence of masses. Owners should be specifically asked if the dog has ever had surgery in the affected area. Owners should also be questioned about the dog's lifestyle and activity level and if it receives sufficient exercise and stimulation for a dog of its type. If the lesion appears particularly proliferative or is growing in size, biopsies would be indicated to rule out neoplasia.

Treatment

There is no single treatment that will cure all cases and clinicians may have to try a number of therapeutic approaches before achieving success. Even then, it can take two to three months before the lesion completely heals. If an underlying cause has been diagnosed, it should be addressed at the same time as the lesion is being treated. In some cases, especially if an underlying cause cannot be found, a permanent cure is not possible.

If there is clinical and/or cytological evidence of staphylococcal infection, treatment should be initiated with systemic antibiotics. Cefalexin is the drug of choice and treatment may need to be continued for up to eight weeks. The lesion should also be washed daily with benzoyl peroxide shampoo, unless this proves to be irritant.

It is also necessary to provide some kind of mechanical barrier to prevent further licking such as an Elizabethan collar, bandage, or sock.

If the clinician believes that infection is not primarily involved, or if the lesion fails to respond completely to antibacterial therapy, topical glucocorticoid therapy is also indicated. This may take the form of a cream, gel or spray. Topical glucocorticoids are useful because they can help to reduce the swelling and thickening of the skin, as well as alleviating pruritus. Suitable choices include betamethasone or hydrocortisone aceponate (Cortavance, Virbac). Topical glucocorticoids should be applied twice daily initially, reducing to once daily when the lesion has shown signs of improvement. Treatment should be continued until the lesion has resolved and the hair has regrown over the affected area.

If the clinician suspects a psychological component to the problem, behaviour modification is indicated. This might include the provision of more walks, more freedom, more human companionship, more canine companionship, more toys, more chews, and removal of obvious sources of stress. In addition, the use of clomipramine (Clomicalm, Novartis) at 1–2 mg/kg every 12 hours can be a helpful adjunctive therapy during the treatment period.

What if it doesn't get better?

If the lesion does not respond to antibiotics and topical glucocorticoid treatment, the clinician can try sub-lesional injections of methylprednisolone acetate (Depo-Medrone, Pfizer). This is only likely to be successful in small lesions, less than 3 cm in diameter. Typically, approximately 0.25–0.5 ml of the solution is injected underneath the lesion every three weeks until it has substantially reduced in size and become non-pruritic. If the problem is thought to be mainly behavioural, and lifestyle changes are not possible or not totally successful, various psycho-active drugs can be contemplated such as fluoxetine, amitriptyline or doxepin. However, these drugs are not licensed for use in animals and are best prescribed by a specialist dermatologist or behaviourist. If medical management fails, other therapies that have been performed with variable degrees of success include acupuncture, radiation therapy, laser therapy, cryosurgery or surgical resection. However, clinicians should approach cryosurgery and surgical excision with great caution, because the procedures can lead to wounds that are difficult to close.

The low-cost option

Clients should be warned that some cases of acral lick dermatitis can be expensive to treat because of the need to search for potential underlying causes and the requirement for prolonged treatment. However, some simple cases may be manageable with a short course of systemic antibiotics, topical application of a glucocorticoid cream and covering with a sock. Prompt treatment of recurrences whilst the lesions are still relatively small in size is also likely to minimise costs.

When should I refer?

Routine cases of acral lick dermatitis should be manageable in general practice. In cases that are refractory or recurrent, especially when an underlying cause has not been found, referral to a specialist dermatologist and/or behaviourist may be advisable.

Peter Hill

Aetiology and pathogenesis

Anal sac problems are very common in dogs but rare in cats. The main conditions recognised are impactions, infections and abscesses. The exact cause isn't known but factors that may be involved include production of excessively thick secretions, too narrow a duct, or changes in the muscle tone surrounding the sac. There is no evidence to indicate that diet plays a major role in the development of anal sac problems. Rarely, tumours may develop in the anal sacs.

History and clinical signs

With anal sac impactions, affected dogs 'scoot' their anus along the ground in an attempt to relieve the uncomfortable sensation. They may lick or chew at the perineum, lumbosacral area or flanks. In some cases, a hot spot (acute moist dermatitis) may develop at the site of self-trauma (see Chapter 21). Anal sac infections can lead to similar signs, but there may be evidence of pain if the area is touched or a sanguinous discharge from the anal sac duct. Anal sac infections may also progress to abscesses, leading to a swelling on the affected side. They are acutely painful, and can make the dog pyrexic and lethargic. Abscesses often rupture, leading to a sinus tract and blood-tinged discharge adjacent to the anus (Figure 23.1). Non-ruptured abscesses need to be differentiated from other causes of lateral perineal swelling, such as tumours or perineal hernias.

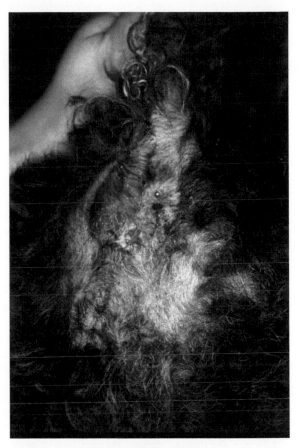

Figure 23.1 **Anal sac abscess in a dog**

Specific diagnostic techniques

The differentiation of anal sac problems is aided by expression of the contents (see below for technique). Normal anal sac secretions vary widely in colour (brown, fawn, yellow), and consistency (watery, creamy, toothpaste-like), and can contain flocculent material. They have a characteristic pungent, 'fishy' odour. In conjunction with typical clinical signs, anal sacs that are full with normal contents are consistent with a diagnosis of impaction. The presence of a

100 Top Consultations in Small Animal General Practice, First Edition
By Peter Hill, Sheena Warman and Geoff Shawcross
© 2011 Blackwell Publishing Ltd

purulent, foul smelling, greenish yellow or reddish discharge tends to suggest infection, as does the presence of blood. If a swelling is present lateral to the anus, careful palpation and a rectal examination are recommended to check for neoplasia and peri-neal hernias.

Treatment

For anal sac impactions, the treatment is to manually express the sacs, either by squeezing on either side of the anus with a 'milking action' (Figure 23.2), or preferably, by inserting a gloved finger into the anus and squeezing each sac individually (Figure 23.3). The latter technique is more effective, especially in large or obese dogs, or when the material is inspissated. In the absence of signs of infection, no antibacterial or anti-inflammatory treatment is warranted. If the scooting behaviour does not resolve after expression (at least temporarily), other causes of peri-anal pruritus should be considered, such as flea allergy, atopic dermatitis, adverse food reactions or *Malassezia* dermatitis.

If infection is present, expression of the sacs and treatment with systemic antibiotics will usually resolve the problem but in some cases, instillation of antibacterial/glucocorticoid preparations into the sac may be beneficial. Sometimes, this can be performed in a cooperative conscious patient, but it may need to be done under sedation or general anaesthesia. Commercially available ear drop preparations are suitable for this purpose; they can be transferred to a syringe and injected through the duct using a lacrimal cannula or 'cut down' tomcat catheter. Care must be taken to avoid traumatising the duct.

Anal sac abscesses are usually too painful to allow palpation or expression at the first visit without seda-tion or anaesthesia. If the abscess is grossly swollen and hasn't burst, drainage under anaesthesia is the preferred treatment option to provide immediate relief. This may require surgical lancing through the perianal skin. Following surgical drainage, or if the abscess has already burst, a 5–7 day course of sys-temic antibiotics is indicated. Suitable choices would be ampicillin, amoxicillin, or amoxicillin/clavulanic acid. Dogs suffering from an abscess should be re-examined after the course of antibiotics to ensure that the anatomy of the anal sac has returned to normal.

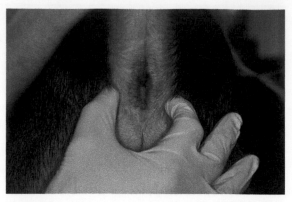

Figure 23.2 **Expression of the anal sacs using an external technique. The anal sacs can be palpated at the 4 and 8 o'clock positions. If they are full, they will feel like firm, spherical swellings. They can be expressed by gently moving the thumb and finger cranial to the sacs and gently squeezing them in a caudal and medial direction, using a 'milking' action. The expressed contents can be caught in the glove or a gauze swab**

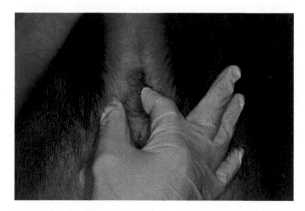

Figure 23.3 **Expression of the anal sacs using an internal technique. A lubricated finger is gently inserted into the anus and the anal sac is palpated between finger and thumb. The sac can then be gently squeezed directly**

What if it doesn't get better?

Anal sac impactions can be a recurrent problem and some owners pay regular visits to the practice to have them expressed. This is a satisfactory solution, as long as it is only required every few months. If the problem is more frequent than this, or if infections or abscesses have occurred on more than one occasion, surgical removal of the anal sacs is indicated. This will be curative, as long as the signs attributed to the anal sac problem have previously responded to conservative management (expression, antibiotics, topical infiltration). Anal sacs should not be removed in an attempt to treat intractable anal pruritus that has not responded to these interventions.

If anal sac infections or abscesses fail to respond to empirical treatment, culture and sensitivity testing is indicated. If the condition has failed to respond to appropriate antibiotic therapy, clinicians should consider other possibilities such as fibrosed abscesses, the entry of grass seeds or the presence of tumours. In such cases, surgical exploration of the sacs is indicated.

The low-cost option

Anal sac problems should not incur high costs unless surgery becomes necessary. If finances are severely limited, owners can be taught how to express anal sacs themselves, but they need to be educated about the signs of infection. Costs can also be minimised by using antibiotics such as ampicillin or amoxicillin.

When should I refer?

Referral of cases suffering from anal sac problems should not be necessary, although anal sacculectomy should be performed by a surgeon who has experience in the procedure, especially if the dog has had recurrent abscesses.

Peter Hill

Aetiology and pathogenesis

Ear infections are very common in dogs in small animal practice. They are less common in cats. Infection of the ear canal is invariably triggered by otitis (inflammation of the ear canal). Otitis may be restricted to the vertical and horizontal ear canals (otitis externa) or it may affect the middle ear cavity (otitis media). This usually occurs when infection spreads through the tympanic membrane into the tympanic bullae. Otitis interna is extremely rare and refers to inflammation that has reached the cochlea or semicircular canals.

As with other types of skin infection, ear infections usually occur secondary to an underlying cause. Figure 24.1 shows the various factors and diseases that contribute to the development of otitis in dogs. The underlying factors are divided into predisposing factors, primary causes and perpetuating factors. Predisposing factors are anatomical, physiological or behavioural factors that make a dog more prone to the development of otitis but do not necessarily cause it. Primary causes are specific diseases or conditions in which otitis is a common manifestation. Perpetuating factors are chronic pathological changes that cause otitis to become recurrent or resistant to treatment. In cats, only ear mites and ear canal masses (polyps and tumours) are common causes of otitis.

Regardless of the underlying cause, the ear canal commonly becomes infected with bacteria or yeasts. Initially, this is likely to be an overgrowth of commensal organisms such as *Staphylococcus intermedius*, *Streptococcus canis* or *Malassezia pachydermatis*. This may progress to involve gram-negative organisms such as *Escherichia coli*, *Proteus spp.* or *Pseudomonas aeruginosa*, especially if inappropriate management is prescribed at the outset.

History and clinical signs

The usual clinical signs are pruritus, pain, head shaking, inflammation of the ear canal, malodour and the presence of a visible discharge (Figures 24.2, 24.3, 24.4 and 24.5). The clinical signs of otitis media are identical to those of otitis externa but they tend to be more persistent and recurrent, and can lead to facial paralysis. Although otitis interna is rare, clinical signs include deafness and vestibular disease (head tilt, nystagmus, ataxia). Further questioning of the owner and a full dermatological exami-

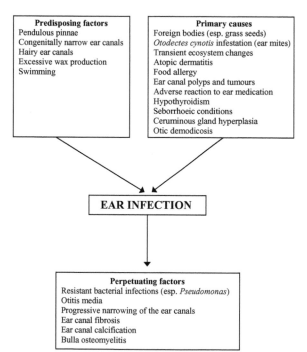

Predisposing factors	Primary causes
Pendulous pinnae	Foreign bodies (esp. grass seeds)
Congenitally narrow ear canals	*Otodectes cynotis* infestation (ear mites)
Hairy ear canals	Transient ecosystem changes
Excessive wax production	Atopic dermatitis
Swimming	Food allergy
	Ear canal polyps and tumours
	Adverse reaction to ear medication
	Hypothyroidism
	Seborrhoeic conditions
	Ceruminous gland hyperplasia
	Otic demodicosis

EAR INFECTION

Perpetuating factors
Resistant bacterial infections (esp. *Pseudomonas*)
Otitis media
Progressive narrowing of the ear canals
Ear canal fibrosis
Ear canal calcification
Bulla osteomyelitis

Figure 24.1   **Underlying causes of otitis**

100 Top Consultations in Small Animal General Practice, First Edition
By Peter Hill, Sheena Warman and Geoff Shawcross
© 2011 Blackwell Publishing Ltd

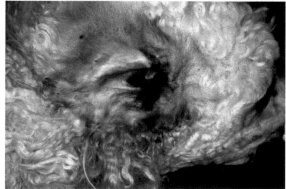

Figure 24.2   **Ceruminous otitis associated with a hairy ear canal**

nation may reveal signs of a potential underlying cause for otitis. For example, acute-onset head shaking is most consistent with a foreign body, whereas a more gradual onset of aural pruritus would be typical of allergic skin disease.

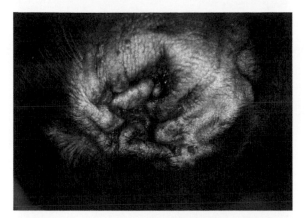

Figure 24.3 **Ceruminous otitis associated with a** *Malassezia* **overgrowth**

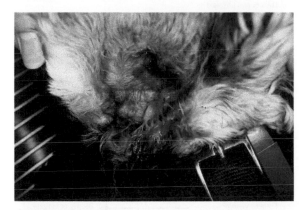

Figure 24.4 **Purulent otitis associated with a** *Pseudomonas* **infection**

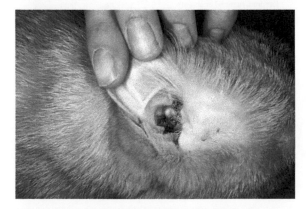

Figure 24.5 **Dry waxy exudate associated with** *Otodectes cynotis* **infestation**

Specific diagnostic techniques

Two specific diagnostic procedures should be performed whenever an ear infection is suspected: otoscopic examination and cytological examination of the discharge. The aim of the otoscopic examination is to detect foreign bodies or ear mites, to assess the condition of the vertical and horizontal canals, to check the appearance and integrity of the tympanic membrane, and to characterise the type of exudate that is present. If the condition is unilateral, clinicians should always examine the good ear first. This prevents the spread of infection from one ear to the other and leaves the most uncomfortable procedure until last. In some cases, the ear canal may be too painful, swollen, or full of exudate to allow a meaningful otoscopic examination to be performed. In these cases, the animal can either be sedated or anaesthetised to allow examination, or a preliminary course of treatment can be given and the ear re-examined a few days later. Which course is taken will depend on the severity of the clinical presentation and the clinician's index of suspicion for the various underlying causes. In either case, it is essential that a full otoscopic examination be performed at some stage.

Cytological analysis of the exudate should be performed on the first and all subsequent visits. This can always be performed, even if the ear is too painful to allow a full otoscopic examination. Cytology allows immediate differentiation of the types of infectious agents that may be present (cocci, rods or *Malassezia*). Detection of cocci or *Malassezia* (Figures 24.6 and 24.7) allows empirical treatment to be prescribed because the sensitivity profile of these organisms can be predicted with reasonable certainty. The presence of rods (Figure 24.8) should prompt the clinician into performing bacterial culture and sensitivity testing because resistance is much more of a problem with gram-negative organisms. Cultures should also be performed on cases that have failed to respond to treatment.

If there are time constraints, the following strategies can help to facilitate the introduction of routine ear cytology into the practice:

* A qualified nurse can be trained to stain and examine the sample whilst the client is waiting
* The dog can be admitted for a short time, allowing the test to be performed when time is available
* The sample can be taken and examined later, when time is available. A sterile swab for

potential culture should be collected at the same time, but only submitted if rods are seen. This approach is less desirable because the information derived from the cytological examination should be used to inform the choice of treatment. Ideally, the client should collect the medication later, when the results of the test are known.

In addition to diagnosing and treating the infection itself, the clinician should also try to determine the underlying cause. This is especially important in any case that has suffered otitis on more than one occasion. If this is not done, many cases will become recurrent or chronic. A summary of the diagnostic approach to acute otitis (animals presenting for the first time) is shown in Figure 24.9.

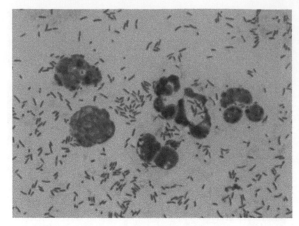

Figure 24.8   **Neutrophilic inflammation with rods**

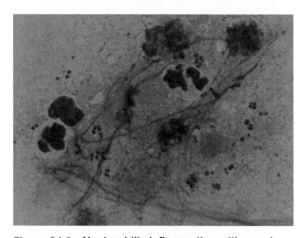

Figure 24.6   **Neutrophilic inflammation with cocci**

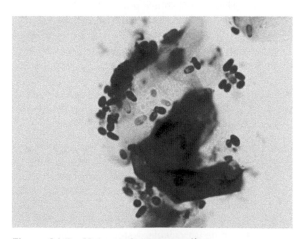

Figure 24.7   *Malassezia* **overgrowth**

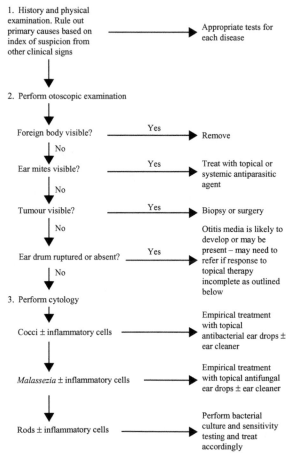

Figure 24.9   **General diagnostic and therapeutic approach to acute otitis externa**

Treatment

Some ear infections occur for no identifiable reason and a single course of treatment can be curative. Such cases are likely to be caused by transient changes to the ecosystem in the ear canal induced by changes in temperature, humidity or microbial population. However, if the ear infection recurs within days or weeks, an underlying cause must be identified and treated to prevent the case from becoming chronic.

Ear infections restricted to the vertical and horizontal canals are treated with commercially available eardrops containing various combinations of antibiotics, antifungal agents and glucocorticoids. Clinicians should base their choice of medication on the organisms that have been seen on cytology, or following culture and sensitivity testing. Treating ear infections without knowing what types of organism are present can lead to the development of resistant bacteria. For pure coccal infections, the most appropriate antibiotics would be fusidic acid (Canaural, Dechra) or polymyxin B (Surolan, Janssen). When rods are seen, possible options (pending results of bacterial culture and sensitivity testing) are neomycin (Panalog, Novartis Animal Health), framycetin (Canaural), polymyxin B (Surolan), gentamycin (Otomax, Schering Plough) or marbofloxacin (Aurizon, Vétoquinol), although the latter two drugs have the widest spectrum of activity against gram-negative organisms. Although any of these agents could be chosen prior to receiving culture results, the final choice of drug may have to be changed as soon as sensitivity results are available. If the tympanic membrane has ruptured, or its integrity cannot be established, gentamycin should be avoided as it carries the greatest risk of ototoxicity. The other topical agents can usually be used safely, but clinicians should be aware that any drug could potentially cause ototoxicity and should consider referring the case if they are particularly concerned.

For pure *Malassezia* infections, resistance is not a problem and all the commercially available antifungal agents in ear drops are likely to be effective, i.e. miconazole (Surolan), clotrimazole (Otomax, Aurizon) or nystatin (Canaural). It is therefore better to base the choice of eardrop on avoidance of potent antibiotics, rather than on the antifungal agent itself. Products containing gentamycin or marbofloxacin in combination with antifungal agents would be best avoided as these agents are important for treating gram-negative infections and indiscriminate use to treat pure *Malassezia* infections may encourage bacterial resistance.

The glucocorticoid component of ear drops is valuable for reducing inflammation and pain, and the type of glucocorticoid does not seem to be important and is not used to inform the choice of treatment. In cases where the ear canal is extremely stenotic, a short course of systemic glucocorticoids can be helpful to reduce inflammation and re-establish the patency of the lumen.

Ear cleaning solutions containing ceruminolytic and drying agents may also be beneficial in the management of otitis. These products are particularly useful for ear canals that are very waxy, or too dirty to allow antimicrobial drops to penetrate, or in the long-term management of chronic ceruminous otitis (see Box 24.1).

Animals being treated for otitis should be re-inspected after 5–7 days to ensure clinical resolution. This is important because clients will be unable to assess whether the infection has resolved in the horizontal canal. Cytology should be used to monitor the response to medication because it is not uncommon for the types of organisms to change following treatment. If the condition has not completely resolved, further treatment should be prescribed. If the nature of the otitis has changed (e.g. different organism present) the treatment should be modified.

If underlying causes are identified, additional management is required. The lack of ventilation and increased humidity associated with predisposing factors can be amenable to maintenance ear cleaning regimes or hair plucking. If this is not successful, and the clinician is certain that these are major contributing factors in a particular case, then surgical alteration of the ear canal by lateral wall resection or vertical canal ablation may be beneficial.

Primary causes require specific treatment. Removal of grass seeds, foreign bodies, ear mites, polyps and tumours can be curative. However, allergic ear disease will require long-term management along with the skin disease (see Chapter 20 on atopic dermatitis). Surgical intervention is not indicated for the treatment of primary causes, with the exception of tumour removal.

Perpetuating factors can be the most troublesome to deal with because they can make the ear infection become recurrent or chronic. If perpetuating factors are allowed to gain momentum, the ear canal can become permanently and irreversibly damaged. If the diagnostic and therapeutic guidelines outlined above are followed carefully, the development of perpetuating factors can usually be avoided. Once they have occurred, however, they require advanced medical and/or surgical intervention to achieve resolution (see below).

Box 24.1   The technique for basic ear cleaning

If successful results are to be obtained, owners must be given a demonstration of this ear cleaning technique. Whilst holding the pinna firmly, the ear canal is flooded with the ear cleaner. The cartilage of the vertical and horizontal canals is then massaged. Owners must be shown how to achieve deep palpation if the technique is to be effective. The appropriate technique produces a characteristic 'squelching' sound. The dog is then allowed to shake its head which removes much of the liquid. Any residual cleaner should then be removed with a slightly moist gauze swab or cotton ball. Cotton buds should be avoided because they can push debris deeper into the ear canal. Owners should be told to inspect the gauze swab carefully to see what comes out. This is very important when ear cleaning is being used on a long-term basis because it can be used to determine the frequency of application. As an adjunct to the treatment of ear infections, the ear cleaner may only have to be used temporarily. However, if longer term use is required, inspection of the gauze swab can determine when the next ear cleaning should be performed. If the swab is very dirty, the ears should be cleaned again the next day. If the swab is completely clean, the ears can be cleaned every other day. If the swab is still clean, twice weekly cleaning may be sufficient, or in some cases, only once weekly. Once the swab starts to look dirty again, the correct frequency of application must be determined.

What if it doesn't get better?

Owners may regard two different outcomes as a 'failure to get better'. First, the initial ear infection may actually respond to treatment, but then recur. In this situation, it is almost certain that an underlying cause has been overlooked or missed. Unless this cause is identified, the problem will never resolve completely. Second, the ear infection may fail to respond to treatment in the first place. This is usually due to the presence of resistant organisms, especially *Pseudomonas aeruginosa*. Culture and sensitivity testing should be performed immediately and appropriate antimicrobial therapy initiated.

The low-cost option

If an obvious and curable cause can be established (foreign body, ear mites, post-swimming ecosystem change), the routine management of an ear infection should not incur high costs. The additional costs associated with performing cytology easily outweigh the risk of embarking on inappropriate treatment that may result in resistant bacteria. Inevitably, higher costs will be associated with management of otitis secondary to lifelong conditions (allergies) or those requiring surgery (ear canal tumours). Very high costs are likely in cases that have developed perpetuating factors such as resistant *Pseudomonas* infections, otitis media or irreversible pathology. In most cases, these costs could have been avoided by initiating prompt and appropriate treatment at the outset.

When should I refer?

Most ear infections associated with predisposing factors or primary causes can be managed in general practice. However, the diagnosis and treatment of perpetuating factors requires considerable experience and expertise. Until clinicians are fully competent at assessing the horizontal ear canal and tympanic membrane, performing and interpreting bulla radiographs or CT scans, managing middle ear disease by bulla flushing, monitoring cases with cytology, and are familiar with the treatment protocols for resistant organisms, these cases are best referred to a specialist dermatologist. Some perpetuating factors represent irreversible pathology and the only form of successful treatment is a total ear canal ablation with a bulla osteotomy. This surgery should only be undertaken by an experienced surgeon. As a general rule, the earlier that a recurrent or chronic ear infection is referred, the more likely it is that surgery can be avoided.

Peter Hill

A number of skin diseases affect the paws of dogs and cats. In some cases, the condition will be restricted to the paws, but it is more common to see pedal disease in conjunction with a more widespread skin disorder. Some of the following conditions are covered elsewhere in this text, so this chapter focuses primarily on the pedal conditions themselves. Multiple aetiologies can be involved and important clues can be obtained by careful assessment of the type of lesions present and the areas of the paws that are affected. Pedal diseases can be pruritic and/or painful, resulting in signs such as licking, chewing or lameness.

Common differential diagnoses

Dogs

Interdigital erythema and pruritus

- Demodicosis
- *Trombicula* infestation
- *Malassezia* dermatitis
- Bacterial overgrowth syndrome
- Atopic dermatitis
- Food allergy
- Contact dermatitis.

Interdigital nodule(s) ± discharging tract(s)

- Demodicosis
- Foreign body
- Bacterial furunculosis and pyogranuloma
- Fungal granuloma
- Traumatic furunculosis (implanted hair shafts)
- Ruptured follicular cyst(s)
- Sterile pyogranuloma
- Neoplasia (sebaceous adenoma, papilloma, plasma cell tumour, histiocytoma, mast cell tumour, sweat gland tumour).

Pad disorders

- Age-related hyperkeratosis (Cocker Spaniel, Beagle, Basset Hound)

- Breed-specific hyperkeratosis (Golden Retriever, Labrador Retriever, Irish Terrier, Norfolk Terrier, Kerry Blue Terrier, Dogue de Bordeaux)
- Keratoma/corn (Greyhound)
- Hepatocutaneous syndrome
- Pemphigus foliaceus
- Zinc-responsive dermatosis
- Lethal acrodermatitis (Bull Terrier)
- Vitiligo (depigmentation).

Claw disorders

- Trauma
- Lupoid onychodystrophy
- Onychomycosis
- Claw-bed tumours (squamous cell carcinoma, keratoacanthoma, melanoma).

Cats

- Cat bite abscess
- Infections associated with FeLV/FIV infection
- Cutaneous viral infections (poxvirus, herpesvirus, calicivirus)
- *Trombicula* infestation
- Demodicosis
- Allergic pododermatitis
- Eosinophilic granuloma
- Dermatophytosis
- Feline plasma cell pododermatitis
- Vitiligo of the pads (depigmentation)
- Claw trauma
- Claw-bed tumours (squamous cell carcinoma, fibrosarcoma, metastatic pulmonary carcinoma / lung digit syndrome)
- Paronychia (bacterial infection, pemphigus foliaceus).

100 Top Consultations in Small Animal General Practice, First Edition
By Peter Hill, Sheena Warman and Geoff Shawcross
© 2011 Blackwell Publishing Ltd

Diagnostic approach

When presented with a case of pedal skin disease, clinicians should first determine if the history and physical examination allow a diagnosis to be made by 'pattern recognition'. This may be possible if an obvious foreign body penetration or *Trombicula* larvae are seen. Experienced clinicians and dermatologists would also be able to recognise vitiligo (a benign depigmentation of the pads), feline plasma cell pododermatitis (a characteristic condition in which the digital pads become swollen, spongy and possibly ulcerated) and lupoid onychodystrophy (a condition in which multiple claws slough for no apparent reason). Important clues to the diagnosis can also be obtained if skin lesions are present in other areas. For example, atopic dermatitis, pemphigus foliaceus, zinc-responsive dermatosis and hepatocutaneous syndrome will all produce characteristic skin lesions at other sites.

The lesions on the paws should be carefully characterised as this has clear implications for the probable diagnosis (see above). In dogs, clinicians should also check for any evidence of anatomical or pathological abnormalities that could be initiating or perpetuating some of the above conditions, especially those resulting in ruptured hair follicles. For example, the conformation of the paws and pads should be examined both in a weight-bearing position and with the paw lifted. Some dogs have abnormal footpad conformations that result in haired skin coming into a weight-bearing position (e.g. the horse shoe pad, Figure 25.1). This can result in traumatic implantation of hair shafts into the dermis, especially in short-coated breeds, resulting in furunculosis and a chronic pyogranulomatous inflammatory reaction. Chronic proliferative changes such as interdigital hyperplasia and fibrosis can lead to further friction, trauma and inflammation.

The next step in trying to establish a precise diagnosis involves microscopic examination of samples taken from the paws. It is essential to rule out demodicosis in any pedal disease that involves the haired skin. Pododemodicosis can occur in the absence of more widespread skin lesions, and in dogs it is often a chronic and stubborn disease to treat. The earlier it is diagnosed, the more likely it is to resolve following treatment. Complicating the diagnosis is the fact that it can present in different ways, including erythema, alopecia, nodules and draining tracts (Figure 25.2). The mites can be detected using either skin scrapings or hair pluckings (see Chapter 18).

Cytological examination of stained tape strips and impression smears is required to identify *Malassezia* dermatitis and bacterial infections (see Chapter 19). These tests can also reveal bacterial overgrowth syndrome, a pruritic condition in which large numbers of organisms are seen without evidence of an accompanying neutrophilic response (Figure 25.3). Recurrent infections in the paws can be caused by numerous underlying disorders, especially allergic skin disease, hypothyroidism, hyperadrenocorticism, chronic glucocorticoid therapy, systemic disease, FeLV/FIV infection and breed-related susceptibility (especially in Bull terriers). If unusual bacteria are seen on cytology (e.g. rods), or a confirmed bacterial infection fails to respond to initial treatment, culture and sensitivity should be performed to check for antibiotic resistance. Cytology is also valuable in the diagnosis of eosinophilic granulomas, plasma cell pododermatitis, dermatophytosis, pemphigus, zinc-responsive dermatosis and neoplasia.

Further investigations will be informed by the clinical signs and the nature of the lesions seen. For red, itchy feet, an allergy investigation or allergy management is indicated once parasitic and infectious causes have been ruled out (see Chapter 20). If significant alopecia is present, tests for dermatophytosis would also be indicated (see Chapter 34). If interdigital nodules ± discharging tracts are present (Figure 25.4), any involvement of foreign bodies, demodicosis or bacterial infection should be dealt with first before embarking on further tests. Once these have been ruled out or dealt with, skin biopsies are indicated to characterise the underlying pathology and reveal the nature of the inflammatory response and the presence or absence of follicular cysts, free hair shafts within the dermis, fungal elements, fibrosis or neoplasia. Biopsies are also indicated for suspected viral infections, and for disorders affecting the pads, unless the change appears to be clinically insignificant (e.g. vitiligo or age-related hyperkeratosis). Suspected tumours can be investigated with fine needle aspirates and biopsies.

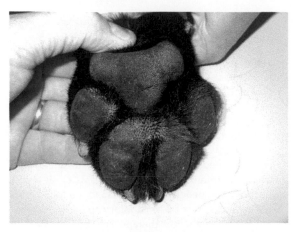

Figure 25.1 A 'horse-shoe pad' in which a bridge of skin connects the two central pads, allowing haired skin to come into a weight-bearing position

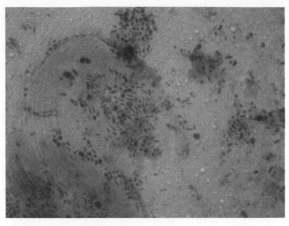

Figure 25.3 Cytological appearance of bacterial overgrowth syndrome

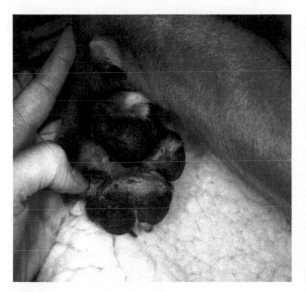

Figure 25.2 Interdigital erythema caused by demodicosis

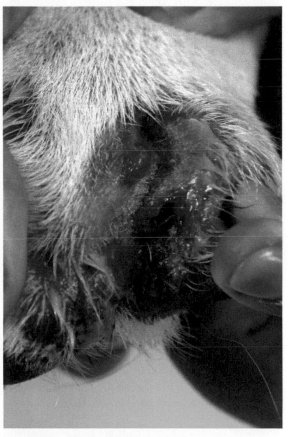

Figure 25.4 Severe pododermatitis comprising interdigital nodules and draining tracts

Treatment

The initial management should be targeted at elimination of any parasitic or infectious causes of the pododermatitis (see Chapters 17–19 and 28). If unusual organisms are detected, or resistance is suspected, antibiotics should be chosen according to sensitivity testing based on culture from a deep discharging tract or skin biopsy. Antibiotic therapy should be continued for as long as improvement occurs, which may require 1–3 months of therapy in chronic cases. In some patients, this may lead to complete resolution of the lesions, while in other cases, some residual pathology may remain. Should this occur, further investigation is required to detect the underlying cause.

Topical therapy with antimicrobial shampoos and creams is a useful adjunctive treatment for true bacterial infections, but can be used as a sole treatment for *Malassezia* dermatitis and bacterial overgrowth syndrome (see Chapter 19). Topically applied fusidic acid (Fucidin) or mupirocin ointment (Bactroban) can be very effective for the treatment of nodules containing deep bacterial infection.

If an underlying allergic skin condition is present, appropriate long-term management should be instituted (see Chapter 20).

The most problematic cases of pododermatitis in dogs are those associated with ruptured hair follicles and multiple follicular cysts resulting in interdigital nodules. These can be associated with significant bacterial infection, but in many cases sterile pyogranulomas persist even after prolonged antibacterial therapy. In these cases, systemic or topical glucocorticoids can be used to dampen down the foreign body reaction and allow resolution of the stubborn nodules. If the problem has arisen due to abnormal footpad conformation, long-term glucocorticoid therapy may be the treatment of choice. Once the lesions are in remission, the lowest possible doses, given on alternate days, should be used. Similar results can be obtained with ciclosporin and/or topical tacrolimus, but these drugs are much more expensive. Daily foot soaks in Epsom salts (a saturated solution of $MgSO_4$) are also useful because they soften the stratum corneum and allow embedded foreign material to be extruded through the skin surface.

Most disorders of the pads are best investigated and treated by specialist dermatologists because the potential causes are very diverse, and an accurate diagnosis is required prior to initiating treatment.

What if it doesn't get better?

There are two situations that owners are likely to interpret as a failure of the animal to get better: problems that are recurrent, or those that are refractory to initial treatment.

The main reason for lesions recurring after apparently successful therapy is the failure to recognise an underlying cause. The most common scenario is recurrent pedal infections secondary to underlying allergic dermatitis, hormonal problems or systemic disease. If an underlying cause cannot be found, but the condition appears to be totally antibiotic responsive, pulse antibiotic therapy can be considered. These cases are best referred to specialists for management.

Pododermatitis may be refractory to treatment if the diagnosis is incorrect or if an underlying cause is not addressed at the same time. In addition, a major problem that occurs in chronic pododermatitis is fibrosis and scarring. This can follow chronic inflammation, infection, furunculosis and foreign body reactions and lead to pathology that can be irreversible.

Specific treatment options for fibrosis and scarring include:

- Glucocorticoids – These can be used to reduce production of fibrous tissue
- Pentoxifylline – This drug has anti-fibrotic effects and is used at a dose of 15 mg/kg TID. Its efficacy is variable but it appears to be beneficial in some cases
- Surgery – Surgical resection of stubborn nodules or focal areas of scarring can lead to resolution of chronic lesions. For solitary or mild lesions, this can be a relatively simple operation. For severe, chronic and scarred interdigital skin, a podoplasty can be performed. This involves removing the diseased interdigital skin and either permanently separating the toes or fusing the weight-bearing pads together. These operations, although potentially curative, carry a high risk of complications and should only be undertaken by surgeons with expertise in the procedures.

The low-cost option

The costs of treating pododermatitis will depend entirely on the diagnosis. A focal lesion caused by a grass seed will be simple and cheap to treat. However, a chronic case of scarring interdigital pododermatitis will involve considerable expense both in the diagnostic and therapeutic phases. Unnecessary costs can be avoided by ensuring that an accurate diagnosis is achieved as soon as possible so that empirically chosen, ineffective treatments are not prescribed.

When should I refer?

Pododermatitis is a common presentation and many cases are treated in general practice. Treatment of parasites and pedal infections should not pose too many difficulties. Referral should be considered for recurrent or refractory cases in which long-term treatments are necessary. The diagnosis and management of pad and claw disorders can be challenging and a specialist opinion may be worthwhile at the outset. Surgical alteration of multiple interdigital spaces should only be performed by specialist surgeons.

Peter Hill

Cutaneous lumps and swellings are a common presenting sign in general practice. They are a source of anxiety to owners because they are either visible or palpable, and may be due to neoplasia. Hence, when presented with such a problem, the clinician's role is to rapidly determine an accurate diagnosis and prognosis.

Common differential diagnoses

Table 26.1 shows the possible causes of cutaneous lumps and swellings in dogs and cats. The diagnosis is based on the type of material that is found within them. This approach is useful because it relates to the diagnostic findings seen on aspiration cytology and/or histopathology.

Table 26.1 Possible causes of cutaneous lumps and swellings in dogs and cats, based on the type of material that is found within them. The conditions in bold are the most common.

Contents of lump	Specific diagnosis	Contents of lump	Specific diagnosis
Blood	**Haematoma** Vascular tumour	Neoplastic or hyperplastic sebocytes	**Sebaceous gland hyperplasia/adenoma** **Tail gland hyperplasia**
Oedema	**Urticaria** **Angioedema**	Mast cells	**Mast cell tumour**
Serum	**Seroma**	Neoplastic epithelial cells	Papilloma **Squamous cell carcinoma**
Pus	**Abscess** Deep bacterial infection Mycetoma Kerion (nodular dermatophyte infection) Deep fungal infection		**Basal cell tumour** **Peri-anal gland tumour** Hair follicle tumours Sweat gland tumours
Inflammatory cells	Sterile nodular panniculitis Sterile nodular granuloma and pyogranuloma Cutaneous histiocytosis Feline plasma cell pododermatitis	Neoplastic spindle cells	**Fibroma/fibrosarcoma** Haemangiopericytoma Neural tumours Vascular tumours
		Neoplastic round cells	Lymphoma **Histiocytoma** Plasma cell tumour
		Melanocytes	**Melanoma**
Anuclear cellular and proteinaceous debris	**Cutaneous cyst**	Calcium	Calcinosis cutis Calcinosis circumscripta
		Mucin	Cutaneous mucinosis
		Hyperplastic tissue	Naevus
Fat	**Lipoma**		Dermatofibrosis

100 Top Consultations in Small Animal General Practice, First Edition
By Peter Hill, Sheena Warman and Geoff Shawcross
© 2011 Blackwell Publishing Ltd

Diagnostic approach

As with other dermatological problems, a history and physical examination are important when presented with a lump. There may be a history of trauma or bite wounds that could have led to haematomas or abscesses. It is also important to determine how rapidly the lump appeared, how long it has been present and whether it is increasing in size. Some lumps may be pruritic or cause the animal discomfort. A general medical history will determine if the animal is showing any other clinical signs.

A general physical examination should be performed to ensure that the animal does not have any evidence of systemic disease, paying particular attention to the regional lymph nodes. A full dermatological examination should be performed to check for the presence of other lumps. It is not uncommon for animals to be presented for examination of a single lump when multiple lumps can be found. In such cases, the masses may be the same or different types. The lump(s) itself should then be carefully examined. Visual inspection should determine the appearance, size, shape, and the presence of any discharging sinuses or ulceration. Palpation should determine the consistency, firmness, depth and attachment to underlying tissues. Although examination of the lump itself is very important, it is critical not to place too much emphasis on this part of the examination. Although with some conditions, it is possible to make a diagnosis on history and examination alone (e.g. haematoma, urticaria, angioedema, abscess, seroma, sebaceous adenoma), in the majority of cases, this is simply not possible. The phrase 'a lump is a lump is a lump' was not born out of ignorance and it is not appropriate for a clinician to feel a mass and tell a client to keep an eye on it to see if it grows.

Unless a specific diagnosis has been made based on the history and physical examination alone, the next step is to perform a fine-needle aspirate. The technique for this is as follows:

1. Spray or wipe the surface of the lesion or mass with alcohol.
2. Hold the mass to fix its position.
3. Insert a 20- or 22-gauge needle into the mass either with or without an attached 5 ml syringe. Move the needle forwards and backwards within the mass a few times, changing the direction slightly each time. If the syringe is attached, the plunger should be pulled back when the needle is actually in the mass. The pressure on the plunger should be released before the needle is withdrawn.
4. Withdraw the needle and remove from the syringe if attached. Immediately fill the syringe with air, re-connect to the needle and forcefully blow the contents out onto a glass slide. This should be performed extremely rapidly (in less than three seconds) so that the material does not dry out inside the needle.
5. Check the slide to see if there is any material on it (it may be a very small amount). If nothing is visible, aspirate the mass again using the alternative technique (either with or without the attached syringe). If there is too much material, smear it out using a second slide.
6. Air-dry the slide before staining with an appropriate in-clinic stain such as Diff-Quik.
7. It is worth collecting more than one aspirate so that an air-dried, unstained slide can be sent away for external analysis if necessary.

The cell-recognition skills required to evaluate fine-needle aspirates are not beyond the scope of general practitioners, and in-house analysis does allow an immediate decision to be made about future management. Some of the conditions have a very characteristic appearance (see subsequent chapters) and with a little practice and experience, the technique can easily become a valuable (and income-generating) component of the practice repertoire. However, if clinicians lack the confidence to examine the samples themselves, they can be sent to an external diagnostic laboratory. Experience can be gained by comparing samples examined in-house with those submitted to an external laboratory.

When examining the sample in-house, the slide should first be scanned on low power to find areas where cellular material has adhered (these will be stained blue). The slide should then be examined using the oil immersion lens (×1000 magnification) to determine the cell types that are present. Fine-needle aspiration cytology may provide a definitive diagnosis, a suspected diagnosis, or no diagnosis. The first objective is to distinguish between inflammation and neoplasia. Inflammation will be characterised by the presence of predominantly neutrophils and macrophages. If this is the case, a search should be made for microorganisms, and further tests (cultures, biopsies) may be required to differentiate the possible causes.

Fortunately, the most common cutaneous neoplasms seen in general practice (cysts, lipomas, sebaceous gland tumours, histiocytomas and mast cell tumours) can all be definitively and easily diagnosed using this technique (see relevant chapters). Fine-needle aspirates may also enable a tumour type to be categorised as epithelial, spindle or round cell, but this requires more expertise and the sample may have to be sent away for an expert opinion. Specific differentiation of these tumour types usually requires histopathology.

If the diagnosis remains uncertain after fine-needle aspiration, a biopsy of the mass, or the whole mass, should be submitted for histopathological analysis. This is also required for some tumours that have already been diagnosed on fine-needle aspiration, in order to allow the mass to be graded and have the tissue margins evaluated. However, fine-needle aspiration should always precede biopsy or surgical excision of a mass as this may render the more invasive technique unnecessary and in some cases (e.g. mast cell tumours) can dictate the extent of the surgery that is required.

Treatment

The treatment of cutaneous lumps and swellings depends on the diagnosis, prognosis and wishes of the client. Depending on the diagnosis, medical or surgical treatment may be necessary. Some conditions require immediate intervention whereas others may be safely left. Benign cutaneous masses such as lipomas, sebaceous adenomas, histiocytomas and cysts are often left alone as long as they are causing no problems for the animal. However, clinicians should bear in mind that surgical resection of masses is much harder at certain body sites than others. For example, tumours on the distal limbs, face or perineal region are best removed before they get too large because skin closure becomes more difficult with time. Benign tumours may also require removal if they lead to self-trauma or become ulcerated.

What if it doesn't get better?

With an accurate diagnosis, it is usually possible to give a reasonably accurate prognosis. Some skin tumours carry a guarded prognosis and can be life-threatening. If a condition does not respond to medical or surgical intervention as expected, clinicians should always re-evaluate the diagnosis.

The low-cost option

Costs can be minimised by making a diagnosis as early as possible using history, physical examination and fine-needle aspiration. This may allow the costs of biopsy, histopathology and surgical excision to be avoided.

When should I refer?

Many of the conditions listed are easily manageable in general practice, either by medical treatment or surgical excision. Referral should be considered if a specific diagnosis cannot be made using the facilities available in the practice. Conditions that might benefit from diagnostic and therapeutic input from a specialist include mycetomas, deep fungal infections, sterile inflammatory diseases (panniculitis and pyogranulomas), mast cell tumours, and any extensive neoplastic process that requires complex medical, oncological or surgical intervention.

Peter Hill

Aetiology and pathogenesis

Urticaria (hives) is a term that refers to the development of multiple cutaneous wheals. A wheal is a well-circumscribed, circular, raised, dome-shaped lesion caused by oedema within the dermis. Wheals are typically 0.5–2.0 cm in diameter. Angioedema refers to gross swelling of an extremity such as a distal limb or the face due to dermal oedema. Urticaria and angioedema are usually caused by acute hypersensitivity reactions, but various non-immunological factors may also be involved in precipitating an episode. Factors that have been reported to cause urticaria or angioedema in dogs are stinging and biting insects, reactions to plants, intestinal parasites, adverse reactions to food, drugs, shampoos, vaccines, allergenic extracts, blood transfusions, snake bites, excessive heat or cold, and oestrus.

History and clinical signs

Most episodes of urticaria or angioedema are acute and are presented as relatively urgent cases (Figures 27.1 and 27.2). The lesions may or may not be pruritic. In some cases, the probable trigger may be obvious because of the temporal association between an event (e.g. vaccine administration, blood transfusion, dog getting stung in the garden) and the development of lesions. In other cases, there may be no obvious cause in the dog's history. Other than the skin lesions, the dogs are usually otherwise well and general physical examination is normally unremarkable. Some cases of angioedema can affect the upper respiratory tract leading to breathing difficulties.

Differential diagnoses

There are few differential diagnoses for urticaria and angioedema. In short-coated dogs, lesions of staphylococcal folliculitis can lead to raised tufts of hair that can be mistaken for urticaria on a cursory examination. In young puppies (3 weeks to 4 months of age), angioedema can be confused with juvenile cellulitis, a disease that causes acute swelling of the face, eyelids, lips and pinna. However,

in this disease, the puppies are systemically unwell, the submandibular lymph nodes are enlarged, there may be a purulent otitis, and the skin contains papules, pustules, draining tracts and crusts. Persistent oedematous swelling of an extremity can also be due to hypoalbuminaemia, right-sided heart failure, vasculitis or lymphoedema, caused by lymphatic obstruction. The latter condition does not have an acute onset and will persist until the underlying cause has been identified and eliminated (primary lymphatic abnormality or obstruction due to neoplasia, surgery or trauma).

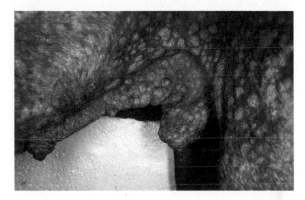

Figure 27.1 **Urticaria in a dog**

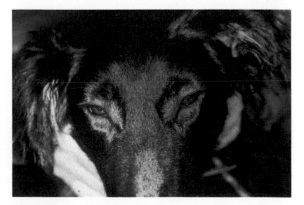

Figure 27.2 **Angioedema in a dog affecting the face and eyelids**

100 Top Consultations in Small Animal General Practice, First Edition
By Peter Hill, Sheena Warman and Geoff Shawcross
© 2011 Blackwell Publishing Ltd

Specific diagnostic techniques

No specific tests are required to confirm a diagnosis of urticaria or angioedema as the history and lesions are pathognomonic. However, a careful dermatological examination is required to ensure that the lesions are actually due to oedema. Wheals and angioedema will pit on pressure.

Treatment

Most dogs presenting with urticaria should be treated with a short course of glucocorticoids, given either orally (prednisolone or methylprednisolone) or by injection (dexamethasone). Antihistamines are ineffective at treating acute reactions because they cannot control the inflammatory reaction that has already occurred. Uncomplicated cases of angioedema showing no other signs can be treated as for urticaria. If there is any respiratory involvement, the dog should be hospitalised, monitored and treated with epinephrine (0.1–0.5 ml of a 1:1000 solution given subcutaneously). Glucocorticoids should also be administered by intravenous injection and followed by a short course given orally or by injection.

What if it doesn't get better?

Rarely, some cases of urticaria and angioedema can become chronic or recurrent. In such cases, a diligent search should be made for precipitating factors, including all those listed earlier in this chapter. This may require investigation for intestinal parasites, exclusion dietary trials and environmental restriction. Urticaria is not a clinical feature of canine atopic dermatitis, but intradermal testing may still be valuable in an attempt to identify potential IgE-mediated plant hypersensitivities. In cases of chronic idiopathic urticaria, antihistamines may be of benefit but a number of different types may have to be tried to find one that is helpful for a particular patient (see Chapter 20 for further details).

The low-cost option

Routine cases of urticaria and angioedema should respond promptly to glucocorticoid treatment and should not incur high costs.

When should I refer?

Referral might be considered in chronic cases in which an underlying cause cannot be found. Identification of an allergic aetiology may require specialist input.

Peter Hill

Aetiology and pathogenesis

Cat-bite abscesses are usually seen in association with fighting. Most occur around the head, base of tail, or limbs but bites to the body can also be seen. Nearly all are associated with infection by *Pasteurella multocida*, an organism that is part of the cat's normal oral flora.

History and clinical signs

The fight is unlikely to have been witnessed by the owner. For bites around the head or tail, owners will either report that the cat is unwell (lethargic and/or inappetent) or will have noticed the lesion itself. Bites to the limbs will present as lameness and can be mistaken as fractures. In the early stages, only the puncture marks may be visible, but these are often hidden by the cat's hair which may be matted over the affected area. The problem may not become apparent for 2–3 days, until the abscess has developed. The abscess normally fills up with pus until it becomes a tense, fluid-filled sac. At some point, the skin overlying the abscess is likely to necrose, allowing it to rupture (Figure 28.1). Variable quantities of pus may then discharge spontaneously. Most abscesses present as prominent swellings that can either be easily seen or palpated, but bites on the legs usually produce a more diffuse cellulitis.

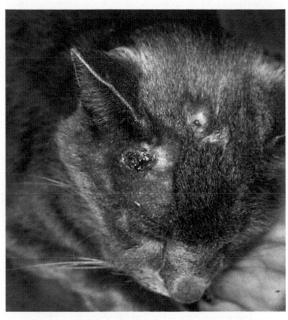

Figure 28.1 **Cat bite abscess on the head of a cat**

Specific diagnostic techniques

The affected area should be examined carefully for evidence of the original bite, such as small crusts, matted hairs, a draining tract or a distinct area of necrosis. The abscess should be palpated to determine if it has 'pointed' (feels fluid-filled). If a tuft of matted hair is found, it might be possible to remove it to expose a drainage hole.

Treatment

The aims of treatment are to provide drainage and treat the bacterial infection. If the abscess has pointed but hasn't already ruptured, it should be lanced. In most cases, this can be achieved without anaesthesia or sedation if the cat is adequately restrained and the procedure performed quickly. The abscess should be immobilised, gently squeezed and a No. 11 blade rapidly inserted into a dependent area. The abscess should be gently massaged until all the pus has been expressed. If the abscess is acutely painful, or the cat very difficult to restrain, the above procedure may need to be carried out under sedation or general anaesthesia but this can be more stressful to the cat than dealing with the problem as an out-patient. As long as adequate drainage has been obtained, there is no need to flush out the interior of the abscess with antiseptic solutions. If the abscess is already draining when it is presented,

100 Top Consultations in Small Animal General Practice, First Edition
By Peter Hill, Sheena Warman and Geoff Shawcross
© 2011 Blackwell Publishing Ltd

the remaining pus should be expressed manually. If the abscess hasn't pointed, and it appears more as a diffuse swelling, lancing isn't necessary.

The cat should then be treated with a 3–5 day course of antibiotics, depending on severity. Suitable choices include ampicillin, amoxicillin, amoxicillin/clavulanic acid or cephalosporins. Long-acting injectable preparations of ampicillin or amoxicillin are just as appropriate as oral tablets. In some cases a single injection may be curative but a repeat dose can be given after 48 hours if necessary. For more severe infections, a single injection of cefovecin could be given if compliance with oral medication is likely to be poor. If deemed necessary, pain relief can be provided by NSAIDs. Castration of male cats may reduce their tendency to fight and develop cat bite abscesses.

What if it doesn't get better?

If the abscess fails to respond to treatment within 3–5 days, the following possibilities should be considered:

- The cat may have a defective immune system (FeLV / FIV infection, systemic illness)
- There might be a foreign body or nidus of infection
- The organism may be resistant to the chosen antibiotic
- There might be an unusual organism present (e.g. *Nocardia* spp., *Actinomyces* spp., mycobacteria, fungi, mycoplasma, *Rhodococcus* spp.).

Further workup and treatment at a second consultation should include:

- Cytology of the exudate to characterise the inflammatory response and organisms
- Culture and sensitivity testing of the organism
- Changing to a different antibiotic.

Blood tests for systemic illness, FeLV and FIV infection, and investigation for foreign bodies (diagnostic imaging or surgical exploration) should also be considered at the second or third consultation.

The low-cost option

The cheapest way to manage the problem is to avoid hospitalisation costs, and to use oral antibiotics such as ampicillin or amoxicillin.

When should I refer?

Referral should be considered when the abscess becomes a chronic draining tract or non-healing wound of unknown cause that hasn't resolved after two or three consultations.

Peter Hill

Aetiology and pathogenesis

Lipomas are very common subcutaneous masses in dogs, but are uncommon in cats. They are benign proliferations of lipocytes of unknown cause.

History and clinical signs

Most owners will notice a lipoma by feeling or seeing a mass, most often on the trunk or upper limbs. They are uncommon on the head or distal limbs due to the lack of fat in these areas. Lipomas are typically well-circumscribed, round or oval in shape, and not firmly attached to underlying tissues. They have a soft, 'springy' feel when palpated. They vary greatly in dimension, but most are between the size of a grape and a golf ball, although masses as large as footballs have been reported in neglected animals (Figure 29.1). Some lipomas are pedunculated, and others may occasionally infiltrate fascial planes.

Specific diagnostic techniques

The mass should be carefully palpated to determine its size, consistency and attachment to underlying tissues. It is important to remember that this examination is most useful in relation to the subsequent treatment of the mass, and does not reveal diagnostically accurate information. Other types of skin tumour can appear and feel identical to lipomas.

In order to confirm the diagnosis, the mass should be aspirated. The material obtained from a lipoma is relatively plentiful compared to other masses and appears as a clear, oily material (Figure 29.2). When placed in alcohol-based fixatives prior to staining, the oily material may dissolve, leaving nothing on the slide. To avoid this, the slide can be heated over a flame and then stained just with the red and blue dyes of the Diff-Quik. Some of the material will still dissolve, but there are usually foci of cells that remain which are sufficient for examination. Microscopically, lipomas consist of morphologically normal lipocytes, which appear as packets of cells with a 'soap bubble' appearance (Figure 29.3). A small nucleus can be seen at the periphery of the cell.

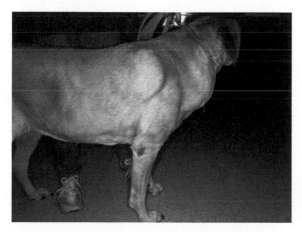

Figure 29.1 **Large lipoma on the side of a dog**

100 Top Consultations in Small Animal General Practice, First Edition
By Peter Hill, Sheena Warman and Geoff Shawcross
© 2011 Blackwell Publishing Ltd

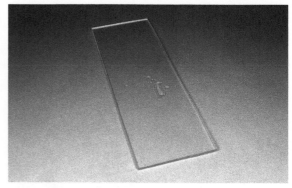

Figure 29.2 **Appearance of the oily material obtained when aspirating lipomas**

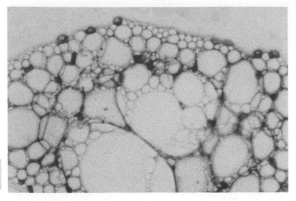

Figure 29.3 Cytological appearance of a lipoma

Treatment

Lipomas can either be surgically removed, or benignly neglected. The option chosen will be determined following discussion with the client. Factors which influence the decision include the size of the mass, its location and its potential for causing future problems should it grow. For example, small masses on the trunk can be safely left, whereas a dog with a larger mass in the axilla may benefit from early surgical resection.

What if it doesn't get better?

Lipomas will not resolve spontaneously so if the owner wants the mass to disappear, it will have to be surgically removed. Post-operative complications are extremely unlikely, but occasional problems can arise due to dead space or trauma to the wound. Lipomas can sometimes recur after resection, and dogs may subsequently develop new tumours at other sites.

The low-cost option

In many cases, it is not essential to remove the mass, eliminating the cost of an operation. If funds are severely limited, the clinician may have to make a clinical judgement of the mass without performing a fine needle aspirate. However, in such cases, the clinician must inform the client that the likelihood of the mass being a lipoma is based purely on probability, and that there is a possibility it could be something more sinister. It then becomes the client's choice not to investigate further, rather than the vet's recommendation.

When should I refer?

Lipomas can be dealt with in general practice and referral is not required.

Peter Hill

Aetiology and pathogenesis

Histiocytomas are benign skin tumours that are seen commonly in dogs but are very rare in cats. They derive from Langerhans cells in the epidermis and probably represent a form of hyperplasia rather than true neoplasia. Their cause is unknown.

History and clinical signs

Histiocytomas are seen most commonly in dogs under 3 years of age. They are usually solitary and rapidly growing. They appear as small (<3 cm), firm, dome-shaped nodules that are typically alopecic and may be ulcerated (Figure 30.1). Histiocytomas occur most frequently on the head, pinnae and limbs, but they can occur anywhere. Rarely, the draining lymph node may be palpably enlarged, but this does not represent malignant metastasis.

Specific diagnostic techniques

Careful palpation of the mass should reveal it to be situated within the dermis. As with any mass, a fine-needle aspirate should be performed to confirm the diagnosis and rule out more sinister causes such as mast cell tumour. Microscopically, histiocytomas consist of large mononuclear cells with the appearance of macrophages (Figure 30.2). Lymphocytes may also be present, and increase in number as the lesion ages. Neutrophils may be seen if the mass is ulcerated. Surgical excision for histopathological analysis is not required, although if performed, will yield a definitive diagnosis.

100 Top Consultations in Small Animal General Practice, First Edition
By Peter Hill, Sheena Warman and Geoff Shawcross
© 2011 Blackwell Publishing Ltd

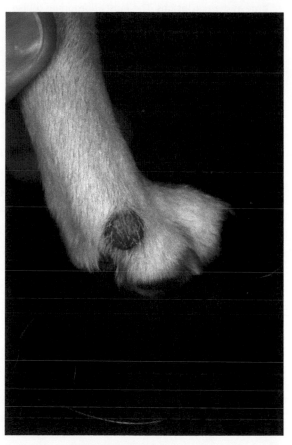

Figure 30.1   Histiocytoma on the leg of a dog

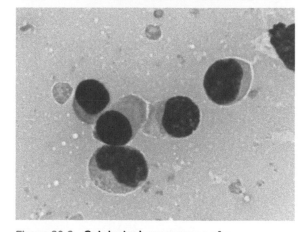

Figure 30.2   Cytological appearance of a histiocytoma

Treatment

The majority of histiocytomas undergo spontaneous resolution within 3 months. If there was an associated lymphadenopathy, this regresses at the same time as the skin lesions. The most appropriate course of action for confirmed cases is therefore observation without treatment. Surgical excision may be appropriate where self-trauma is occurring.

What if it doesn't get better?

Occasionally, histiocytomas do not regress within 3 months. In such cases, surgical excision and histopathological analysis is recommended. This would normally be curative.

The low-cost option

Costs can be minimised by recognising that the lesion is a histiocytoma, thereby avoiding the need for surgical excision and histopathological diagnosis. If the history and appearance is completely typical, some owners may decline fine-needle aspiration and choose to wait and see what happens. This is an appropriate approach as long as the case is carefully monitored and re-evaluated if the lesion has not regressed within 3 months.

When should I refer?

Routine histiocytomas can be dealt with in general practice and referral is not required.

Peter Hill

Aetiology and pathogenesis

Mast cell tumours are very common in dogs, and are occasionally seen in cats. They are caused by a neoplastic proliferation of dermal mast cells, but the precise trigger for their formation is unknown. A genetic tendency to develop mast cell tumours is suggested by strong breed predispositions (Boxers, Bulldogs, Boston Terriers, Staffordshire Bull Terriers, Rhodesian Ridgebacks, Pugs, Beagles, Weimaraners, Labrador Retrievers and Golden Retrievers).

History and clinical signs

Mast cell tumours have been reported in animals as young as four months of age, but they typically occur in older animals with a mean age at presentation of eight years. Their appearance can vary dramatically, depending on whether they are benign or malignant. Benign mast cell tumours are typically solitary lesions that present as a slowly growing cutaneous nodule (Figure 31.1). They may be firm or very soft, and some may become ulcerated. They can occur anywhere on the body. Occasionally, multiple mast cell tumours can be seen in the same patient. This usually represents simultaneous development of individual tumours, rather than systemic metastatic disease. Some mast cell tumours release histamine locally, causing oedema and fluctuations in their size and degree

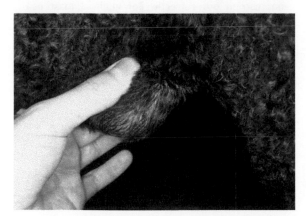

Figure 31.1 **Mast cell tumour in the skin of a dog**

100 Top Consultations in Small Animal General Practice, First Edition
By Peter Hill, Sheena Warman and Geoff Shawcross
© 2011 Blackwell Publishing Ltd

of redness. More aggressive mast cell tumours may grow rapidly and diffusely infiltrate surrounding tissues. Rarely, chronic release of histamine into the circulation may cause gastro-duodenal ulceration and clinical signs such as anorexia, vomiting, anaemia and melaena.

Specific diagnostic techniques

Suspected or confirmed mast cell tumours should be palpated with care in order to prevent degranulation and histamine release. If malignant, mast cell tumours usually metastasise via the lymphatics, so careful palpation of the draining lymph nodes is indicated.

As with any cutaneous mass, a fine needle aspirate should be performed before contemplating benign neglect or surgical excision. This is critical for mast cell tumours as a cytological diagnosis will inform the nature of the subsequent surgery. Mast cell tumours can be easily identified on Diff-Quik stained cytology and appear as a monomorphic population of large round cells with a central nucleus and cytoplasm that contains purple-staining granules (Figure 31.2). Eosinophils may also be seen, because they are attracted to sites of high mast cell density. If enlarged, the draining lymph node should also be aspirated.

Mast cell tumours submitted for histopathological analysis are usually graded as 1, 2 or 3, with grade 1 being a well-differentiated tumour, grade 2 being an intermediate stage, and grade 3 being a poorly differentiated tumour. In dogs, these categories correlate with prognosis after treatment, with typical survival times of 3–4 years being seen with grades 1 and 2, compared to less than a year with grade 3 mast cell tumours. In contrast, feline cutaneous mast cell tumours nearly always follow a benign course, regardless of their histological grade, and very rarely result in death of the cat.

The extent and prognosis of malignant mast cell disease (i.e. animals with a grade 3 tumour or involvement of the local lymph node) can be assessed by further staging. This involves performing radiography and ultrasonography of the chest and abdomen. Examination of bone marrow aspirates can also be performed, although infiltration of the bone marrow is a rare sequel to mast cell metastasis.

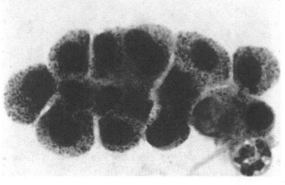

Figure 31.2 **Cytological appearance of a mast cell tumour. Note that the amount of granularity can vary considerably**

Treatment

The optimal treatment protocol and prognosis of mast cell tumours depends on the histological grade, size of the mass, anatomical site and stage of disease. After diagnosis by cytological examination, the first step is to determine what histopathological grade of tumour is present. For solitary cutaneous nodules in areas amenable to routine surgical resection, complete excision is the treatment of choice and allows the whole mass to be submitted for histopathological analysis. A 2-cm margin around the edge of the mass, and one fascial plane beneath it are now regarded as acceptable margins for the removal of mast cell tumours. For grade 1 or 2 masses, this treatment is very likely to be curative. If the mass is not amenable to easy surgical excision with appropriate margins due to its size or location, a biopsy should be obtained to allow histological grading.

Grade 3 tumours and grade 2 tumours that have not been completely removed will require adjunctive treatment to improve the prognosis. Potential options include radiation therapy, chemotherapy and subcutaneous injection of de-ionised water. Radiation therapy is considered most useful for solitary mast cell tumours that cannot be completely excised due to their anatomical location (such as on a distal limb). Chemotherapy is only used for the management of mast cell tumours that have already metastasised, or when dealing with grade 3 tumours. In this context it can be used as an adjunct to surgery, or as a sole treatment if the mass is non-resectable. There are no optimised chemotherapeutic regimes for the management of mast cell tumours, but prednisolone, vincristine, vinblastine, lomustine, tyrosine kinase inhibitors or combinations of these have all been used with some success. Clinicians unfamiliar with protocols involving these drugs should seek advice from a specialist oncologist. Injection of deionised water into the tumour site following removal of mast cell tumours has been reported to destroy residual tumour cells and reduce the rate of recurrence, but this is regarded by oncologists as a controversial treatment due to lack of definitive evidence for its efficacy.

What if it doesn't get better?

Most grade 1 and 2 mast cell tumours can be cured by performing complete resections on the first occasion. Problems arise when skin tumours are removed without having previously performed a fine needle aspirate, and thus not allowing the adequate margins of excision required for mast cell tumours. The prognosis will be greatly reduced if the first operation is not carried out correctly. For grade 3 mast cell tumours, the prognosis is inherently worse, and owners must be warned that remission following surgery, with or without adjunctive treatment, may only be temporary.

The low-cost option

The lowest cost option following diagnosis by cytological examination is benign neglect, without surgical resection or histological grading. Some grade 1 tumours may remain in situ for years without growing or metastasising and when finances are severely limited, or in a very elderly dog, some owners may choose this course of action. However, this approach carries considerable risk because the biological behaviour of the tumour cannot be predicted based on its cytological appearance, so owners have to accept the risk that the tumour may grow or metastasise and result in death of the dog.

To prevent escalating costs, mast cell tumours should be removed completely on the first occasion using the principles outlined above. If this is not done, further surgery or referral to an oncologist may be subsequently required. If radiation treatment or chemotherapy is not an option, the cheapest post-surgical adjunctive treatment when clean margins have not been obtained is to inject deionised water into the tumour site. Advice should be obtained from an oncologist before performing this procedure.

When should I refer?

Removal of mast cell tumours from areas where there is plenty of surrounding skin can be easily achieved in general practice. If a mast cell tumour is detected on a distal limb, or other area where adequate surgical margins are difficult to obtain, referral to a specialist surgeon or oncologist may be advisable. Following histological analysis, grade 3 tumours, or incompletely removed grade 2 tumours, would benefit from referral to an oncologist who could advise on the suitability of the patient for radiation treatment or chemotherapy.

Peter Hill

Aetiology and pathogenesis

Sebaceous adenomas are benign skin tumours that are seen commonly in dogs but rarely in cats. They derive from sebaceous gland cells and sometimes represent a form of hyperplasia rather than true neoplasia. Many clinicians refer to sebaceous adenomas as warts, but this is not an appropriate term because warts are viral-induced papillomas and are uncommon in dogs. Follicular cysts (sometimes called epidermal inclusion cysts) are common in dogs but rare in cats. They are epithelium-lined swellings that contain keratin and lipids. They probably derive from hair follicles that have sealed over for unknown reasons.

History and clinical signs

Sebaceous adenomas and follicular cysts are seen most commonly in middle- to old-aged dogs. Both can be solitary or multi-focal and are usually noticed by owners whilst the dog is being stroked or groomed. Sebaceous adenomas are most common in Poodles, Cocker Spaniels, Beagles, Dachshunds and Miniature Schnauzers. They have a characteristic appearance and can usually be recognised grossly. They appear as small (usually less than 1 cm), cauliflower-like masses which project above the skin surface (Figure 32.1). Sometimes they have a morphological appearance that resembles a tiny brain or walnut. Sebaceous adenomas occur most frequently on the trunk and limbs, but they can occur anywhere. In most cases, they are asymptomatic but some dogs find them irritating, especially if they are on the distal limbs.

Follicular cysts are dermal in location and appear as well-circumscribed, palpable nodules that range in size from 0.5–5 cm in diameter (Figure 32.2). Some follicular cysts are 'open' and have a tiny pore through which a caseous, grey, yellow or brownish 'toothpaste'-like material may be discharged. Follicular cysts may rupture and discharge their contents into the dermis, resulting in a foreign body reaction and secondary infection. The lesions

may then become painful and cause irritation. They are most common on the head, neck and trunk. Occasionally they may occur in the interdigital region, but they are not the usual cause of the lesions frequently referred to as 'interdigital cysts'. The latter lesions are normally pyogranulomas caused by foreign bodies, deep infections or traumatically implanted hair shafts.

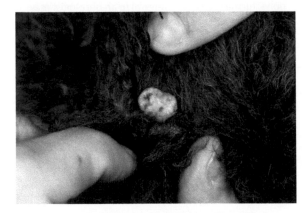

Figure 32.1 **Sebaceous adenoma on the skin of a dog**

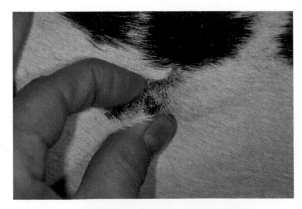

Figure 32.2 **Follicular cyst on a dog, draining a thick, caseous, blood-tinged material**

100 Top Consultations in Small Animal General Practice, First Edition
By Peter Hill, Sheena Warman and Geoff Shawcross
© 2011 Blackwell Publishing Ltd

Specific diagnostic techniques

Sebaceous adenomas and 'open' follicular cysts are rare examples of skin masses that can be diagnosed on gross appearance alone, as long as they appear as described above. It is tempting to squeeze follicular cysts that have a pore, but although this helps to confirm the diagnosis, it should be done very gently to avoid rupturing the wall and spilling the contents into the dermis. In cases where there is some doubt (i.e. unusual appearance of mass or a follicular cyst that has no pore), a fine needle aspirate can be performed. Microscopically, sebaceous adenomas appear as clumps of large, mononuclear cells that contain large numbers of lipid vacuoles surrounding a central nucleus (Figure 32.3). Follicular cysts contain non-nucleated keratinocytes embedded in a proteinaceous and lipid background (Figure 32.4). Surgical excision for histopathological analysis is not required, although if performed, will yield a definitive diagnosis.

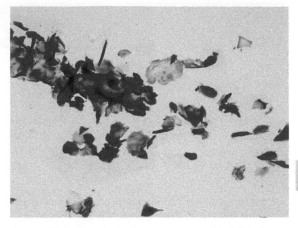

Figure 32.4 **Cytological appearance of a follicular cyst**

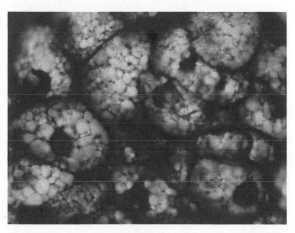

Figure 32.3 **Cytological appearance of a sebaceous adenoma**

Treatment

The treatment of choice for both sebaceous adenomas and follicular cysts is either surgical excision or observation without treatment. Masses that are causing irritation are best removed.

What if it doesn't get better?

Sebaceous adenomas and follicular cysts will not resolve spontaneously and will persist unless surgically removed. If the lesions appear to be enlarging, or multiple lesions are appearing, confirmation of the diagnosis by cytology and histopathology is indicated.

The low-cost option

Costs can be minimised by recognising that the lesion is a sebaceous adenoma or follicular cyst, thereby avoiding the need for surgical excision and histopathological diagnosis.

When should I refer?

Sebaceous adenomas and follicular cysts can be dealt with in general practice and referral is not required.

Peter Hill

The appearance caused by loss of hair is known as alopecia. It can range from partial, in which the hair density is merely reduced, to total, in which the area of affected skin is completely bald. Various mechanisms can cause alopecia:

- Self-trauma, most often due to pruritus (conditions causing this are covered in the Chapters 15 and 16 on itchy dogs and cats)
- Folliculitis, most often caused by bacteria, fungi or parasites
- Disruption of hair follicle cycling, resulting in most hairs being in the telogen phase, typically due to endocrine or metabolic diseases
- Anatomical abnormalities of the hair follicle, such as congenital alopecias or follicular dysplasias.

Common differential diagnoses

Spontaneous hair loss in dogs typically occurs in one of three patterns, which are significant because they influence the differential diagnosis:

1. A single patch of alopecia at a single site is most often caused by demodicosis, dermatophytosis, scars, subcutaneous steroid injections or topical application of medications (Figure 33.1).
2. Multi-focal alopecia (in which the coat appears 'moth-eaten' and the lesions appear as multiple, patchy, approximately circular areas of alopecia scattered over the body) is typically caused by demodicosis, dermatophytosis or staphylococcal folliculitis (Figure 33.2).
3. A symmetrical or diffuse pattern of alopecia may be caused by the generalised forms of demodicosis or dermatophytosis, but this pattern is also seen with endocrine diseases (hypothyroidism, hyperadrenocorticism, gonadal sex hormone alopecia, pituitary dwarfism, cyclic flank alopecia), follicular dysplasias (congenital alopecia, colour dilution alopecia, black hair follicular dysplasia,

breed-related follicular dysplasias, pattern baldness) and sebaceous adenitis (Figure 33.3).

Spontaneous hair loss in cats is rare and is not covered in this chapter. The most common reason for hair loss in cats is excessive licking, which is covered in Chapter 16.

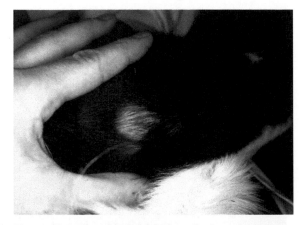

Figure 33.1 Focal patch of alopecia on a dog's face due to demodicosis

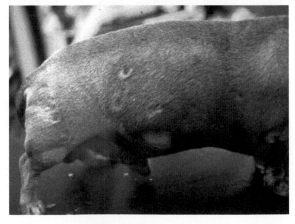

Figure 33.2 Multi-focal patches of circular alopecia in a dog with staphylococcal folliculitis

100 Top Consultations in Small Animal General Practice, First Edition
By Peter Hill, Sheena Warman and Geoff Shawcross
© 2011 Blackwell Publishing Ltd

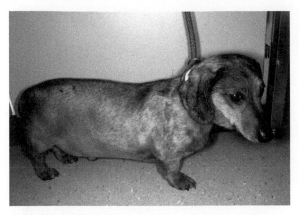

Figure 33.3 Symmetrical alopecia in a dog with hypothyroidism

Diagnostic approach

The first step is to determine if the hair loss is a clinically relevant problem. Some dogs are presented for excessive hair loss when in fact they are just shedding heavily. In these dogs, there will be no visible alopecia and although the hairs can be easily epilated by gentle pulling, continued removal will not leave a bald patch.

In dogs with alopecia, clinicians should first determine if the history and physical examination allow a diagnosis to be made by 'pattern recognition'. This may be possible with injection site reactions, sites of trauma or scars, sites of medication application, congenital alopecias, pituitary dwarfism, black hair follicular dysplasia, alopecia due to testicular tumours or cyclic flank alopecia. The latter condition is the only form of alopecia that appears and disappears in relation to the climatic seasons.

If a diagnosis is not immediately apparent, a careful examination of the skin and coat can provide clues to help prioritise the differential diagnoses. The hairs around the areas of alopecia should be carefully assessed to see if they are easily epilated (as in endocrine diseases) or if they are broken off at the skin surface (as in dermatophytosis). Comedones may be seen with demodicosis, hypothyroidism and hyperadrenocorticism. Follicular casts are a common feature of demodicosis and sebaceous adenitis. If hyperpigmentation is present, a diffuse blackening of the skin may suggest endocrine disease whereas a slate-grey pigmentation is more suggestive of demodicosis. The skin thickness should also be assessed because it can appear thin in hyperadrenocorticism or thicker at sites of pruritus or self-trauma.

Although these clues can be helpful, they will not provide a definitive diagnosis and further investigation of the cause will require diagnostic tests. The first step in all cases of canine alopecia is to rule out demodicosis by examining hair plucks (trichogram) or skin scrapings (see Chapter 18). Further tests for dermatophytosis should be performed if the history and skin lesions are consistent with this diagnosis (see Chapter 34). The multi-focal pattern of alopecia that can be seen with staphylococcal folliculitis can be diagnosed by assessing the response to appropriate antibiotic therapy (see Chapter 19).

To investigate endocrine diseases as a cause of symmetrical alopecia, clinicians should first rule out hypothyroidism and hyperadrenocorticism. There may be obvious clues from the history and physical examination that suggest one of these conditions (see Chapters 73 and 74). A routine haematology and biochemistry profile can also provide pointers towards one condition or the other. However, definitive diagnosis will require thyroid or adrenal function tests.

In cases of unexplained alopecia, referral to a dermatologist is likely to be the most cost-effective option. Skin biopsies and additional blood tests, such as sex hormone profiles, may be helpful in some cases, but correlation of the laboratory findings with the clinical picture is essential for making a diagnosis.

Treatment

The management of alopecia is entirely led by diagnosis. Non-specific attempts to stimulate hair growth with hormones or other treatments in the absence of a definitive diagnosis is never indicated.

What if it doesn't get better?

The prognosis for hair regrowth varies dramatically depending on the underlying cause. Conditions such as demodicosis, dermatophytosis, staphylococcal infections, hypothyroidism and hyperadrenocorticism should respond well to appropriate treatment. Reasons why they may not are given in the relevant chapters. Removal of neoplastic testicles will usually resolve gonadal sex hormone alopecia, as long as there are no functional metastases. However, in some conditions such as congenital alopecias and follicular dysplasias, there is little to no hope of hair regrowth.

When should I refer?

Referral should be offered if a definitive diagnosis cannot be reached within the practice. There are a number of causes of alopecia that are too rare to be covered in this chapter but will be familiar to veterinary dermatologists. Early referral may prevent unnecessary tests from being performed because dermatologists will be familiar with all the breed-related syndromes and may be able to make a diagnosis by 'pattern recognition'. Dermatologists will also be able to explain to the owner the various treatment options that are available for the less common entities.

The low-cost option

The main way to minimise costs is to establish a diagnosis as quickly as possible. Repeated visits, performance of unnecessary tests and prescription of trial therapies can all waste valuable resources. Clinicians must follow a thorough and logical approach when investigating alopecia and only perform tests to confirm or rule out differential diagnoses they are actively considering. Paradoxically, referral to a specialist may ultimately save the client money because an accurate diagnosis and prognosis is likely to be achieved in the shortest possible time with a minimum number of tests. The costs associated with treating alopecia will depend on the cause identified.

Peter Hill

Aetiology and pathogenesis

Dermatophytosis is a follicular, and rarely epidermal, skin disease caused by infection with fungi of the genera Microsporum or Trichophyton. Two species cause the vast majority of cases in dogs and cats: *Microsporum canis* and *Trichophyton mentagrophytes*. *Microsporum persicolor* (from voles) and *Trichophyton erinacei* (from hedgehogs) are also isolated occasionally. Dermatophytes are not part of the normal resident flora in cats and dogs, although they can occasionally be isolated from the coats of clinically normal animals. In such cases, spores have usually been picked up by the coat but have not caused an active infection.

Infection occurs when spores from an infected animal or from the environment (e.g. brushes, combs and bedding) gain access to the skin of a susceptible animal. Factors that make infection more likely include young age, no previous exposure, pre-existing skin damage, a compromised immune system (e.g. systemic disease, immunosuppressive drugs) and warm/humid climates. Once infection is established, the spores germinate and produce hyphae that invade the cuticle of the hair shaft causing weakening and breakage above the skin surface. Owners and veterinary staff should be warned that dermatophytosis is a zoonosis, with children and immunocompromised people being most at risk.

History and clinical signs

Most cases of dermatophytosis lead to alopecia with varying degrees of scaling and inflammation. Pruritus is variable and may or may not be present. Dermatophytosis may present as focal or multifocal patches of alopecia (Figure 34.1), a regional alopecia with marked scaling and a well-demarcated border (more likely with *Trichophyton* infections, Figure 34.2) or more diffuse, patchy alopecia with scaling (Figure 34.3).

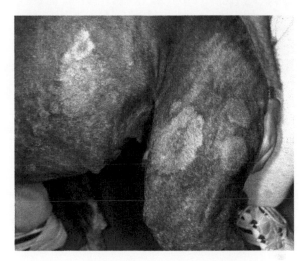

Figure 34.1 Multi-focal patches of circular alopecia in a dog with *Microsporum* dermatophytosis

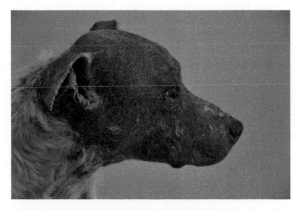

Figure 34.2 Complete alopecia affecting the head of a dog with *Trichophyton* dermatophytosis

100 Top Consultations in Small Animal General Practice, First Edition
By Peter Hill, Sheena Warman and Geoff Shawcross
© 2011 Blackwell Publishing Ltd

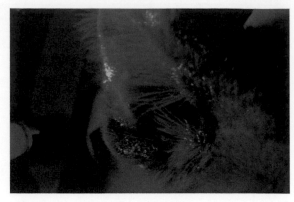

Figure 34.4 **Apple green fluorescence of hairs infected with *Microsporum canis***

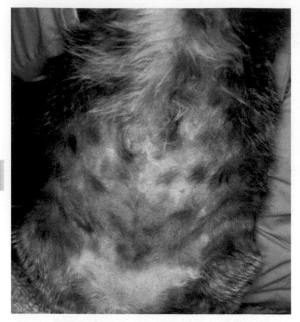

Figure 34.3 **Diffuse, patchy alopecia in a cat with** *Microsporum* dermatophytosis

Specific diagnostic techniques

Three diagnostic tests are useful in the diagnosis of dermatophytosis: Wood's lamp examination, microscopic examination of hairs, and fungal culture. Dermatophytosis can also be diagnosed on skin biopsy, but this procedure should not be necessary if the other techniques are carried out correctly.

The Wood's lamp is an ultraviolet lamp that can detect the fluorescence associated with the metabolites produced by some strains of *Microsporum canis*. It is not useful for detection of other species of dermatophytes. The lamp should be allowed to warm up for a few minutes before use to allow the UV emittance to stabilise. The entire coat of the animal should then be examined in a darkened room. A positive result is seen as an apple-green fluorescence of infected hair shafts (Figure 34.4). A blue–purple iridescence is often seen, associated with dust particles or fabric fibres. Some ointments can appear green under the Wood's lamp but they do not fluoresce. If a positive result is obtained, the finding should be confirmed by either direct microscopy or fungal culture. A negative Wood's lamp result does not rule out the possibility of dermatophytosis.

Hairs that fluoresce under the Wood's lamp, or broken, stubbly hairs from around the periphery of lesions, can be plucked, suspended in mineral oil or potassium hydroxide solution and examined directly under a microscope (a trichogram). Infected hairs are covered in spores (Figure 34.5). This technique requires some practice and, as with the Wood's lamp, a negative result does not rule out dermatophytosis.

A fungal culture is the only way to confirm the diagnosis if Wood's lamp and microscopic examinations are negative. If the latter tests are positive, fungal culture can still be helpful because it allows speciation of the dermatophytes involved. This can be helpful in determining the likely source of infection which may be of interest to certain clients. The most reliable method of collecting a sample is the 'toothbrush' technique. This involves brushing the hair coat and lesions for 1–2 minutes with a new toothbrush. This picks up fungal spores, even if the level of infection is fairly low. Plucking individual hairs is less sensitive because infected hairs might be missed. The bristles on the toothbrush are then used to inoculate the fungal culture medium. Some practices do this in-house using Dermatophyte Test Medium, a Sabouraud's-based medium that contains an antibiotic and a colour indicator. The colour indicator changes from orange to red if dermatophytes grow, but stays the same colour if saprophytic fungal contaminants are present. This test can be reliable in experienced hands, and it can save costs, but it is usually preferable to send the sample to a microbiology laboratory that has expertise in culturing and identifying fungi.

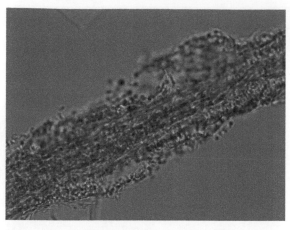

Figure 34.5 Infected hair covered in fungal spores

Treatment

Successful treatment of dermatophytosis is best achieved with a combination of systemic and topical therapy. For systemic therapy, itraconazole or griseofulvin are the treatments of choice. In the UK, itraconazole is the only drug licensed for use in cats. There are no licensed treatments for dermatophytosis in dogs. In cats, itraconazole is administered orally at a dose of 5 mg/kg every 24 hours on a one-week on, one-week off basis. Treatment should be given on weeks 1, 3 and 5 and not in weeks 2 and 4. In dogs, a similar protocol could be used, but continuous daily dosing has also been described. If itraconazole is not effective, or is poorly tolerated, griseofulvin can be used. It is administered orally at a dose of 25–50 mg/kg every 12 hours for at least 4 weeks, or until the lesions have completely resolved. The lower dose rate should be used initially and increased if there is not a satisfactory response after a few weeks. The absorption of griseofulvin is increased if it is given with a high fat meal (a teaspoon of vegetable oil can be added to the food). Griseofulvin is highly teratogenic and should not be handled by pregnant women. Glucocorticoids should not be used concurrently in any case of dermatophytosis as they will inhibit the body's ability to clear the infection and may lead to recurrence.

For topical therapy, a miconazole/chlorhexidine shampoo (Malaseb), enilconazole solution (Imaverol) or lime sulfur dips (LimePlus Dip) are appropriate choices. A once-weekly bath is usually sufficient. Clipping the hair coat removes infected hairs and reduces environmental contamination but does not hasten resolution and should be regarded as optional. The environment should be cleaned thoroughly by vacuuming and the dust bag destroyed by burning. Hard surfaces can be decontaminated with bleach.

What if it doesn't get better?

Clinicians should first ensure that the diagnosis has been definitively established. If it has, they should check that the owner has been administering the treatment properly and carrying out any other recommendations. Dermatophytosis may fail to resolve in animals with a defective immune system. Cats should be checked for FeLV and FIV infection, and other immunosuppressive diseases should be ruled out. In rare situations, the organism may be resistant to the treatments used, and alternative drugs or higher dosages may need to be tried.

The low-cost option

In otherwise healthy animals, dermatophytosis typically resolves spontaneously after 3–4 months. In situations where there are no other susceptible animals or people at risk, some clients may elect to decline treatment and wait for spontaneous recovery.

When should I refer?

The management of dermatophytosis is easily accomplished in general practice. Referral to a dermatologist may be considered in refractory cases, or when advice is required for more complex management scenarios such as cattery outbreaks.

Sharon Redrobe and Peter Hill

The approach to skin problems in animals such as small mammals and birds is essentially the same as it is in dogs and cats. However, unless the animal is particularly cherished, valuable or insured, owners may not be willing to spend as much money on tests and treatments as they would for dogs and cats. This limits the clinician's ability to diagnose and treat skin problems optimally.

Common skin diseases and symptoms in rabbits

Ectoparasites

- *Cheyletiella parasitovorax* – causes scaling and crusting over the dorsum with mild pruritus
- *Sarcoptes scabei/Notoedres cati* – cause pruritus
- *Psoroptes cuniculi* – causes irritation, inflammation and crusty exudate within the ears (Figure 35.1)
- Fleas – cause irritation and pruritus
- Maggots – cause fly strike, resulting in ulcers and tissue damage, usually around the perineum.

Skin infections

- Staphylococci – cause subcutaneous and mammary gland abscesses, necrotizing dermatitis, septicaemia. Outbreaks of exudative staphylococcal dermatitis can cause high morbidity and mortality in young rabbits
- *Pasteurella multocida* – can be involved in abscesses, cellulitis and limb dermatitis
- *Pseudomonas aeruginosa* – occurs secondarily to wetting, leading to a blue discolouration of the fur
- *Treponema cuniculi* – rabbit syphilis, causes crusting at mucocutaneous junctions
- Dermatophytosis – caused by *Trichophyton mentagrophytes*, *Microsporum canis* or *Microsporum gypseum*, resulting in alopecia and scaling
- Myxomatosis – caused by myxoma virus, resulting in swelling of the eyelids and genitalia
- Ulcerative pododermatitis – caused by poor flooring and inactivity, with secondary bacterial infection.

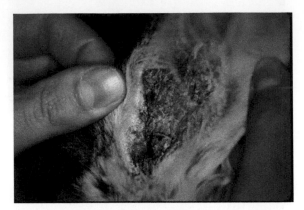

Figure 35.1   Thick, crusty exudate in a rabbit with psoroptic otitis

Other problems

- Urine scald – should be differentiated from dermatitis and eosinophilic granuloma
- Mammary tumours or cysts – should be differentiated from engorged mammary glands due to pseudopregnancy
- Dacryocystitis – caused by an infected or blocked nasolacrymal duct, resulting in facial scald and sometimes corneal oedema or ulceration. Often associated with dental disease
- Sebaceous adenitis.

Common skin diseases and symptoms in hamsters

- Abscesses – caused by bite wounds, trauma, tooth root infections
- Demodicosis – causes alopecia and scaling
- Epitheliotropic T cell lymphoma/mycosis fungoides – causes alopecia and scaling (Figure 35.2)
- Hyperadrenocorticism – causes symmetrical alopecia of the flanks and ventrum.

Common skin diseases and symptoms in Guinea pigs

Ectoparasites (often exacerbated by hypovitaminosis C)

- *Trixacarus caviae* – causes intense pruritus, self-trauma and occasionally seizures

100 Top Consultations in Small Animal General Practice, First Edition
By Peter Hill, Sheena Warman and Geoff Shawcross
© 2011 Blackwell Publishing Ltd

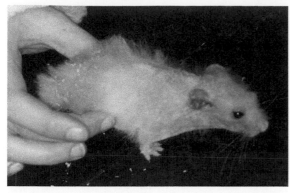

Figure 35.2   Epitheliotropic lymphoma in a hamster

- *Chirodiscoides caviae* – can cause pruritus and hair loss with heavy infestations in debilitated animals
- *Cheyletiella parasitovorax* – causes dorsal scaling in Guinea pigs living with infested rabbits.

Skin infections

- Abscesses – caused by fighting and trauma, with infection by staphylococci, streptococci, *Pseudomonas, Pasteurella, Corynebacterium*
- Cervical lymphadenitis/'lump disease' – caused by *Streptococcus zooepidemicus*.
- Pyoderma – caused by staphylococci and occasionally other bacteria
- Ulcerative pododermatitis/bumble foot – infection with *Staphylococcus aureus* due to various underlying factors such as obesity, poor hygiene, ageing, hypovitaminosis C or poor flooring
- Dermatophytosis – caused by *Trichophyton mentagrophytes*, resulting in alopecia and scaling.

Other problems

- Cystic ovaries (entire females) – cause symmetrical alopecia over the flanks and ventrum
- Hypovitaminosis C – causes a rough coat and scaling of the pinnae
- Fur chewing and barbering – occurs in groups of Guinea pigs.

Common skin diseases and symptoms in caged birds

Ectoparasites

- *Cnemidocoptes pilae* – causes scaling and crusting on the cere, beak and feet
- *Dermanyssus gallinae* – causes skin irritation
- Feather and quill mites – usually asymptomatic, but can cause self-mutilation with heavy infestations or in debilitated hosts.

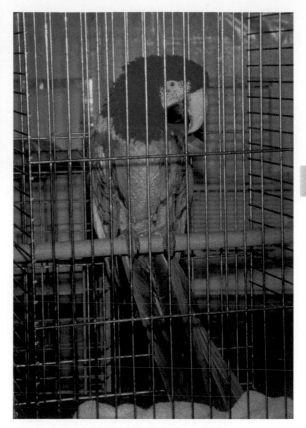

Figure 35.3   Feather plucking in a parrot

Skin infections

- Ulcerative pododermatitis/bumblefoot – infection with staphylococci or *E. coli* due to various underlying factors such as obesity, poor perch design (equal diameters or covered in sandpaper) or hypovitaminosis A
- *Aspergillus fumigatus* – causes fungal dermatitis in immunocompromised birds
- Psittacine beak and feather disease virus (PBFD) – may result in sudden death without feather changes or a chronic form with feather changes that is fatal in months/years. The chronic form can lead to dystrophic feathers, changes in feather colour, loss of powder down, deformed beak and nails
- Polyoma virus – causes dystrophic feathers and feather loss. A chronic form in budgerigars appears restricted to loss of flight feathers and some contour feathers.

Feather plucking

This is a multi-factorial problem with many causes, some of which are medical (including nutritional) and some which are behavioural (Figure 35.3).

- Medical causes
  - Poor feather quality – occurs due to poor diet, classically in seed-fixated parrots
  - Skin or feather mites leading to overpreening and feather chewing
  - Clipped or damaged feathers. The bird will become frustrated when trying to preen broken or damaged feathers, which may lead to chewing and self trauma or plucking of abnormal feathers, progressing to plucking of healthy feathers
  - Allergic skin disease
  - Respiratory disease- often the plucking starts over the back (lung areas) but can be anywhere on the body
  - Giardiasis
  - Liver disease, including Chlamydophila (psittacosis)
  - Poor air quality/pollution, due to aerosols, smoke, perfumes
  - Hypothyroidism
  - Polyomavirus
  - PBFD
  - Lead or zinc poisoning
  - Hypocalcaemia leading to poor or no featherdown, resulting in poor feather maintenance, frustrated preening, and chewing and plucking (it is important to measure ionised calcium, not just total calcium, in these patients)
  - Skin tumours
- Behavioural causes
  - Boredom or stress – wild parrots spend a lot of time searching for food and interacting with other birds. Cage-confined animals may begin to self-mutilate due to lack of normal lifestyle stimulation. A change in approach to care such as training, time out of the cage, or a more varied diet, is essential. If all other diseases have been excluded, then referral to a parrot behaviourist and/or trainer is required
  - Anxiety caused by separation from the owner
  - Sexual frustration, caused by the parrot bonding to the owner
  - Moving the cage to a different room
  - Inability to preen. Birds that were weaned away from adult birds at a very young age may not have developed good preening behaviour. Gentle misting will encourage preening, and allowing the bird to see other birds preen can be useful.

Other problems

- Hypovitaminosis A – causes hyperkeratosis of the skin and white plaques in the oral cavity.

General diagnostic approach to skin disease in non dog/cat species

In all skin conditions in non dog/cat species, it is important to consider the animal's husbandry and systemic health as possible contributing factors. The following are all important considerations to be explored in the history:

- Diet – An inappropriate diet can lead to clinically relevant vitamin deficiencies in many species. A poor diet can also lead to general ill-health which may predispose to other conditions such as ectoparasite proliferation and skin infections. Small mammals in particular need a good source of fibre to maintain gastro-intestinal and general health, and a deficiency can lead to barbering or other skin disorders
- Environment – An inappropriate environment can lead to many health problems, including cutaneous abnormalities. Poor flooring or perches can lead to pedal and foot problems in small mammals and birds. Lack of bedding and poor hygiene can increase the risk of skin infections. Abnormal temperatures or humidity may cause stress, or predispose to respiratory conditions, which can ultimately lead to the development of skin problems
- Social interactions – Overcrowding small mammals can lead to problems such as barbering or fighting. Bringing in new animals can introduce parasites or infectious diseases. In contrast, solitary confinement can be a problem, especially in social animals such as parrots. This can contribute to conditions such as feather plucking as mentioned above
- General health – Skin problems are common in sick animals, or those suffering from stress. It is important to consider the animal's age and other symptoms in addition to the skin signs. If systemic illness is considered a possibility (for example in feather-plucking birds), it is essential to investigate this first rather than attempting to treat the skin problem empirically. As in dogs and cats, blood profiles, radiographs and ultrasonography can be used to investigate the animal's organ function.

Following on from the above considerations, the possible role of parasites and infections should be explored, especially in small mammals, in which these conditions are common. These may be primary diseases, or secondary to some other debilitating condition. A good example is demodicosis in hamsters, which is often associated with systemic illnesses. Even parasites that would normally be considered as contagious may not cause any symptoms until the animal suffers some form of stress or other illness. This may occur with hypovitaminosis C, leading to clinical Trixacariasis in Guinea pigs. If suspected, parasites can be detected using the same techniques as used for dogs and cats, such as tape strips, skin scrapings and hair plucks. If bacterial or fungal infection is suspected, useful diagnostic tests include cytological examination and cultures. Culture samples need to be obtained with care in these species because open wounds are often contaminated with resident flora or environmental organisms. Sampling of primary lesions such as pustules or draining pus, and correlating the culture results with cytological findings, can help to maximise the diagnostic value of the technique. For abscesses, a sample of the wall is most valuable because the centre of the lesion is often sterile. Some infections require more specialised tests such as serology (*Aspergillus*, *Chlamydophila*) or PCR (PBFD, *Chlamydophila*).

Skin biopsies are rarely indicated in these species to establish a diagnosis. In most cases, careful attention to the above approaches will yield greater diagnostic success than skin biopsies. Biopsies are indicated for suspected neoplastic conditions (e.g. cutaneous lymphoma in hamsters) or endocrine disorders.

General therapeutic approach to skin disease in non dog/cat species

The following represent the most common treatment strategies for these species:

- Correction of inadequate husbandry
- Treatment of systemic illnesses
- Treatment of parasites – the most useful treatment is systemic ivermectin
- Treatment of infections – this can involve topical and systemic antimicrobial agents
- Surgical resection of tumours or abscesses.

For further details of these treatments, including drug formularies, see Chapters 93–6.

Placing a collar on a bird to prevent feather plucking should not be considered until a very through diagnostic work-up and investigation has excluded treatable disease, as there is a significant welfare problem associated with placing a collar on a bird.

What if it doesn't get better?

In most cases, failure to see an improvement following treatment would indicate that the original diagnosis was either incorrect, or associated with another problem that had not been identified. Some conditions carry an inherently poor prognosis. These include myxomatosis, ulcerative pododermatitis, cutaneous lymphoma, some abscesses, PBFD, conditions associated with old age or organ failure, and feather plucking, if a treatable cause cannot be identified.

The low-cost option

Most parasitic problems and skin infections can be treated at relatively low cost. If a more severe problem is present and finances do not allow further investigation, empirical treatment may have to be prescribed on the basis of a tentative diagnosis. When this is done, the welfare of the animal should be paramount. With severe symptoms, euthanasia should be considered if a prompt and satisfactory improvement is not seen.

When should I refer?

In many cases, referral of small mammals will not be an option. However, some owners might consider this if there were a specialist within an appropriate distance. Owners of birds (particularly valuable ones) are more likely to be keen on an early referral to a specialist. Referral should be considered if a diagnosis can't be made with the expertise and facilities available within the practice, or if the pet is not responding to treatment as expected. Any illness in these animals would benefit from being diagnosed and treated by a clinician with specific expertise and facilities for dealing with these species.

Section 4
Gastrointestinal problems

Norman Johnstone

Aetiology and pathogenesis

Dental problems may be congenital, such as abnormal bites, malocclusion and retained deciduous teeth, or acquired, such as calculus, gingivitis, periodontal disease, resorptive lesions, tooth root abscesses, dental attrition, and tooth fractures. Acquired dental disease becomes more common as animals age, and small breeds (<5 kg) and brachycephalic types suffer from more severe dental disease earlier in life than other breeds. Dental disease is very common in dogs and cats. Calculus, a form of mineralised plaque, affects 20–25% of dogs and cats seen in general practice, with 15–20% of those suffering from varying degrees of gingivitis (inflammation of the gums). Periodontal disease (a progression from simple gingivitis), is the most common infectious disease found in dogs and cats. It affects the attachments of the teeth to the mouth, resulting in progressive loosening of the teeth. If left untreated, the infection commonly spreads through the body via the bloodstream, the lymphatics or by being swallowed, resulting in sub-clinical organ damage or systemic illness.

Tooth trauma or caries can lead to damage to, and probably infection of, the pulp cavity. The pulp then undergoes inflammation and usually necrosis. If toxins and bacteria leak out from the root apex, tooth root abscesses or granulomas can form. This process can occur quickly over days or slowly over months.

Dental abrasion (abnormal wearing of the teeth) is usually caused by stone or ball chewing. Attrition is caused by abnormal contact between teeth. Tooth fractures are often caused by stone or bone chewing, but also occur with rawhide strips and hard nylon chews. Current thinking is that any object that cannot be pitted with a finger nail should not be recommended.

Tooth resorption is only seen *commonly* in cats, but can affect up to 75% of the population at some point in their lives. There is a complex classification system for these lesions based on severity and location of the defects. The severity is graded from Stage 1 (mild enamel loss), progressing through Stage 4 (extensive hard tissue loss with most of the tooth having lost its integrity) to Stage 5 (remnants of hard tissue completely covered by gingiva and only visible as irregular radiopacities on radiographs). Radiographically, the lesions are classified as Types 1, 2 and 3 (see below).

History and clinical signs

Despite the high prevalence of dental disease, dogs and cats rarely show overt signs of oral pain and owners rarely present their pets because of a concern with the mouth. Animals with dental disease may be asymptomatic, or they may show various presenting signs such as loss of appetite, anorexia, weight loss, depression, halitosis, dysphagia, excessive salivation, chattering jaws, difficulty in closing or opening the mouth, or facial swelling. Tooth root abscesses affecting the upper premolars or molars can result in a maxillary swelling and discharging sinus below the eye (Figure 36.1). This is known as a malar abscess. Canine tooth root abscesses can cause a unilateral nasal discharge, or discharging sinus high on the oral mucosa above the tooth.

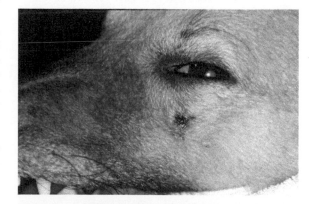

Figure 36.1 **Dog with sinus in the malar area**

100 Top Consultations in Small Animal General Practice, First Edition
By Peter Hill, Sheena Warman and Geoff Shawcross
© 2011 Blackwell Publishing Ltd

Specific diagnostic techniques

It is important that clinicians thoroughly examine the oral cavity whenever they perform a full clinical examination (to detect pathology that the owner may not be aware of) and also when an oral problem is suspected. Firstly, the outer surface of the head should be visually inspected and palpated for pain, sensitivity, heat, or swelling, along with the sub-mandibular lymph nodes. The lips should then be examined and retracted to reveal the inner surfaces of the lips, the buccal mucosa, the rostral surfaces of the incisors and the buccal surfaces of the canines, premolars and molars. The mouth should then be opened to allow examination of the floor of the mouth, the tongue, the inner aspects of the teeth and gingiva, the palate, the oropharynx and tonsils. Clinicians should check for changes in colour, inflammation, ulceration, hyperplasia, bleeding, unusual swellings, tumours and foreign bodies.

When specifically examining the teeth, clinicians should look for, and assess the severity of, calculus (Figure 36.2), gingivitis, periodontal disease (Figure 36.3), malocclusion (Figure 36.4), and, in cats, tooth resorption lesions (Figures 36.5 and 36.6). Other abnormalities that may be found include delayed eruption, persistent deciduous teeth, dental attrition, enamel abnormalities, root or furcation exposure, caries, 'missing teeth' and fractured teeth.

A more detailed oral examination (performed under sedation or general anaesthesia) may be necessary if an oral problem is detected, or if the animal is unwilling or unable to open its mouth. This allows periodontal and dental charting, assessment of sulcus depth and detection of infected periodontal pockets. Accurate diagnosis of periodontal disease requires subgingival probing for sulcus depth. Normal maximum sulcus depth findings are 3 mm for dogs and 1 mm for cats. Careful evaluation of the teeth may also reveal areas where caries or pulp exposure may be suspected (often seen initially as black spots on incisal edges or occlusal pits).

Dental radiography can be very valuable for determining the diagnosis, prognosis and treatment of many dental problems, including periodontal disease (Figure 36.7), endodontic disease and tooth resorption. Teeth surrounded by sulcus depths or pockets deeper than 4 mm should be radiographed to allow optimal assessment of severity. Accurate distinction between Types 1, 2 and 3 tooth resorption lesions in cats can only be made on the basis of dental radiographs:

- Type 1 – focal or multifocal radiolucency is present in the tooth with otherwise normal radiopacity and normal periodontal ligament space (Figure 36.8).
- Type 2 – narrowing or disappearance of the periodontal ligament space in at least some areas and decreased radiopacity of part of the tooth (Figure 36.9).
- Type 3 – features of both type 1 and type 2 are present in the same tooth.

Clearly, in order to offer a good standard of dentistry, practices should purchase an appropriate dental X-ray machine, and clinicians should master the techniques required to obtain good oral radiographs.

Routine blood tests are indicated in some animals with dental disease to investigate the possibility of concurrent systemic disease, and because many dental patients fall into high-risk categories for anaesthesia (e.g. geriatrics, breeds weighing less than 5 kg, animals with chronic periodontal disease, and those that are generally debilitated). Bacterial culture is rarely helpful for evaluating dental disease because there is a large and diverse oral flora in both healthy and diseased mouths. The exception to this rule is feline chronic gingivitis/stomatitis syndrome. This condition is complex and multifactorial in origin, but cultures from these cases typically reveal a pure culture of *Pasteurella multocida*. While this finding is significant for the patient, there are likely to be other aetiological factors present, such as feline calici virus, genetic and environmental influences.

If a mass if found in the mouth, biopsy is required for precise diagnosis.

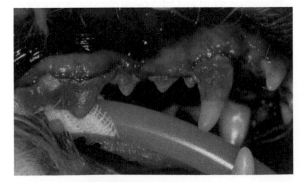

Figure 36.2 **Extensive accumulation of calculus and gingival inflammation**

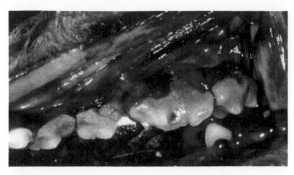

Figure 36.3 **Extensive periodontal disease, deep gingival cleft and fracture of main cusp**

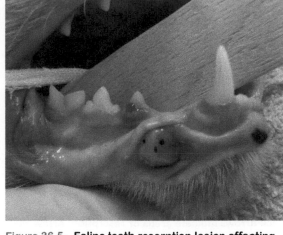

Figure 36.5 **Feline tooth resorption lesion affecting a lower premolar**

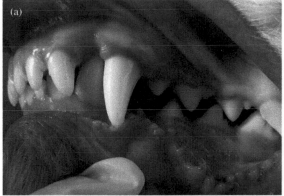

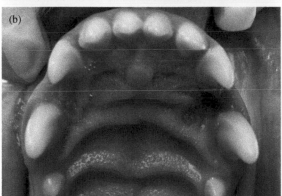

Figure 36.4 **(a) A 6-month-old Italian Spinone with severe mandibular brachygnathism (class 2 bite). Note occlusion of left lower permanent canine into hard palate. (b) Image of hard palate in same dog. Note infected pits from traumatic occlusion of lower canines**

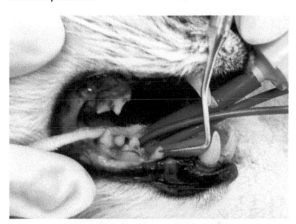

Figure 36.6 **Feline tooth resorption lesions affecting premolars and molars**

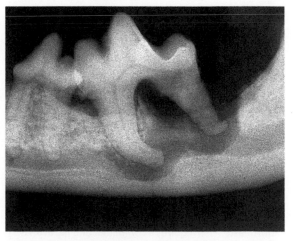

Figure 36.7 **Radiograph of tooth (left lower molar 1) with extensive attachment loss due to advanced periodontal disease**

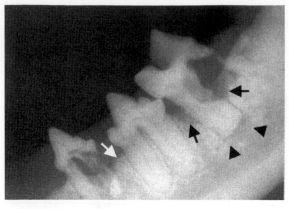

Figure 36.8   Radiograph of Type 1 resorptive lesion. Black arrows indicate areas of resorption. Arrow heads indicates lucent area at apex of root. White arrow indicates periodontal disease

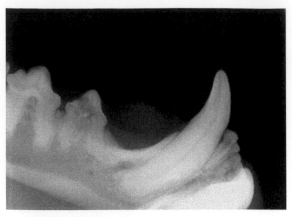

Figure 36.9   Radiograph of Type 2 resorptive lesion affecting lower premolar 3. Note complete replacement of root by bone

Treatment

Calculus, gingivitis and periodontal disease

The optimal time to intervene is when gingivitis is present, but before periodontal disease and attachment loss has commenced. At this stage, the gingival inflammation is reversible if scaling, polishing and daily homecare is performed. Once periodontal disease has developed, there will be ever-increasing loss of attachment of the teeth to underlying bone, which will ultimately result in tooth loss. If periodontal disease is present, treatment should be considered mandatory. The teeth should be scaled/polished and, if possible, radiographed to determine the optimal treatment plan and prognosis. Teeth that are loose, or have over 50% attachment loss, are best extracted. It is possible to salvage teeth with less than 50% attachment loss, but specialised techniques are required and referral to a veterinary dentist would be advised. Depending on the severity of the periodontal disease, systemic antibiotics may be required. In advanced cases, these should be started 5 days before the dental procedures take place; in less severe cases, a post-operative course may be sufficient. Clindamycin, metronidazole and doxycycline are considered to be the most effective. Long-term prophylaxis can only be achieved by recommending daily tooth brushing with veterinary toothpaste. This requires a committed and motivated owner, and a compliant pet. Teaching and encouraging tooth brushing is an important role for a veteri-

nary practice. Human toothpaste should never be used in animals because they contain detergents, foaming agents and fluoride, which is toxic when swallowed on a long-term basis (dogs and cats cannot spit and rinse). Many rinses, chews and other additives sold on the market as aids in the removal of dental plaque come with little or no meaningful science behind the claims made by the manufacturers. Care and due diligence is advised before recommending or selling these to clients.

Tooth root abscesses

These are treated by identifying the tooth involved, preferably by dental radiography. Surgical extraction of the affected tooth is curative, but root canal treatment can be performed in dogs and cats, particularly for canines and carnassials.

Worn or fractured teeth

If the pulp cavity is not exposed, attempts should be made to prevent continued trauma and the teeth should be monitored twice yearly. If the pulp cavity is exposed, pulpitis and pulp necrosis will follow. These teeth should either be extracted, or undergo root canal treatment to remove and replace the infected or necrotic pulp. No fractured tooth with pulp exposure should be left to 'see what happens.'

Tooth resorption in cats

Correct radiographic typing of these lesions is required to ensure optimal treatment, but all affected teeth will need to be removed. Teeth with Type 1 lesions still have organic components capable of inducing inflammation and necrosis. They need to be removed in a conventional manner, ensuring that all the roots are extracted. This extraction is often difficult due to the loss of integrity of the tooth structure, and a flap may need to be raised to allow complete removal. Teeth with Type 2 lesions no longer demonstrate a periodontal ligament or pulp and are integrating with the surrounding bone. Conventional extraction is not indicated for these lesions because the roots are ankylosing with bone and this doesn't act as a source of ongoing pain. A coronectomy (controlled crown removal via a small envelope flap) and intentional retention of roots is the accepted treatment for these lesions. Teeth classified as Type 3 require a combination of the treatments used for Type 1 and 2 lesions, such as conventional removal of one root and retention of the other.

Persistent deciduous teeth

Deciduous teeth should be removed if they are traumatising soft tissues, or if they persist after the permanent tooth has erupted. These teeth are fragile and have long roots, so extreme care is required in their removal. Usually a mucogingival flap is required for good access and to prevent damage to the successor permanent tooth.

Abnormal bite/malocclusion

The most common painful defect is an overshot bite (short mandible/normal maxilla), also known as mandibular distoclusion or brachygnathism. Often, the lower canine teeth occlude onto the hard palate, causing pain. Treatment should be performed as soon as possible. For deciduous teeth, surgical removal of the lower canine(s) is required. For permanent teeth, a range of options is available including surgical extraction, crown amputation coupled with pulp capping, or orthodontic tipping.

What if it doesn't get better?

Removal of calculus should result in an immediate resolution that the owner can see. Following extractions, or treatment for periodontal disease, the animal should show a marked improvement within a few days. If there is still evidence of oral pain, it is likely that diseased teeth may have been missed, or roots may have been left in situ. Dental charting helps identify areas of concern and dental radiography can be used to detect such problems.

The low-cost option

Dentistry in dogs and cats will always incur the cost of general anaesthesia. Other costs can be minimised by keeping dental procedures as simple as possible, such as extracting diseased teeth rather than attempting salvage procedures. Encouraging the owner to undertake regular daily tooth brushing at home may also extend the intervals between professional intervention.

When should I refer?

Basic dental procedures such as scaling and simple extractions are within the scope of general practice. Referral to a specialist veterinary dentist should be offered if advanced procedures are required such as root canal treatment or oral surgery. In addition, teeth affected by pathology such as root resorption can present a real challenge without radiographs and specialist equipment.

Geoff Shawcross

Retching and gagging are unproductive attempts to vomit (retching) or to clear the pharynx (gagging). They are common presenting signs and usually represent an important, and sometimes serious, underlying condition. It is usually easy to differentiate between retching and gagging from the clinical signs, or from the owner's description.

Common differential diagnoses

- Pharyngeal foreign body – usually grass seeds, needles, fishhooks or bones
- Pharyngeal wounds – usually caused by stick injuries or bones
- Pharyngeal tumours such as tonsillar tumours (e.g. melanoma, squamous cell carcinoma) or eustachian tube polyps (cat)
- Tonsillitis
- Lymph node enlargement – especially the retropharyngeal lymph nodes, associated with malignancy or abscessation
- Tracheal foreign body – may be inhaled, or aspirated material from the oesophagus
- Tracheal inflammation caused by infection (e.g. infectious tracheobronchitis) or parasitism (e.g. *Oslerus osleri*)
- Oesophageal disease – especially foreign bodies (usually irregular bones, and often stuck at the level of the base of the heart) or oesophagitis. Mega-oesophagus can sometimes cause retching and gagging but is more commonly associated with regurgitation.
- Vomiting on an empty stomach (see Chapter 38)
- Gastric dilatation and volvulus (GDV) – this represents a very serious cause of (usually) non-productive retching (see Chapter 44)
- Cardiac disease (dogs) – a severe coughing bout is often followed by retching a small amount of phlegm
- Breed-related malformations such as prolongation of the soft palate or fleshy enlargement of the fauces.

100 Top Consultations in Small Animal General Practice, First Edition
By Peter Hill, Sheena Warman and Geoff Shawcross
© 2011 Blackwell Publishing Ltd

Diagnostic approach

The rate of onset of signs and the demeanour of the animal are important factors when investigating these cases. The signs caused by foreign bodies are usually acute in onset and cause the animal considerable distress. Salivation (may be blood-stained) and pawing at the mouth is frequently seen when there is an oro-pharyngeal foreign body present. Animals are usually reluctant to eat, although they may try to drink. The initial, severe signs will often improve after 24 hours, so care should be taken when interpreting the response to any empirical treatment that may be given. The signs associated with tumours or congenital malformations generally have an insidious onset, which gets steadily worse as the pathology progresses; in such cases, the appetite usually remains good.

The head, throat and neck should be palpated for symmetry and evidence of pain. Particular attention should be paid to the lymph nodes in the region. The oral cavity should be examined but opening the mouth may be resented if it is painful. When there is a high index of suspicion of an oro-pharyngeal foreign body, examination of the area needs to be thorough and this requires good illumination and often a general anaesthetic. Even if the diagnosis can be made in the conscious patient, treatment to remove the foreign body usually requires general anaesthesia. The examination should include a search of the tonsillar crypts and behind the soft palate. Any pharyngeal wounds or sinus tracts should be carefully searched for foreign material. The base of the tongue should be examined for the presence of an abscess, which would suggest an embedded foreign body.

Radiography will usually demonstrate the presence and position of metallic objects, such as needles and fishhooks, but will not readily demonstrate grass seeds, wood or fish bones, which are common oro-pharyngeal foreign bodies. An ultrasound scan of the area may be able to demonstrate soft tissue enlargements, displacements and cavitations that would be suggestive of a migrating or embedded foreign body. Evaluation under anaesthesia will also demonstrate the presence of pharyngeal/laryngeal malformations and tumours.

When a pharyngeal lesion is not demonstrated, radiographs of the neck and thorax should be included, as these may reveal mega-oesophagus or an oesophageal obstruction/foreign body.

In the dog, gagging and retching are often associated with prolonged bouts of coughing which may be caused by respiratory tract disease or cardiac disease, typically congestive heart failure (CHF). Auscultation of the heart and lungs should readily identify a cardio-respiratory cause of the clinical signs. Thoracic radiographs, cardiac ultrasonography, and tracheal and oesophageal endoscopy may be required to reach a diagnosis.

Retching that is the result of persistent vomiting should be obvious from the history and the cause of the vomiting needs to be investigated (see Chapter 38). GDV is invariably associated with retching and readily identifiable from the clinical signs (for more information, see Chapter 44).

Treatment

Appropriate treatment can only follow a diagnosis. The majority of cases are associated with pharyngeal disease and will require evaluation under general anaesthesia so that the pharynx, trachea and oesophagus can be fully evaluated. General anaesthesia will also facilitate radiography and ultrasonography, if required. If a foreign body is removed, or there is a pharyngeal wound, a short course of a broad-spectrum antibiotic is appropriate, together with an anti-inflammatory drug to control pharyngeal oedema.

In dogs in which acute tracheobronchitis is suspected, antibiotics may help speed up resolution of clinical signs (see Chapter 54). Where chronic coughing is the cause of the retching, suitable treatment should be instituted for cardiac or respiratory disease as appropriate (see Chapter 53). Equally, where the signs are associated with persistent attempts to vomit, suitable measures should be taken to investigate the cause of the vomiting (see Chapter 38).

What if it doesn't get better?

Signs associated with a foreign body should resolve quickly after its removal. Most complications arise where there has been a severe stick injury, a migrating grass-seed foreign body or an oesophageal foreign body. Stick injuries and retropharyngeal abscesses can be difficult to manage and may require extensive surgery. An oesophageal foreign body may result in necrosis at the site of impaction some days after an apparently successful removal, leading to catastrophic pneumothorax and respiratory distress. Respiratory tract infection and CHF should respond to appropriate treatment.

The low-cost option

When the index of suspicion is high for an oro-pharyngeal foreign body, tumour or malformation, a thorough examination under general anaesthesia will result in an accurate diagnosis, prognosis, and treatment protocol, without wasting resources on empirical treatment. When appropriate (based on history and physical examination findings), trial medication for respiratory tract infection or CHF can be instigated without recourse to extensive investigations. Similarly, where vomiting is the cause of the signs it may be appropriate to control the underlying symptoms with anti-emetics.

When should I refer?

Referral should be offered when a diagnosis cannot be made with the equipment and expertise available within the practice. Referral should also be offered for complex procedures such as removal of oesophageal foreign bodies (thoracotomy may on occasion be required following failed attempts at endoscopic or fluoroscopic removal). The anatomy of the pharynx and neck is complex and surgery in this area is best performed by an appropriately experienced surgeon. Other cases may warrant referral for specialist medical management, e.g. chemotherapy.

Sheena Warman

Vomiting is a common presenting sign in small animal practice. It is important to differentiate vomiting (forceful expulsion of material from the stomach and/or small intestine) from regurgitation (expulsion of material from the pharynx or oesophagus) as this will affect the diagnostic approach and treatment. Unlike vomiting, regurgitation is a relatively passive action, does not involve signs of nausea or retching, and there should be no bile in the material produced. In some patients, it is difficult to distinguish between the two. In many circumstances vomiting is a protective mechanism for the gastrointestinal tract, but it can also be a sign of serious systemic disease.

Common differential diagnoses

- Gastrointestinal disease – dietary indiscretion, obstruction, inflammatory disease (e.g. acute gastroenteritis, or more chronically as a manifestation of inflammatory bowel disease), infectious disease such as parasitism, parvovirus or *Giardia* (often associated with diarrhoea), ulceration, neoplasia
- Extra-gastrointestinal abdominal disease – pancreatitis, hepatic disease, renal failure, pyometra, peritonitis, prostatitis
- Metabolic/endocrine disorders – feline hyperthyroidism, hypercalcaemia, hypoadrenocorticism, diabetic ketoacidosis
- Drugs/toxins
- Motion sickness
- CNS disease – vestibular disease, brain tumour.

Diagnostic approach

An initial aim is to establish whether the vomiting is likely to be caused by gastrointestinal or systemic disease. A full history should be obtained to establish, in particular, whether the dog is truly vomiting, how often, for how long it has been happening, and whether there is any pattern (for example, in relation to feeding). Further information should be sought regarding the appearance of the vomitus, whether there has been any associated diarrhoea or weight loss, and whether there have been any other recent signs, such as changes in thirst, appetite, or demeanour. Some vomiting pets will drink more than normal to replace lost fluids, whilst others will not drink at all and be more at risk of becoming dehydrated. Polydipsia prior to onset of vomiting suggests systemic disease, such as diabetes mellitus, renal failure, pyometra, or hypercalcaemia (see Chapter 6). The owner should also be asked about any dietary changes or indiscretions such as stone-chewing or scavenging behaviour, or any access to medications or toxins. Blood in vomitus can appear fresh or semi-digested ('coffee grounds', Figure 38.1). If the owner reports acute non-productive retching, gastric dilation and volvulus should be considered (Chapter 44).

A thorough physical examination should be performed, with particular attention paid to abdominal palpation. It is important to note that gastric foreign bodies and some intestinal foreign bodies will not be palpable. Linear foreign bodies can be particularly challenging to diagnose. The mouth should be examined carefully for foreign objects such as thread which can become hooked around the base of the tongue, particularly in young cats. Abdominal palpation under sedation or anaesthesia is rewarding in some cases. The patient should be carefully examined for any signs of systemic disease, e.g. pyometra (entire bitches), uraemic ulcers, goitre (cats), or prostatitis (entire male dogs).

Acute vomiting and diarrhoea in dogs is often associated with dietary indiscretion, but other causes such as foreign bodies or pancreatitis should be considered. Foreign bodies are less common in cats but

100 Top Consultations in Small Animal General Practice, First Edition
By Peter Hill, Sheena Warman and Geoff Shawcross
© 2011 Blackwell Publishing Ltd

can still occur. Persistent vomiting in older pets is more likely to reflect serious underlying disease.

The need for further investigation will depend on the individual case. Cases of motion sickness, intoxication, or vestibular disease will usually be identified with a thorough history and physical examination. In other cases the approach will vary depending on the severity and chronicity of the vomiting, and any associated signs.

Mild, acute vomiting

If the patient is otherwise well, and foreign body ingestion considered unlikely, symptomatic treatment and re-examination in 2–3 days (or before if patient deteriorates) is appropriate.

Severe, acute vomiting

The initial aim in these cases is to establish whether the vomiting is due to gastrointestinal or non-gastrointestinal disease, and whether medical or surgical management (to treat e.g. intestinal foreign body) is appropriate. Haematology, biochemistry (including urea, creatinine, liver enzymes, bilirubin, albumin, globulin, glucose, sodium, potassium, chloride, calcium ± amylase and lipase) ± urinalysis should be performed to investigate non-gastrointestinal causes and to help assess the severity of any dehydration or electrolyte changes that can occur as a consequence of vomiting. Rectal palpation of the prostate should be performed in entire male dogs. Abdominal radiographs (right lateral and ventrodorsal views) should be obtained to help identify foreign bodies or other causes of intestinal obstruction which may require surgical intervention; the presence of a 'gravel sign' (a collection of small mineral densities in an area of the intestines due to accumulation of ingesta) and distended loops of small intestine are highly suggestive of obstruction. If there is uncertainty regarding the presence of an intestinal obstruction, a barium study can be performed. Abdominal ultrasound can help diagnose pyometra (Chapter 70), peritonitis, and pancreatitis (Chapter 43). Assessment of serum levels of species-specific pancreatic lipase immunoreactivity (PLI) is useful if pancreatitis is suspected (Chapter 43). If haematemesis is a consistent feature, investigations should consider the likelihood of gastrointestinal ulceration (particularly due to NSAIDs), neoplasia, or a bleeding disorder. Endoscopy is useful to identify (and often remove) gastric foreign bodies, and to identify and biopsy mucosal lesions in the stomach and duodenum.

Chronic or recurring vomiting

Haematology, biochemistry and urinalysis should be performed as above, and abdominal imaging performed (radiography ± ultrasound). It is appropriate to perform a bile-acid-stimulation test to assess liver function, and an ACTH-stimulation test (dogs) to exclude atypical hypoadrenocorticism, as these diseases may not be detected on routine biochemistry. In cats, FeLV/FIV testing and thyroxine (T4) assay should be performed. If non-gastrointestinal causes have been excluded, in many chronic or recurring cases it is appropriate to institute a strict dietary exclusion trial with a novel protein and carbohydrate source prior to invasive procedures. Although serology is available for the diagnosis of dietary allergies, the significance and interpretation of the results is controversial and there is no effective substitute for a strict dietary trial. Further investigation of gastrointestinal causes of vomiting usually requires endoscopy or laparotomy for collection of multiple biopsies.

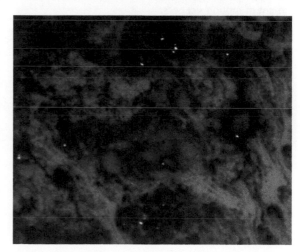

Figure 38.1 Coffee grounds in the vomitus of a dog (photo courtesy of Ed Hall)

Treatment

Symptomatic treatment of **mild, acute vomiting** consists of a short (24-hour) period of starvation, followed by introduction of small quantities of a highly digestible, low-fat diet. The animal should be encouraged to drink little and often; oral electrolyte solutions are often palatable and can be offered in addition to plain water. Anti-emetics (maropitant or metoclopramide) can be given if gastrointestinal obstruction has been excluded. Patients should be re-examined within 2–3 days if there is no improvement, or before if they deteriorate. Anti-parasitic treatment should be considered, particularly in puppies and kittens; if vomiting is persistent then oral dosing may be problematic and an alternative preparation required. Antibiotics are not indicated for the routine treatment of acute gastroenteritis.

Patients with **severe, acute vomiting** may be benefit from intravenous fluid therapy to correct dehydration and any associated electrolyte abnormalities, whilst further investigations are undertaken. If haematemesis is a feature, gastroprotectants (sucralfate and omeprazole or an H_2-blocker such as cimetidine) should be provided.

Treatment of **chronic or recurrent vomiting** depends on identification of the underlying cause. Maropitant tablets are licensed in dogs for the treatment of motion sickness.

What if it doesn't get better?

If there is no response to initial therapy, or if problems recur, then the patient should be re-evaluated and further investigations performed as outlined above.

The low-cost option

Managing cases as out-patients whenever possible will help to minimise costs. However, the importance of re-assessment if there is no improvement must be emphasised to the owner. In acute, severe cases abdominal radiography should be a priority to help rule out a disorder requiring urgent surgical intervention. In chronic cases, priority should be given to performing blood tests for biochemistry (and T4 in cats) to rule out common systemic causes of vomiting. Investigations can be performed in a step-wise approach; it is important not to overlook the possibility of non-gastrointestinal causes of vomiting. Treatment trials with anti-parasitic drugs or exclusion diets can be considered prior to further, more expensive, investigations; however the owner should be warned that parasites and food allergies are relatively uncommon causes of vomiting and that further investigations are likely to be required.

When should I refer?

Referral should be considered if a diagnosis is not established following tests which can be performed within the practice, or if there is an inadequate response to treatment for the suspected disease. Endoscopy is best performed by an experienced endoscopist in order that both the stomach and duodenum are thoroughly examined and biopsies obtained from both. Obtaining biopsies by endoscopy is less risky for the patient than exploratory laparotomy, and referral for endoscopy should be discussed with owners if facilities or expertise are not available within the practice.

Sheena Warman

Diarrhoea means the passage of faeces containing excessive water, which results in increased frequency, volume, and/or fluidity of the faeces. It can be caused by gastrointestinal or non-gastrointestinal disease and is a common presenting sign in small animal practice, particularly in dogs. Most cases of diarrhoea are of primarily small or large intestinal origin. Small intestinal (SI) diarrhoea results in only a slight increase in frequency of defaecation, with increased volume and no mucus or tenesmus. Melaena (partially digested blood) may be a feature. Chronic SI diarrhoea will result in weight loss and sometimes polyphagia. Vomiting is more commonly associated with SI diarrhoea than with large intestinal diarrhoea. Large intestinal diarrhoea often causes marked increase in the frequency of defaecation, with small volumes produced at a time. Haematochezia (unaltered blood), mucus and tenesmus are often features of large intestinal diarrhoea, whereas weight loss or polyphagia would not be expected.

This chapter will concentrate on SI diarrhoea; large intestinal diarrhoea (colitis) in dogs is discussed in Chapter 41.

Common differential diagnoses

Acute small intestinal diarrhoea

- Dietary factors – dietary indiscretion, intolerance or allergy
- Infectious disease – roundworms, viral infections (parvovirus, coronavirus), bacterial infections (*Campylobacter, Salmonella, Clostridia*), protozoal disease (*Giardia*)
- Intestinal tract disease – haemorrhagic gastroenteritis (see Chapter 40), partial obstruction (intussusception, foreign body), inflammatory bowel disease, hepatic disease, pancreatitis (although more commonly causes vomiting and large intestinal diarrhoea)
- Metabolic/endocrine diseases – acute renal failure, hypoadrenocorticism
- Drug administration/toxin ingestion.

100 Top Consultations in Small Animal General Practice, First Edition
By Peter Hill, Sheena Warman and Geoff Shawcross
© 2011 Blackwell Publishing Ltd

Chronic small intestinal diarrhoea

- Dietary – intolerance or allergy
- Infectious disease – roundworms, protozoal infections (*Giardia*; *Tritrichomonas* in cats usually causes large intestinal diarrhoea), diseases associated with FIV, FeLV or FIP infection in cats
- Intestinal tract disease – inflammatory bowel disease, antibiotic-responsive enteropathy, chronic intussusception, lymphangiectasia, exocrine pancreatic insufficiency, hepatic disease, neoplasia (lymphoma, adenocarcinoma)
- Metabolic/endocrine – hypoadrenocorticism, hyperthyroidism (cat).

Diagnostic approach

A full history should be obtained, paying particular attention to dietary history, the appearance of the faeces, identification of diarrhoea as of small or large intestinal (or mixed) origin, and any associated vomiting, inappetence or weight loss. A complete physical examination should be performed, including assessment of general demeanour, body condition score, hydration status, and thorough abdominal palpation.

Acute SI diarrhoea

Most cases of acute diarrhoea in patients that are otherwise well are due to dietary indiscretions. They respond to symptomatic management and do not require further investigation. However, if patients are systemically unwell, the diarrhoea is severe, there is evidence of melaena, or the problem is recurrent, then further investigations are warranted.

In severe acute cases, infectious causes are more common. Enteric pathogens can be detected in a number of ways including culture, parasitological tests, ELISA or PCR. The latter technique can now be used to isolate multiple infectious agents from a faecal sample (e.g. *Giardia, Cryptosporidium, Salmonella, Clostridium perfringens* enterotoxin A gene, enteric coronavirus, plus for dogs, parvovirus and distemper, and for cats, *Tritrichomonas foetus*, *Toxoplasma,* and panleukopenia). Faecal ELISA is available for parvovirus testing in dogs. Note that *Campylobacter* can be isolated from the faeces of many asymptomatic dogs, so the clinical significance is not always certain; however, in a symptomatic dog it is usual to provide specific treatment if *Campylobacter* is isolated (see below). Faecal analysis is not a particularly sensitive test for *Giardia*, so a PCR test or a therapeutic trial with a 3–5 day course of fenbendazole at 50 mg/kg is often justified. Haematology, biochemistry (to include urea, creatinine, albumin, globulin, liver enzymes, glucose, sodium, potassium, calcium and cholesterol) and urinalysis should be performed to investigate extra-intestinal causes and assess the degree of dehydration. An abdominal radiograph should be obtained to investigate any evidence of partial obstruction which may require surgery. Further investigation of suspected pancreatitis is discussed in Chapter 43.

Chronic SI diarrhoea

Similarly, in chronic cases of SI diarrhoea, faecal culture, parasitology or a PCR panel should be performed (if not already done). At this stage, in many cases, it is also appropriate to institute dietary trials with an exclusion diet, and to consider a treatment trial with a 2–3 week course of oxytetracycline or metronidazole in case of antibiotic-responsive diarrhoea.

If there is no improvement, the problem recurs, or the patient is systemically unwell, haematology, biochemistry and urinalysis should be performed to exclude non-gastrointestinal causes. In cats, FIV and FeLV testing and T4 assays should be performed, and in dogs a bile acid stimulation test and ACTH stimulation test should be considered to exclude hepatic dysfunction and hypoadrenocorticism (not all cases have abnormal electrolyte concentrations). If chronic pancreatitis is suspected, PLI should be performed (see Chapter 43). Trypsin-like immunoreactivity (TLI) should be tested to rule out pancreatic insufficiency. Measurement of serum folate and cobalamin concentrations can be helpful but is not essential; elevated folate and low cobalamin suggests bacterial overgrowth; low folate suggests proximal SI disease, and low cobalamin suggests severe distal SI disease. Although serological assays are available to investigate cases of food allergy, studies have shown that results of these do not correlate with results of dietary trials, and their use is not recommended.

Depending on the clinician's index of suspicion, radiography may be performed before or after the blood tests. An abdominal radiograph should be obtained to rule out a partial obstruction; a contrast study with barium-impregnated-polyspheres may be useful if there is any uncertainty. Abdominal ultrasound performed by a competent clinician can help identify extra-intestinal causes of diarrhoea and can be used to assess intestinal wall thickness, mesenteric lymph nodes, and to help identify focal lesions. If melaena is a feature, consideration should be given to causes of upper gastrointestinal bleeding (ulceration or neoplasia) or bleeding disorders.

If an answer is not derived from the previous tests, further investigation of chronic diarrhoea requires endoscopy or exploratory laparotomy to obtain multiple small intestinal biopsies. Endoscopy is best performed by clinicians who have received specialist training in the use of the equipment and in biopsy acquisition.

Treatment

Symptomatic treatment of *mild, acute SI diarrhoea* consists of a short (no more than 24-hour) period of starvation, followed by introduction of small quantities of a highly digestible, low-fat diet. Antibiotics are not indicated in these cases. Products are available which contain probiotics, prebiotics, kaolin and pectin; these are widely used although there is limited published evidence regarding their efficacy. Anti-spasmodics such as butylscopolamine are useful if there is abdominal discomfort, although more serious causes of diarrhoea such as obstruction should be considered in these cases. Patients should be re-examined within 2–3 days if there is no improvement. Anti-parasitic treatment should be considered, particularly in puppies and kittens.

Severe, acute cases may require intravenous fluid therapy to treat dehydration. If melaena is a feature, gastroprotectants (sucralfate and omeprazole or an H_2-blocker such as cimetidine) should be provided. Further treatment will depend on the underlying cause of the diarrhoea. *Campylobacter* infection in symptomatic animals should be treated with enteric-coated erythromycin tablets, and owners should be warned of the zoonotic potential and advised to maintain good hygiene. Dogs with parvovirus infection often require intensive treatment with intravenous fluids (sometimes including colloids and/or blood products), intravenous antibiotics to reduce the risk of bacterial translocation if haemorrhage is present, anti-emetics, gastroprotectants, and adequate nutritional support. Recombinant feline interferon-omega has been shown to reduce mortality in dogs with parvovirus. Cases with infectious disease should be barrier nursed. Hypoglycaemia can occur quickly in puppies and kittens with diarrhoea and should be treated with oral and intravenous glucose supplementation.

In cases with *chronic or recurring SI diarrhoea*, in which dietary and parasitic causes have been excluded, treatment will depend on identification of the underlying disease.

What if it doesn't get better?

As many cases of diarrhoea are not life-threatening, most clinicians adopt a step-by-step approach to investigation and treatment, as outlined above. Although this is a medically prudent and cost-effective approach, it does mean that some cases will persist after an initial treatment has been recommended. Owners should be warned about this possibility in advance so that they know further investigations may be necessary. Such cases will not resolve completely until an accurate diagnosis has been made and appropriate treatment instigated.

The low-cost option

The step-by-step approach outlined above inherently keeps cost to a minimum, rather than recommending that all the tests are performed at the same time. Acute, mild cases should be managed inexpensively as out-patients with simple advice regarding dietary management. However, dehydrated and systemically unwell animals will inevitably incur costs associated with intravenous fluid therapy and supportive care. In chronic cases, sequential dietary trials and treatment trials with anti-parasitic drugs or antibiotics such as oxytetracycline or metronidazole can be cost-effective, and in many cases will result in resolution of signs without the need for expensive investigations. As mentioned earlier, owners should be warned that further investigations may be necessary, and these will incur additional costs.

When should I refer?

Referral should be discussed if a patient has chronic or recurrent diarrhoea that does not respond to treatment as outlined above, or if a diagnosis cannot be achieved using the facilities available. Obtaining biopsies by endoscopy is less risky for the patient than exploratory laparotomy, and referral for endoscopy should be discussed with owners if facilities or expertise are not available within the practice. Focal or sub-mucosal lesions can be missed by endoscopy; however, thorough investigations prior to endoscopy will usually identify patients in which exploratory laparotomy is likely to be of more benefit. Endoscopy is best performed by an experienced endoscopist in order that as much of the intestines as possible is thoroughly examined and biopsies obtained from multiple sites.

Sheena Warman

Aetiology and pathogenesis

Haemorrhagic gastroenteritis (HGE) describes a specific syndrome seen most commonly in small-breed, middle-aged dogs, although it can affect dogs of any age or breed. The precise aetiology is unknown, but it may represent a Type I hypersensitivity reaction or could be a consequence of enterotoxin production by *Clostridium perfringens*.

History and clinical signs

Affected dogs present with acute, profuse, haemorrhagic diarrhoea with large quantities of fresh blood and sometimes sloughed intestinal mucosa in the faeces. Additional clinical signs include depression, vomiting, haematemesis and abdominal pain. Pyrexia is uncommon, and some patients are hypothermic. In severe cases, blood and fluid loss into the small intestine can be dramatic, with patients presenting with signs of hypovolaemic shock and/or dehydration. Sepsis is possible due to translocation of bacteria across the intestinal wall, resulting in clinical signs of tachycardia, pale mucous membranes, slow CRT and a weak pulse.

Important differential diagnoses

The most important differential diagnosis for this condition is parvovirus infection, and patients should be barrier-nursed until parvovirus is confirmed or excluded. Other differential diagnoses include:

* Salmonellosis
* Intussusception
* Intestinal tumours
* Dietary indiscretion
* Administration of cytotoxic drugs
* Coagulopathy.

100 Top Consultations in Small Animal General Practice, First Edition
By Peter Hill, Sheena Warman and Geoff Shawcross
© 2011 Blackwell Publishing Ltd

Specific diagnostic techniques

A full history should be obtained, ensuring there has been no known dietary indiscretion, that vaccinations are up-to-date, and that there has been no known exposure to parvovirus-infected dogs. Physical examination should concentrate on assessing the degree of hypovolaemia (pulse rate and quality, mucous membrane colour) and dehydration (skin turgor, tackiness of mucous membranes). The abdomen should be thoroughly palpated (as far as possible in the presence of abdominal pain) and an estimation made of bladder size, to help with ongoing monitoring of urine output in a hypovolaemic patient.

Haematology should be performed. These patients are characteristically haemoconcentrated (PCV ≥ 55%, and often >65%) despite blood loss, due to fluid shifts into the small intestine. Total protein concentrations are usually normal. A presumptive diagnosis is usually made on typical history and clinical signs, in combination with the presence of haemoconcentration. White cell count is usually normal compared to the leukopenia which occurs in about 65% of dogs with parvovirus infection. Parvovirus testing should be performed as a priority, especially in young or unvaccinated animals. In-house 'snap' tests for faecal ELISA are considered reliable in acute cases. Alternatively, faecal samples can be submitted to external laboratories for ELISA or PCR analysis. Faecal cytology may demonstrate the presence of clostridial spores.

Measurement of total serum proteins or total solids can be used in conjunction with PCV to help guide fluid therapy. Total solids can be measured with a refractometer on the serum portion of a spun microhaematocrit blood sample, and in many cases further biochemistry analysis is not necessary. However, in moribund cases, further biochemistry should be performed to assess renal function, glucose, proteins and electrolytes.

Further investigations are not usually necessary. Radiographs may demonstrate intestinal ileus, and imaging can be used to rule out foreign bodies and intussusceptions.

Treatment

Barrier-nursing precautions should be put in place in case of parvovirus infection. Aggressive IV fluid therapy is required to replace the circulating blood volume and fluid losses. Lactated Ringer's solution is administered initially as shock boluses of 20–30 ml/kg (to a maximum total dose of 90 ml/kg in the first hour), until cardiovascular parameters are normal, then continued at 2–4 ml/kg per hour. Monitoring of PCV and total solids helps guide fluid therapy. If total solids drop precipitously (<35–40 g/l), colloidal therapy may be required. Supplementation with potassium chloride in maintenance fluids is recommended once the patient has been treated for hypovolaemia and dehydration. Ideally, serum potassium should be monitored and supplemented according to standard guidelines. Broad-spectrum IV antibiotics (e.g. amoxicillin/clavulanic acid) are usually given to reduce the risk of sepsis secondary to bacterial translocation. In severely affected animals, urine output and renal parameters should be monitored to detect acute renal failure secondary to hypovolaemia. Antiemetics may be required if vomiting is persistent. Oral feeding should be initiated as soon as vomiting is controlled and the patient will eat, with frequent small meals of a highly digestible, low-fat diet. Owners can be advised that the prognosis is usually good and that full recovery can be expected in most cases (although relapses may occur).

What if it doesn't get better?

Most patients with HGE improve dramatically within a few hours of starting fluid therapy, and most make a full recovery within 2–4 days. If there is no improvement, the differential diagnoses should be reconsidered. A test for parvovirus should be performed if not already done. Diagnostic imaging should be performed along with bacterial culture for faecal pathogens. If the symptoms are still unexplained, endoscopy or exploratory laparotomy may have to be considered to look for neoplasia.

The low-cost option

The diagnosis of HGE is based on clinical presentation and simple laboratory tests, and is relatively inexpensive. However, treatment invariably requires hospitalisation, aggressive fluid therapy and appropriate nursing care, which is associated with significant expense. It is not appropriate to manage cases of HGE as out-patients because of the high morbidity and risk of mortality.

When should I refer?

It would be unusual to need to consider referral for these cases, as treatment should be within the scope of any small animal practice. However, if the patient does not respond to treatment, or relapses are frequent, then there may be an additional ongoing disease process and referral for further investigations should be discussed.

Sheena Warman

Aetiology and pathogenesis

Colitis is the term used to describe inflammation of the colon, resulting in clinical signs of large intestinal diarrhoea. Acute colitis is common in dogs but uncommon in cats. Dietary causes (indiscretion or hypersensitivity) are usually self-limiting. Infectious causes (e.g. *Salmonella, Campylobacter, Clostridium perfringens, Giardia, Cryptosporidium*) usually require specific treatment, although spontaneous recovery can occur in some cases. Chronic colitis is less common. It can be caused by dietary hypersensitivity, infections (*Giardia*, hookworms, *Tritrichomonas* in cats) or inflammatory bowel disease (lymphoplasmacytic or eosinophilic). Histiocytic ulcerative colitis in young Boxers (and occasionally other breeds) is now thought to be due to intracellular infection with attaching and invading *E. coli*. Physical obstruction due to intussusceptions, foreign bodies or tumours can occasionally cause colitis. Pancreatitis can be associated with signs of colitis, due to the physical proximity of the inflamed pancreas to the colon.

History and clinical signs

Clinical signs of colitis include increased frequency of defaecation, often with only small quantities produced each time. Mucus and fresh blood (haematochezia) are frequently present, and urgency followed by tenesmus is common (Figure 41.1). In patients with acute colitis, there may be a history of dietary indiscretion. Patients are usually bright, alert and systemically well, with a normal appetite. Cases with chronic colitis often have intermittent recurring signs.

Important differential diagnoses

Acute colitis

- Colo-rectal obstruction – foreign body, intussusception
- Rectal tumour

- Haemorrhagic gastroenteritis
- Perianal disease, including anal sac disease.

Chronic colitis

- Neoplasia – lymphoma, adenocarcinoma
- Functional disorder – 'irritable bowel syndrome'.

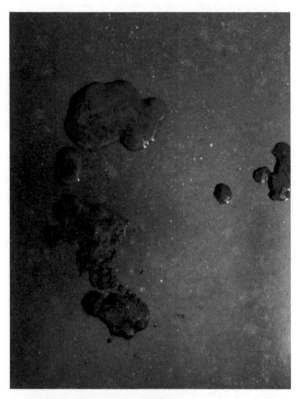

Figure 41.1 Haemorrhagic diarrhoea in a dog with colitis (photo courtesy of Ed Hall)

100 Top Consultations in Small Animal General Practice, First Edition
By Peter Hill, Sheena Warman and Geoff Shawcross
© 2011 Blackwell Publishing Ltd

Specific diagnostic techniques

Acute colitis is characterised by the recent onset of clinical signs of large intestinal diarrhoea. There may be a history of dietary indiscretion. Physical examination should be thorough to exclude the uncommon possibility of colo-rectal obstruction causing large intestinal diarrhoea, and must include digital rectal palpation, although this may be painful. Infected anal sacs can cause tenesmus and blood on faeces. Dogs with acute colitis are usually systemically well, unlike patients with haemorrhagic forms of gastroenteritis (e.g. parvovirus; haemorrhagic gastroenteritis).

In patients with *chronic or recurring colitis*, a full history should also be obtained, paying particular attention to any association with diet. A full physical examination and rectal palpation should be performed. The peri-anal region should be examined as chronic colitis can occur in association with peri-anal fistulae. Further investigation should include faecal culture, parasitology and/or a PCR diarrhoea panel (typically containing *Giardia*, *Cryptosporidium*, *Salmonella*, *Clostridium perfringens* enterotoxin A gene, and enteric coronavirus, plus for dogs, parvovirus and distemper; and for cats, *Tritrichomonas foetus*, *Toxoplasma* and panleukopenia). Trial treatment with fenbendazole can be considered in case of occult giardiasis, and strict dietary trials with a high-fibre diet, preferably using a novel protein and carbohydrate source. If there is no improvement, haematology, biochemistry, abdominal radiographs and endoscopic examination with biopsies are indicated. In cats, FeLV and FIV testing should be performed.

Treatment

Most cases of *acute colitis* are self-limiting and respond to symptomatic management with a short (12–24 hour) period of starvation followed by introduction of a bland, fibre-supplemented diet. Fibre can be supplemented using ispaghula granules or powder. If fresh blood is a feature, many clinicians will choose to treat with a short course of broad-spectrum antibiotics (e.g. amoxicillin/clavulanic acid) or metronidazole due to the increased risk of bacterial translocation. If there is no improvement, faecal analysis and a treatment trial with fenbendazole (for occult giardiasis) is indicated. Specific bacterial infections usually require antibiotic treatment if the patient is symptomatic. *Campylobacter* is treated with enteric-coated preparations of erythromycin. The zoonotic implications should also be discussed and effective hygiene emphasised. Metronidazole or ampicillin is usually effective against *Clostridium* spp. infection.

In many cases of *chronic colitis*, dietary manipulation with highly digestible, good-quality diets can result in improvements in faecal quality. Some patients will benefit from commercially available high-fibre diets, while others will respond to prescription hydrolysed hypoallergenic diets, or exclusion diets containing a novel protein and carbohydrate source. Infectious causes of chronic colitis should be treated with antiparasitic or antibacterial therapy as outlined above. *Tritrichomonas foetus* most commonly affects young cats and kittens from rescue centres or multi-cat households. Most cases are self-limiting but take an average of 9 months to resolve, so many owners will opt to treat. Unfortunately, the only effective treatment currently available is ronidazole, which is not licensed for cats; specialist advice should therefore be sought.

Cases diagnosed with lymphoplasmacytic colitis should also have dietary trials with hypoallergenic and high-fibre diets, before resorting to immunosuppressive drugs. Metronidazole is often useful both for its antibacterial and immunomodulatory properties. In refractory cases, treatment with prednisolone or sulfasalazine may be necessary. If sulfasalazine is used, the owner should be aware of the risk of development of keratoconjunctivitis sicca (KCS). Eosinophilic colitis usually responds to hypoallergenic diets but may require additional use of immunosuppressants. Histiocytic ulcerative colitis in Boxers usually responds to treatment with fluoroquinolones.

What if it doesn't get better?

Acute colitis usually responds to symptomatic treatment within 48 hours. If there is no improvement, faecal analysis and additional treatment should be considered as outlined above. If the patient is systemically unwell, simple acute colitis is unlikely and further investigations (including abdominal radiographs) should be undertaken.

Cases with chronic or recurrent colitis should be investigated and treated as outlined above. Exclusion of infectious disease and strict dietary management will result in good control in many cases, and efforts should be made to ensure good owner and patient compliance with treatment regimes. If there is no response to appropriate management, other differentials such as neoplasia should be considered and investigated, especially in older animals that have previously been well.

When should I refer?

Referral should be considered if there is inadequate response to treatment or the diagnosis remains uncertain following investigations performed in the practice. In chronic cases which do not respond to dietary manipulation or treatment of infectious disease, further investigation including biopsies is indicated. Endoscopic biopsies are preferred over full-thickness biopsies obtained during exploratory surgery as these are less risky for the patient. Referral should be recommended if facilities and expertise are not available to undertake this procedure within the practice.

The low-cost option

Treatment of acute colitis is inexpensive. If finances are limited, dietary changes followed, if necessary, by empirical treatment with antiparasitic drugs is appropriate. Antibacterial therapy should ideally be restricted to patients in which an infectious process has been confirmed on faecal analysis. However, in some cases (particularly those in which fresh blood is present) empirical treatment will be necessary and ampicillin or metronidazole would be appropriate choices. Antibiotics should not generally be used as first-line treatment for patients with non-specific colitis. Erythromycin is not licensed for dogs or cats and its use should be reserved for patients with confirmed *Campylobacter* infection.

In patients with chronic colitis, dietary trials and exclusion of infectious disease should be the priority prior to more expensive investigations. If owners decline further tests, empirical treatment with courses of metronidazole and/or sulfasalazine may help. Empirical treatment with prednisolone should only be undertaken as a last resort.

Sheena Warman

Aetiology and pathogenesis

Liver disease is relatively common in dogs and cats and can be caused by a range of primary and secondary disorders. It is a differential diagnosis for many non-specific clinical signs (see below). In some cases, liver disease is suspected following results of blood tests indicating elevations in liver enzymes and/or bile acids.

Common differential diagnoses

It is important to consider the common differential diagnoses for liver disease as outlined below, and in particular to be aware of the possibility of secondary hepatic involvement with a more significant disease in another organ.

Dogs

- Hepatitis
  - Drugs (e.g. phenobarbitone, NSAIDs, potentiated sulphonamides)
  - Toxins (e.g. mycotoxins, pesticides, heavy metals)
  - Infectious agents (e.g. leptospirosis, infectious canine hepatitis)
  - Breed-associated disorders (e.g. Bedlington Terrier, Cocker Spaniel, Doberman Pinscher)
  - Idiopathic (chronic active hepatitis), aetiology unknown, possibly immune-mediated.
- Nodular regeneration and cirrhosis – can result from chronic hepatitis
- Steroid-induced hepatopathy
- Congenital portovascular disorders (e.g. portosystemic shunt)
- Neoplasia (e.g. hepatocellular carcinoma, metastases)
- Hepatic nodular hyperplasia – a common, benign, incidental finding in older dogs
- Secondary hepatic disease (due to e.g. pancreatitis, sepsis, hyperadrenocorticism, diabetes mellitus).

Cats

- Suppurative (neutrophilic) cholangitis – probably due to ascending infection from the duodenum

- Lymphocytic cholangitis – possibly immune-mediated; often associated with pancreatitis and inflammatory bowel disease ('triaditis')
- FIP
- Hepatic lipidosis – primary, or secondary to any disease causing a period of anorexia, leading to massive fat deposition within the liver and cholestasis
- Acute toxic hepatopathy
- Congenital portosystemic shunt
- Neoplasia (e.g. biliary carcinoma or adenoma, metastases)
- Secondary hepatic disease (due to e.g. pancreatitis, hyperthyroidism, diabetes mellitus, sepsis, systemic infectious diseases).

Diagnostic approach

Historical and clinical features of liver disease can be vague, e.g. inappetence, lethargy, weight loss, vomiting and diarrhoea. More specific (but not pathognomonic) signs include jaundice, ascites, and polyuria/polydipsia. In severe cases there may be bleeding associated with coagulopathies, or neurological signs associated with hepatic encephalopathy. In animals with suspected liver disease, the owner should be questioned regarding any access to medications or toxins, vaccination history, concurrent diseases, and familial history. Thorough abdominal palpation is important to assess for hepatomegaly, discomfort, ascites or abnormalities in other organs.

In cats, the index of suspicion of the most common liver disorders is guided by the clinical presentation (Figure 42.1). Suppurative cholangitis usually occurs in middle-aged to older cats which present acutely ill with pyrexia, anorexia, jaundice and abdominal pain. Lymphocytic cholangitis usually occurs in younger cats which are often bright and eating well, but jaundiced. Clinical signs associated with hepatic lipidosis are initially vague, progressing to jaundice and encephalopathy.

Patients with portosystemic shunts usually exhibit poor growth, with a history of poor appetite and intermittent vomiting and diarrhoea. They may have signs of lower urinary tract disease due to the presence of ammonium urate uroliths. Cats sometimes

100 Top Consultations in Small Animal General Practice, First Edition
By Peter Hill, Sheena Warman and Geoff Shawcross
© 2011 Blackwell Publishing Ltd

have distinctive copper-coloured irises. Older patients presenting with signs of liver failure are more likely to have hepatic neoplasia or cirrhosis.

Haematology, biochemistry and urinalysis should be performed in all patients with suspected liver disease. Haematology may show non-specific changes such as a stress leukogram. In patients with chronic gastrointestinal blood loss or portosystemic shunts, microcytosis may be evident.

Biochemistry is central to the diagnosis of liver disease, and is used to assess hepatocellular damage, cholestasis and liver function. Liver enzyme elevations (ALT and AST) indicate hepatocellular damage. ALT is more liver-specific. Elevations of ALP and GGT indicate cholestasis. ALP can also be elevated following corticosteroid administration, with bone disease, or in young animals. GGT is particularly useful in cats as it tends to be elevated in cholangitis but not in hepatic lipidosis. It must be remembered that elevations in liver enzymes are common with many secondary hepatic disorders, and mild-to-moderate elevations may not always reflect primary hepatic disease. It should also be noted that hepatic nodular hyperplasia is often associated with mild-to-moderate elevations in ALP, although this is of no clinical significance. Markers of reduced hepatic function include hypoalbuminaemia, elevated bilirubin (see Chapter 9) and elevated bile acids; bilirubin and bile acids may also be elevated with cholestasis.

If liver disease is suspected following initial biochemistry tests, the most useful way of assessing hepatic function is to perform a bile acid stimulation test. This is performed by fasting the patient for 12 hours, taking a serum sample for fasted bile acid concentrations, feeding the patient a high-fat meal, then taking a second blood sample 2 hours later for postprandial bile acid concentrations. A concentration above 25 μmol/L indicates impaired liver function. Patients with portosystemic shunts usually have markedly elevated bile acids, normal or mildly elevated liver enzymes, and normal bilirubin. Urinalysis might show evidence of bilirubinuria or ammonium urate crystals.

Leptospirosis antibody titres should be measured if there is a possibility of this infection, e.g. in unvaccinated animals with acute onset of clinical signs.

It is important to consider the possibility of hepatic involvement and elevated liver parameters as a consequence of disease elsewhere. In patients with secondary hepatic disorders, signs of the primary disease usually predominate. However, these may be similar to signs which can be associated with liver disease, which can lead to confusion. Pancreatitis and endo-crine disorders (particularly diabetes mellitus, hyperadrenocorticism and hyperthyroidism) should be considered and investigated where appropriate clinical and laboratory abnormalities are detected (see relevant chapters).

Further investigations for hepatic disease can include radiology, ultrasound and biopsy. Radiology is useful to assess hepatic size and the presence of abdominal masses. If ascites is present, radiographs are of limited value. Ultrasound allows visualisation of the hepatic parenchyma and biliary tract, and can be used to confirm the presence of abdominal fluid. In experienced hands, it is very useful for identification of portosystemic shunts. Ultrasound alone can rarely be used to make a diagnosis of neoplasia within the liver as nodular lesions can represent benign nodular hyperplasia, abscesses, haematomas or neoplastic lesions. Also, a normal ultrasonographic appearance does not rule out hepatic disease. Biopsies are not usually performed in acute cases unless there is no improvement following initial management, but they can be used to achieve a definitive diagnosis in chronic cases. Biopsies can be obtained during exploratory laparotomy, via laparoscopy or with ultrasound guided Tru-cut needles (see below).

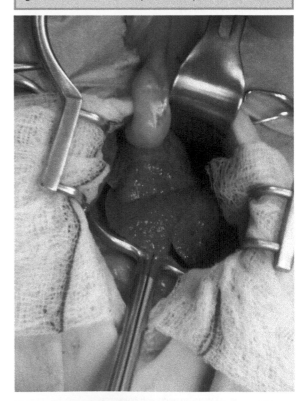

Figure 42.1 Liver of a cat with cholangiohepatitis (photo courtesy of Catherine Bovens)

Treatment

Initially, it is usually appropriate to provide supportive treatment to patients with liver disease. Intravenous fluid therapy may be required if the patient is dehydrated. Adequate nutrition should be provided and, although prescription hepatic diets are useful, it is more important that inappetent patients eat something than specifically insisting on a hepatic diet. In patients which have been inappetent for more than a few days, particularly cats, use of appetite stimulants and/or naso-oesophageal tube feeding may be required (see Chapter 4). Anti-emetics and analgesia should be provided if necessary. Dogs with suspected leptospirosis should be barrier-nursed and receive appropriate antibiotic therapy (e.g. amoxicillin/clavulanic acid).

Cats with suppurative cholangitis should receive broad-spectrum antibiotics (e.g. amoxicillin/clavulanic acid), ideally tailoring therapy on the basis of bile culture results (although gall bladder sampling would not be routinely performed in general practice). Lymphocytic cholangitis requires treatment with prednisolone, initially at an immunosuppressive dose, then tapering off over 6–12 weeks.

Anti-oxidants, which may reduce ongoing hepatic damage, can be provided in the form of S-adenosyl methionine (SAM-e). Ursodeoxycholic acid (UDCA) can be useful to improve biliary flow, but it should not be used in patients with complete biliary obstruction. These drugs may be beneficial in any form of hepatitis, including the two forms of cholangitis in cats.

The mainstay of treatment of hepatic lipidosis is aggressive nutritional support, usually requiring tube feeding. L-Carnitine, taurine, vitamin E, vitamin B1, vitamin K1, and vitamin B12 are sometimes supplemented, as early provision of these is thought to improve clinical outcome. Intensive monitoring of these cats is recommended, as complications such as gastric stasis, hepatic encephalopathy, hyperkalaemia and hypophosphataemia (causing haemolytic anaemia) can occur.

Patients with portosystemic shunts and hepatic encephalopathy can be managed surgically (shunt ligation) or medically. Medical treatment comprises a low-protein diet, lactulose (orally or as an enema in severely depressed patients), and amoxicillin or ampicillin.

What if it doesn't get better?

If there is no improvement following supportive treatment, the diagnosis of a primary liver problem should be reconsidered. Definitive treatment of liver disease depends on correct identification of the underlying disease process, followed by specific treatment when appropriate (particularly with infectious diseases). This may involve more specialised procedures such as ultrasonography or hepatic biopsy. If owners decline referral, then an educated 'guess' must be made as to the probable underlying disease, and treatment can be provided as outlined above. However, it is important that owners are aware that this may be suboptimal and, on occasion, even harmful to the patient.

Clotting times (PT and APTT) should be assessed prior to obtaining biopsy samples, and parenteral vitamin K supplementation provided for a few days if clotting times are prolonged. Small samples can be collected by fine needle aspiration, ideally with ultrasound guidance. Cytology can be useful to suggest hepatic lipidosis in cats, or detect neoplasia such as lymphoma or mast cell tumours, but it is of limited value in inflammatory hepatitis. It is usually preferable to obtain larger samples by 'Tru-cut' techniques or via laparoscopy/laparotomy.

Dogs with idiopathic chronic hepatitis can be treated with commercially available diets designed for dogs with liver disease, anti-oxidants such as SAM-e, bile acid modifiers such as UDCA, and anti-inflammatory doses of prednisolone. It should be noted that, apart from prednisolone, there is little published evidence of the efficacy of these treatments in dogs, although in theory they should be beneficial. If there is evidence of neutrophilic inflammation, particularly in the periportal areas, broad-spectrum antibiotics should be administered.

Some liver disorders such as neoplasia or cirrhosis inherently carry a poor prognosis.

The low-cost option

Financial limitations will sometimes prevent investigation of liver disease beyond initial laboratory work. In dogs, if inflammatory liver disease is considered likely, supportive care can be provided with dietary modifications, anti-oxidants and UDCA, if finances allow. Trial treatment with broad-spectrum antibiotics can be prescribed, but is rarely beneficial. In cats, assuming reasonable caloric intake, initial treatment with broad-spectrum antibiotics can be given. If there is no improvement after 4 weeks of antibiotics, consideration can be given to adding anti-inflammatory doses of prednisolone in case of lymphocytic cholangitis. Owners should be made aware of the potential risks associated with giving prednisolone, both in terms of side-effects and if there is undiagnosed infectious disease. Management of severe hepatic disease is expensive, and euthanasia may need to be considered in some cases.

When should I refer?

Many cases of liver disease may benefit from the expertise of a medicine specialist. Referral should be discussed if the facilities and expertise are not available to reach a definitive diagnosis, if advanced diagnostic evaluation is required (ultrasonography and/or Tru-cut biopsies), if intensive care facilities are not available for acutely ill patients, if treatment advice is required for chronic cases, or for confirmation and surgical management of a portosystemic shunt.

Sheena Warman

Aetiology and pathogenesis

Pancreatitis is a common problem in dogs, and is increasingly being recognised in cats. It is probably under-diagnosed because of the non-specific clinical signs and, until recently, the lack of reliable in-house tests. It can occur as an acute, chronic or relapsing problem in both species. The underlying cause is not known but in dogs, acute episodes are sometimes associated with ingestion of fatty food. In cats, it sometimes occurs as part of an inflammatory 'triaditis' (inflammatory bowel disease, cholangitis and pancreatitis), possibly due to the anatomical association between the cat's pancreatic and bile ducts.

History and clinical signs

Dogs with acute pancreatitis usually present with sudden onset vomiting and signs of cranial abdominal pain. Some dogs adopt a 'praying position', presumably due to abdominal discomfort (Figure 43.1). Some dogs have signs of large intestinal diarrhoea due to the anatomic proximity of the transverse colon to the inflamed pancreas. Jaundice may occur if pancreatic swelling is severe enough to cause obstruction of the bile duct. Severe pancreatitis can cause signs of dehydration, shock and rarely, disseminated intravascular coagulation (DIC). Dogs with chronic pancreatitis usually present with intermittent anorexia and lethargy, with or without vomiting or signs of abdominal discomfort.

Cats with severe (often acute) pancreatitis present with variable signs of lethargy, anorexia, dehydration and hypothermia. Only about 30% of patients vomit or show signs of abdominal pain. An abdominal mass can occasionally be palpated. Mild (often assumed to be chronic) pancreatitis in cats usually presents with vague, non-specific signs such as mild lethargy and/or inappetence. Jaundice will be noted if obstruction of the common bile duct has occurred due to pancreatic swelling or concurrent cholangitis.

Patients with chronic disease can have acute flare-ups. With severe or end-stage disease, additional problems such as diabetes mellitus or exocrine pancreatic insufficiency, occasionally occur.

Important differential diagnoses

Acute disease

- Gastrointestinal foreign body
- Acute gastroenteritis
- Gastric ulceration
- Acute hepatic disorders
- Pancreatic neoplasia.

Chronic disease

Any disease causing intermittent lethargy and inappetence such as chronic gastrointestinal disease (e.g. inflammatory bowel disease), chronic hepatic disease, hypoadrenocorticism or neoplastic diseases.

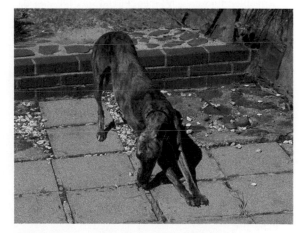

Figure 43.1 A whippet demonstrating the 'praying position' commonly associated with cranial abdominal pain such as that caused by pancreatitis

100 Top Consultations in Small Animal General Practice, First Edition
By Peter Hill, Sheena Warman and Geoff Shawcross
© 2011 Blackwell Publishing Ltd

Specific diagnostic techniques

Thorough abdominal palpation is important to check for cranial abdominal discomfort or abdominal masses. Haematology may show a neutrophilia and non-regenerative anaemia. Leukopenia can occur and has been associated with a poorer prognosis in cats.

Interpretation of biochemistry requires care, as pancreatitis can cause various abnormalities which may lead to a misdiagnosis. Pancreatitis often causes a mild to moderate elevation of hepatic enzymes, without there being significant hepatic disease. Cholestasis (characterised by elevated ALKP, bilirubin and bile acids) is common. Acute cases can have severe pre-renal azotaemia, hyperglycaemia (due to reduced insulin production), hypokalaemia (due to inappetence) and occasionally hypocalcaemia (due to saponification of fat and soft tissues). Serum amylase and lipase are of limited sensitivity and specificity in the dog, but can be helpful in the acute case if markedly elevated (more than three times the top of the reference range). Amylase and lipase are not helpful in the cat.

The most sensitive indicator of pancreatitis is an elevation in species-specific serum PLI. This test is available commercially (Spec cPL and Spec fPL, Idexx). There is also an in-house test for dogs (SNAP cPL, Idexx) which gives a positive or negative result at a relatively low cut-off for cPL levels. Thus the in-house test appears to have good sensitivity but may result in some false positives, and a positive result should ideally be followed up with a Spec cPL test.

Abdominal radiographs often show poor detail in the mid-cranial abdomen and displacement of the duodenum and/or colon due to the presence of an enlarged pancreas. Dilated loops of intestine might be visible. Abdominal radiography is particularly useful for ruling out other differential diagnoses, such as foreign bodies. Ultrasonography of the pancreas is very useful but requires considerable expertise.

Treatment

Mild cases of pancreatitis can be managed as out-patients. Vomiting should be controlled with anti-emetics (e.g. maropitant or metoclopramide). Dogs should be starved for 24 hours before introducing a bland, low-fat diet. As cats rarely vomit with pancreatitis, and development of hepatic lipidosis is a concern, starvation should NOT be recommended and the cat should continue to be fed.

More severe cases require admission for intravenous fluid therapy to treat dehydration or shock and to provide ongoing maintenance requirements. Analgesia is essential, with pethidine, methadone or buprenorphine being most appropriate (buprenorphine has a significantly longer action). NSAIDs should be avoided in acute cases, due to the increased risk of gastrointestinal and nephrotoxicity in hypovolaemic/dehydrated patients. Pancreatitis is rarely associated with bacterial infection in the dog and antibiotic therapy is only indicated when bacterial infection or abscessation is suspected, or in cases with signs of shock or DIC where bacterial translocation from the intestines becomes a concern. Severe neutrophilia with toxic changes, or marked pyrexia, would suggest an infective process, although both of these can also be caused by a severe sterile inflammatory response. Complications such as diabetes mellitus will require additional treatment, but in acute cases with no prior history of diabetes mellitus it is appropriate to monitor any hyperglycaemia and only treat if it is persistent or if there is evidence of ketoacidosis (e.g. ketones on urine dipstick).

Many cases of severe pancreatitis make a good recovery. Dogs with a history of pancreatitis should always be fed a low-fat diet, and owners should be warned that recurrence is likely. If signs of shock or DIC are apparent then the prognosis must be guarded, even with aggressive management.

In cats, the management is similar except for the following:

- Starvation is not necessary and dietary intake should be encouraged with whatever food the cat will eat. Appetite stimulants such as cyproheptadine or mirtazipine can be helpful. Feline patients which remain anorexic should be fed by naso-oesophageal tube. There is little evidence that a low-fat diet is beneficial in cats
- Broad-spectrum antibiotics such as amoxicillin/clavulanic acid are more commonly given to cats due to the possibility of ascending bacterial infection and cholangitis
- Hypocobalaminaemia is common in cats with pancreatitis and supplementation with vitamin B12 is indicated.

What if it doesn't get better?

If mild cases do not improve after conservative management, the diagnosis should be reconsidered and further investigation recommended. If severe cases do not respond to a short period of starvation, anti-emetics and appropriate fluid therapy, further investigation (including abdominal radiography) is essential, to ensure that a surgical problem, such as an intestinal foreign body, has not been missed.

The low-cost option

A presumptive diagnosis is often made in dogs based on clinical signs of vomiting and cranial abdominal pain, and many cases can be managed as out-patients. In mild cases, a single dose of an anti-emetic and buprenorphine, followed by a 24-hour fast and reintroduction of a low-fat diet, may be adequate. Cases showing signs of shock or DIC require aggressive treatment; if this is not an option then euthanasia should be considered.

When should I refer?

Most cases of pancreatitis are manageable in general practice, but referral should be offered in the following situations:

- If the practice doesn't have facilities for management of severe, acute cases with signs of shock which do not respond quickly to aggressive management. These cases may require intensive care
- Chronic or recurring cases in which the diagnosis is uncertain and specialised investigative procedures may be required.

Section 4

Gastric dilatation and volvulus (GDV) is characterised by distension of the stomach with gas and fluid, which then rotates on its axis. GDV is one of the few real emergencies in small animal practice: it is a life-threatening condition where successful management depends on a prompt diagnosis, and appropriate medical and surgical treatment.

Aetiology and pathogenesis

The cause of GDV is not fully understood but a number of 'risk-factors' have been identified:

- Large, deep-chested dogs are most commonly affected with the Doberman Pinscher, German Shepherd dog, Great Dane, Saint Bernard, Standard Poodle, Weimeraner, Irish and Gordon Setters being predisposed. Although GDV is rare in small dogs, the Dachshund is over-represented
- The incidence increases with age, being most common in dogs 7–10 years old
- The condition often occurs when vigorous exercise is taken after a large meal
- There is a greater risk if large volumes of food or water are ingested at one time, and if the food is of a small particle size
- Feeding from elevated food bowls also increases the risk of GDV.

Dilatation is due to the accumulation of gas within the stomach. The gas forms by a combination of aerophagia, release of carbon dioxide after the reaction of hydrochloric acid with bicarbonate, and bacterial fermentation of the stomach contents. It is likely that some degree of dilatation precedes the torsion. In patients with GDV, there is a fundamental problem with gastric emptying as normal gastric function should allow the gas and fluid to move out of the stomach before it becomes problematic. The nature of this problem has yet to be elucidated. Neoplasia, pyloric stenosis and a foreign body are all tangible reasons for impaired gastric emptying but are rarely found in cases of GDV. As the stomach swells, the duodenum becomes

100 Top Consultations in Small Animal General Practice, First Edition
By Peter Hill, Sheena Warman and Geoff Shawcross
© 2011 Blackwell Publishing Ltd

compressed against the abdominal wall, further compromising gastric emptying. In addition, as dilatation increases, there is an increase in intra-abdominal pressure, resulting in a reduced venous return to the heart, reduced tissue perfusion and increased pressure on the diaphragm, which makes breathing difficult.

When torsion occurs, the stomach usually rotates 90–360° clockwise about the distal oesophagus when viewed from behind. The pylorus is displaced to the left of the midline, the duodenum becomes trapped between the distal oesophagus and the stomach, and the spleen becomes displaced because of its attachment to the greater curvature of the stomach. When the volvulus is greater than 180°, the distal oesophagus becomes occluded and there is no longer the possibility of spontaneous gastric decompression. The blood supply to the stomach and spleen can be severely compromised, possibly resulting in necrosis of a large segment of the stomach wall and splenic rupture. Endotoxaemia, hypoxaemia, metabolic acidosis, and hypotension all predispose to the development of DIC.

History and clinical signs

There is usually a history of a recent meal and exercise. The first clinical signs reflect abdominal discomfort, characterised by restlessness and excessive salivation, but owners who are unaware of this condition may miss their significance. The condition progresses extremely quickly with the development of the pathognomonic signs of GDV, which are repeated non-productive retching and regurgitation of white, frothy saliva, and rapidly developing abdominal tympany. Usually, by the time the dog is presented for examination, clinical signs have deteriorated further to include signs of hypovolaemic shock. The dog is usually reluctant or unable to stand, exhibiting tachypnoea or dyspnoea, rapid and weak arterial pulses, pale or sometimes blue–grey mucous membranes, and prolonged CRT. Cardiac arrhythmias are frequently present, characterised by an irregular heart rate and associated pulse deficits.

Important differential diagnoses

The initial contact with the owner will usually alert the clinician to the probability of GDV having occurred. The presentation of GDV is so typical that it unlikely to be confused with any other disease. Unproductive retching with small amounts of frothy saliva may be seen with oesophageal and pharyngeal problems. Abdominal distension, especially associated with discomfort and restlessness, can be associated with conditions such as ascites and late pregnancy. However, the lack of abdominal tympany and the speed of progression of the distension should alert the clinician to the probability of GDV.

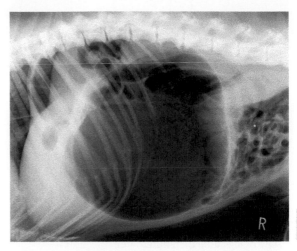

Figure 44.1 **Radiograph of a dog with severe GDV, demonstrating the 'double bubble' effect**

Specific diagnostic techniques

It should be possible to make a diagnosis confidently based on a clinical examination. Haematology and blood biochemistry (a minimum of PCV, platelet count, total solids, urea, creatinine, glucose, electrolytes, plus ideally acid–base analysis and coagulation times) should be taken to allow proper supportive management of the case. Measurement of serum lactic acid concentrations can assist in determining prognosis. Values above 6.0 mmol/L are associated with gastric necrosis and increased mortality. Initial treatment should not be delayed pending the results. The results will reflect the effects of systemic hypotension and the development of pre-renal azotaemia, with increases in serum urea, creatinine and phosphorus concentration. After decompression, when blood that had sequestered into the splanchnic bed and posterior muscle masses re-enters the general circulation, there is an increase in AST and creatine kinase (CK) owing to striated muscle damage and cell membrane injury.

Radiography can be useful to differentiate simple gastric dilatation from gastric dilatation with volvulus. Surgical gastropexy is still recommended in patients with dilatation without volvulus, but immediate surgical intervention is not required assuming decompression via stomach tube is successful. Radiography should not be undertaken in preference to aggressive stabilisation of the patient. The first abdominal radiographs should be taken in right lateral recumbency because the gas-filled pylorus is usually identifiable dorsal and cranial to the gas-filled gastric fundus in this projection. Torsion results in a shelf of soft tissue being apparent within the stomach in the right lateral view, known as a reverse C sign or 'double bubble' (Figure 44.1).

Treatment

There are four elements to the management of GDV:

Stabilisation of the patient's condition

These cases represent a high anaesthetic risk and hypovolaemic shock should be treated quickly and aggressively. One or more short, large-bore intravenous catheters should be placed in cephalic or jugular veins. Saphenous catheters should not be used as venous return will be obstructed. Shock doses (60–90 ml/kg) of isotonic crystalloids should be given in boluses of 20–30 ml/kg as required IV in the first hour of treatment, and then the rate adjusted, based on clinical response and the need to maintain adequate blood pressure and cardiac output. Dogs in severe shock may benefit from the use of hypertonic saline (4 mL/kg over 5–10 min) or colloidal fluids (e.g. gelatins or starch-based solutions), followed by isotonic fluids as indicated above, until clinical signs of shock have improved. Oxygen therapy should be provided by face-mask, flow-by or nasal prongs. Because endotoxaemia frequently complicates the disease process, broad-spectrum IV antibiotics should be administered (e.g. amoxicillin/clavulanic acid) and continued for 3–5 days after surgery. Administration of glucocorticoids is contraindicated.

Metabolic acidosis frequently accompanies GDV but adequate fluid therapy and gastric decompression generally correct this problem. Electrolyte abnormalities should be addressed if present.

Decompression

Gastric decompression must be accomplished as soon as possible, after cardiovascular stabilisation has been initiated. Initially, an attempt should be made to pass a well-lubricated orogastric (stomach) tube. If sedation is required, an opioid–benzodiazepine mixture probably offers the best compromise between adequate sedation and patient safety as this combination is relatively safe in critically ill animals. The opioid component (morphine 0.2–0.4 mg/kg IM, or pethidine 2–4 mg/kg IM) is given first, and usually produces little if any sedative effect. Satisfactory sedation usually results when either diazepam (0.25 mg/kg) or midazolam (0.25 mg/kg) is given by slow IV injection 10 minutes later.

In order to reduce the risk of pushing the stomach tube through a devitalized stomach wall, the distance from the incisors to the xiphoid should be measured and marked by a piece of tape on the stomach tube. The dog can be positioned in either sternal or lateral recumbency and the mouth should be wedged open with a gag or a roll of bandage. As the stomach tube is advanced, some resistance is usually felt as the tube passes through the cardiac sphincter. It should be possible to overcome this resistance by gently rotating the tube whilst it is being advanced. Undue force may tear the oesophagus. Once the tube enters the stomach, gastric gas readily escapes. After the stomach has been decompressed, it should be lavaged with 5–10 ml/kg warm water or saline to remove any remaining food, but great care must be taken to avoid aspiration. It is very important to appreciate that successful passage of a tube does not rule out concurrent gastric volvulus.

If a tube cannot be passed, decompression may be achieved by inserting a 12–18-gauge needle or 'over the needle' catheter into the stomach percutaneously. An area (10 × 10 cm) on the abdominal wall over the area of maximum distension and tympany, caudal to the last rib and ventral to the transverse vertebral process, should be shaved and prepared in an aseptic fashion. Before the needle is inserted, the area should be percussed to avoid accidental puncture of an overlying spleen. Gastric decompression generally facilitates the passage of a stomach tube and lavage of the stomach.

Surgical correction

Surgical correction should be carried out as soon as the patient's condition is stable. Once the stomach and spleen have been repositioned, the stomach should be fixed to the abdominal wall (gastropexy), to reduce the possibility of the condition recurring. Various different techniques are described, and the reader is advised to consult appropriate surgical textbooks for further information. During surgery, the integrity of the stomach and spleen must be fully evaluated but gastric wall resection or splenectomy is only necessary when there is evidence that tissue viability has been compromised. Splenic congestion generally resolves after the stomach has been repositioned. The value of pyloromyotomy and pyloroplasty in an effort to promote gastric emptying has not been substantiated.

Post-operative management

Food should be withheld for 12 hours after surgery and then small amounts of a low fat food can be introduced. Fluid therapy and analgesia should be maintained, but NSAIDs should be avoided. The patient should be monitored for signs of haemorrhage, sepsis, peritonitis, cardiac arrhythmias, aspiration pneumonia and DIC. Cardiovascular and respiratory parameters, urine output, blood pressure, and basic laboratory parameters (PCV, total solids, electrolytes) should be monitored. Potassium supplementation may be required. Ventricular arrhythmias are common, especially 12–36 hours post-operatively, due to the effects of myocardial ischaemia, and electrolyte and acid–base imbalances. In most cases, these resolve spontaneously once the factors that predispose to ventricular arrhythmias have been addressed. If the arrhythmia persists and results in haemodynamic compromise, is multiform, has a rate greater than 160–180 bpm, or shows R-on-T phenomenon (when complexes are inscribed on the T-wave of the previous complex), it should be treated with IV lidocaine and monitored by electrocardiography. Anti-emetics should be administered if necessary. Broad-spectrum antibiotics that were given peri-operatively should be continued for a further 3–5 days.

In the long term, dogs that have recovered from GDV, and breeds that have a predisposition to GDV, should be fed small meals frequently over the course of the day. Excessive exercise should be discouraged to reduce the risk of volvulus occurring, and the consumption of large volumes of water after exercise should be prevented to avoid gastric distension. Use of elevated feeding bowls is not recommended.

What if it doesn't get better?

If treatment of GDV is not initiated quickly enough, or the condition managed appropriately, it is likely that death will result. Even with surgical management, there is a 15% mortality rate. If the serum lactate is over 6 mmol/L, mortality rates increase to 30%. If the patient is not making a satisfactory recovery from surgery, it is likely that there is a post-operative complication. Patients need to be carefully monitored and evaluated to ensure that these are not missed. Undetected problems such as hypokalaemia, anaemia, acidosis, peritonitis, gastric ulceration, DIC or ventricular arrhythmias may all complicate the recovery. Following a successful recovery from GDV surgery and gastropexy, the risk of recurrence is less than 10%.

When should I refer?

Because there are severe time constraints during which treatment must be instigated, referral is not likely to be practicable when a case of GDV first presents. If the practice does not have the surgical and supportive facilities necessary to manage a case of GDV, the patient should be properly stabilised, decompressed and then referred for corrective surgery and gastropexy at the earliest opportunity. In such cases, further advice should be obtained from the referral centre.

The low-cost option

GDV is an expensive condition to manage, involving major surgery and aggressive pre- and post- operative medical treatment. The client should be given a realistic estimate of the likely cost involved, after taking into account the possible intra- and post-operative complications. Even with prompt and aggressive therapy, a successful outcome is far from certain and this should be fully explained to the client. If there are financial constraints, the option of euthanasia should be broached before embarking on treatment. Medical treatment alone by orogastric decompression and lavage may be temporarily successful but the recurrence rate is very high.

Geoff Shawcross

Obstipation is a condition in which an animal finds it extremely difficult or impossible to defaecate, usually because of a colonic or rectal obstruction. Megacolon is characterised by distension of the colon with the accumulation of faecal material that becomes difficult or impossible to void.

Aetiology and pathogenesis

Obstipation in the dog is most commonly the result of dietary indiscretion such as the ingestion of indigestible material (e.g. bones, sand) or, occasionally, a sharp object such as a needle. It can also develop secondarily to any condition that constricts or compresses the distal colon or rectum, such as prostatic enlargement, perineal hernias or rectal diverticula, intra-pelvic tumours or narrowing of the pelvic canal following pelvic fractures. In the cat, obstipation usually results from narrowing of the pelvic canal as a consequence of poorly managed pelvic fractures, or from a stricture at the colo-rectal junction caused by a carcinoma. Obstipation can occur in hospitalised patients because of a change in their routine, pain following surgery or as the side-effect of some drugs (e.g. opiates).

Slowed transit time through the colon results in faecal material becoming dry, hard and impacted. This makes it increasingly difficult to defaecate and, if the underlying condition is one which develops slowly, the diameter of the colon will increase with time to accommodate the faecal material, resulting in megacolon. This distension, however, will usually resolve or improve when the underlying condition is corrected. The most usual cause of megacolon in the cat is an idiopathic form which is either neurogenic in origin or, more commonly, the result of impaired colonic smooth muscle function. Obstipation and the associated megacolon have also been associated with Key–Gaskell Syndrome (feline dysautonomia) and spinal nerve injury.

History and clinical signs

The presenting signs depend on the cause, severity and chronicity of the obstipation but in most cases, the owner will report some degree of unproductive rectal straining, discomfort and possibly signs of rectal bleeding. The owner may be aware that their pet has not defaecated for several days, even in the absence of rectal straining. In cats, some owners are unaware of the lack of defaecation and the pet is presented for lethargy or vomiting.

- Obstipation that results from eating bones or sharp objects presents as an acute syndrome, characterised by frequent bouts of straining to pass faeces and is often extremely painful (rectal tenesmus). The dog may pass small amounts of faecal-stained fluid which has by-passed the obstruction, and may be confused with diarrhoea by the owner. This will be blood-stained if the rectal wall is lacerated. The dog is usually anorexic and may even vomit. Signs of endotoxaemia can develop if the condition is not resolved quickly
- Obstipation caused by narrowing of the rectum (e.g. intra-pelvic mass, narrowing of the pelvic canal) is characterised by straining to defaecate but is not usually painful until the condition is advanced. The character of the faecal mass is usually altered; it may be narrowed in diameter as it is forced through the constricted rectum and often has a 'toothpaste' consistency. Colo-rectal tumours may result in fresh blood being present around the anus if the blood vessels in the stricture are torn
- Obstipation resulting from a perineal hernia is not usually painful and straining is intermittent. As the dog strains, a swelling lateral to the anus is usually visible owing to loss of muscular support allowing displacement of the rectum
- Obstipation resulting from idiopathic megacolon may go un-noticed for a considerable time, especially in cats that spend time outdoors and do not use a litter tray. Affected cats develop a general malaise and often have periods of straining to defaecate, followed by long periods when they make no attempt. Abdominal distension is commonly seen in chronically affected cats, caused by the gross distension of the colon.

100 Top Consultations in Small Animal General Practice, First Edition
By Peter Hill, Sheena Warman and Geoff Shawcross
© 2011 Blackwell Publishing Ltd

Specific diagnostic techniques

A thorough abdominal palpation will usually identify an enlarged colon and reveal the extent of the impaction. A rectal examination is generally possible in the dog and will reveal conditions such as a perineal hernia, rectal diverticulum, intra-pelvic mass, skeletal deformity, splintered and impacted bones, or rectal foreign body. Blood may be present on the examination glove even if it was not evident clinically. The clinician should appreciate that this examination may be extremely painful and resented by the patient.

Plain abdominal radiographs will demonstrate the extent of the impaction, the nature of the faecal material and any anatomical abnormalities that have contributed to the obstipation. Additional imaging techniques such as contrast radiography and ultrasonography should be considered if the cause of the obstipation is obscure.

Haematology and biochemistry are rarely abnormal but may yield additional information that will be helpful in managing cases that have to be hospitalised because of clinical signs of illness (e.g. vomiting or signs of endotoxaemia).

Treatment

The aim of treatment is to facilitate the passage of the faecal mass and then correct the underlying cause, wherever this is possible.

Mild cases

Many cases can be treated as out-patients. Treatment with a sodium citrate micro-enema (Micralax, Pharmacia) may be adequate in some cases. Animals should be well hydrated before laxatives are given, otherwise their dehydration will be exacerbated. Owners should encourage fluid intake and provide a wet, high-fibre or low-residue diet. If this is unsuccessful, attempts should be made to soften the faecal mass and lubricate its passage by giving lactulose or liquid paraffin by mouth. Liquid paraffin is tasteless and thus does not always stimulate normal swallowing if given orally, increasing the risk of lipid pneumonia. It should therefore be added to food and not be syringed orally. Paraffin paste is available and in many cases can be administered by applying it to food or the paws and allowing the pet to lick it. Stimulant laxatives should not be given in cases of rectal obstruction until the faecal mass is soft enough to pass.

Severe or non-responsive cases

Manual removal of rectal obstructions and faecal boluses with the use of enemas is indicated in these cases. This can be coupled with trans-abdominal manipulation of the colon to disrupt the faecal mass. Enemas should be warmed to body temperature and infused slowly via a suitably sized catheter. Plain water, saline and soapy water are all satisfactory. Proprietary phosphate enemas are toxic to cats and should not be used. Administration of an enema and the subsequent manipulation may not be possible in a conscious animal, in which case hospitalisation and general anaesthesia are required. General anaesthesia also permits better manipulation, and more convenient use of enemas. Faecoliths can also be broken down by careful use of forceps introduced through the anus. Because colonic tissue can become devitalised, and there is a risk of perforation and endotoxaemia developing, broad-spectrum antibiotic cover should be given. Several anaesthesias may be necessary before the obstipation is resolved and consequently attention must be paid to the hydration status and electrolyte balance of the patient.

Long-term management of recurrent cases or idiopathic megacolon

Many of the drugs used for the long-term management of obstipation and megacolon are not licensed (in the UK) for veterinary use (see Table 45.1). Bulking laxatives, such as sterculia (Peridale) granules or high dietary fibre supplements, will usually help in the long-term management of recurrent obstipation as they encourage bowel movement and keep the faeces soft. However, some experimentation may be required to establish an effective regime and maintain palatability. Some cases are best managed with a highly digestible diet that results in a low faecal residue. Weight control and increasing the pet's activity levels (e.g. encouraging a sedentary cat to play games) can be helpful. Lactulose (a poorly absorbed polysaccharide) is an effective laxative that is convenient to use and well tolerated over the long term by both dogs and cats. Liquid paraffin should not be given frequently because it limits the absorption of fat-soluble vitamins. Megacolon in the cat can often be effectively managed using an appropriate diet (high fibre or low residue), weight control, increased activity and drugs such as docusate sodium/dantron combinations (Normax).

Table 45.1   Medical treatments for obstipation and megacolon. Further information and doses available in formularies.

	Example	Brand name	Notes
Enemas	Sodium citrate micro-enema	Microlax	Mild constipation or out-patient use
	Bisacodyl	Dulcolax	Available as rectal suppository
	Docusate sodium	Various	Can be used orally or as an enema. Do not use with mineral oil.
	Warm tap water or soapy water		
	Warm isotonic saline		
	Liquid paraffin		
	Lactulose	Lactulose	
Oral laxatives			
Bulk-forming laxatives	Sterculia granules	Peridale	Add to moist food
Lubricant laxatives	Paraffin	Katalax	Liquid paraffin should not be given orally due to risk of aspiration; paraffin paste is preferred (and will often be licked by the animal if applied to paws).
Hyperosmotic laxatives	Lactulose	Lactulose	
Emollient laxatives	Docusate sodium	Normax	Mixed with dantron, a mild stimulant for the lower bowel. Do not use with mineral oil. Hepatotoxicity and carcinogenesis reported in rats.
Stimulant laxatives	Bisacodyl	Dulcolax	Available as tablets
Prokinetic drugs	Ranitidine	Zantac	Of limited effect
	Cisapride		No longer available in UK

What if it doesn't get better?

Colotomy and removal of the faeces should be considered, but only if the use of laxatives, enemas and manual removal of faecal material fails to relieve the obstipation. Corrective surgery of perineal hernias, pelvic abnormalities and any condition causing colorectal compression will have to be considered if the problem is not to recur. Subtotal colectomy is successful in the majority of cats that suffer from megacolon that are unresponsive to medical management, although some cats may then have soft stools indefinitely.

The low-cost option

Hospitalisation, anaesthesia, imaging and corrective surgery are all expensive, so costs will be reduced if the case can be managed by the owner as an outpatient. Attention to diet and the frequent administration of laxatives by the owner will reduce the need for veterinary intervention in chronic or recurrent cases. Owners can be taught to manage the faecal obstruction resulting from perineal hernias.

When should I refer?

The management of obstipation is commonly undertaken in general practice and referral is rarely required. Referral should be considered if corrective surgery is required that is beyond the scope of the practice (such as sub-total colectomy or pelvic fracture repair).

Section 5
Musculoskeletal problems

Martin Owen

Aetiology and pathogenesis

Most orthopaedic problems in young, growing, dogs occur due to abnormalities of skeletal development (bones, joints or soft tissues). Immature dogs are also susceptible to a number of inflammatory and traumatic disorders of the skeleton that cause pain and lameness.

Common developmental abnormalities and breed predispositions:

- Hip dysplasia – Medium/large dogs and some smaller breeds, e.g. spaniels, bulldogs
- Osteochondrosis of the shoulder, hock or stifle – Medium/large dogs, spaniels and English Bull Terriers
- Elbow dysplasia complex (comprises fragmentation of the ulnar coronoid process ± medial humeral condylar lesion ± ununited anconeal process) – Medium/large dogs
- Patellar luxation – Small breed dogs, Labradors and occasionally large breeds, e.g. Great Danes
- Aseptic necrosis of the femoral head (Legg–Calvé–Perthes) – Terriers.

Inflammatory disorders:

- Panosteitis – German Shepherd dogs, medium/large dogs
- Hypertrophic osteodystrophy (metaphyseal osteopathy) – All dogs, but especially Collies, Great Danes, Weimaraners. Often occurs following vaccination.

Traumatic injuries:

- Bone fractures (see Chapter 51)
- Growth plate fractures
- Angular deformities due to premature growth plate closure – Medium/large breed dogs following minor trauma, chondrodystrophoid breeds without trauma.

100 Top Consultations in Small Animal General Practice, First Edition
By Peter Hill, Sheena Warman and Geoff Shawcross
© 2011 Blackwell Publishing Ltd

History and clinical signs

Hip dysplasia

Dogs with hip dysplasia generally have stiffness and lameness of both hind limbs, and are reluctant to exercise and play. They may *have* a very upright hind limb conformation (particularly Labradors), the hind-quarters may appear wobbly, and they may 'bunny hop' instead of trotting. Physical examination generally identifies poor hind limb muscle development, and pain on extension and sometimes abduction of the hips. Crepitation or clunking of the hip (due to subluxation or reduction of the joint) may be detected during manipulation.

Osteochondrosis

Osteochondrosis causes significant joint pain and often marked effusion that is detectable as a 'puffy' joint by careful digital palpation. Pain can be elicited on forced flexion of the joint. Osteochondrosis is often bilateral, although lameness is often lateralised because one joint is more uncomfortable than the other. If bilateral disease is present, bilateral pain is usually evident on physical examination.

Elbow dysplasia

Elbow dysplasia causes pain and lameness in one, or both forelimbs. Owners may report stiffness, reluctance to play or a tendency to lie down. The front paws are often externally rotated when the dog is sitting or standing, presumably as this relieves pressure and pain from the medial side of the elbow. Poor forelimb muscle mass may be evident in chronic cases. Severely affected dogs have palpable effusion, detected as a puffy, fluid-filled component on the caudolateral elbow. Pain is evident both on extreme elbow flexion (so that the carpus touches the shoulder) whilst supinating the paw, and forced extension (forcibly stressing the joint beyond its natural end point).

Aseptic necrosis of the femoral head

Aseptic necrosis of the femoral head is markedly painful and affected dogs are either severely lame or non-weight-bearing. Hip manipulation is extremely uncomfortable, especially on extension. Chronic lameness often results in visible and palpable loss of muscle mass in the affected limb. This disease is usually unilateral but it can be bilateral, though in such cases, generally, one limb is more severely affected than the other.

Patellar luxation

Patellar luxation is not usually painful on physical examination. Initially, the problem is intermittent and when the patella luxates during locomotion, the affected limb is carried in flexion for a few steps resulting in a skipping lameness. With time, many dogs are presented with a persistent lameness because the patella is luxated most of the time. When patellar luxation occurs in young growing dogs, the medial displacement of the patella can lead to growth deformity and genu recurvatum.

Panosteitis

Panosteitis most commonly causes forelimb lameness but it can affect the hind limbs. Affected dogs have long bone pain, due to inflammatory changes within the medullary cavity. It can be detected in the ulna, radius, humerus, femur or tibia. Often the lameness is episodic and it can affect different bones at different times, resulting in a cyclic or shifting lameness. There is marked pain when firm digital pressure is applied to the affected bones. Occasionally, affected dogs may be inappetent and mildly pyrexic. It is much more common in males than in females.

Hypertrophic osteodystrophy

Hypertrophic osteodystrophy causes lameness, often on all four limbs. Affected dogs are pyrexic, dull and depressed. Markedly painful and swollen distal long bone metaphyses (radius/ulna and tibia/fibula) are evident. Gentle pressure on the metaphysis elicits a pain response that can be differentiated from joint pain by careful localisation. Affected dogs often become severely ill and clinicians should anticipate significant morbidity.

Physeal fractures

Physeal (growth plate) injuries are common in puppies and are generally caused by minor trauma, such as jumping down from furniture or being dropped from the owner's arms. Affected dog are generally non-weight-bearing on the affected limb(s) and there is marked pain of the injured region(s), often with soft tissue swelling. Growth plate injuries occur both with and without marked displacement. Trauma to the growth plate can result in premature closure and cessation of growth at the physis, resulting in relative shortening of the affected bone. For the paired bones, premature closure of the ulnar or fibular growth plates results in a valgus (outward) deformity whereas premature closure of the radial or tibial growth plate results in a varus (inward) deformity. The distal ulnar physis is most commonly affected and presents as external rotation of the paw, valgus deformity and cranial bowing of the radius. Affected dogs are often lame because the length discrepancy between the paired bones results in joint pain (normally the elbow joint). Clinicians should be aware that premature physeal closure can occur even if a radiograph of the affected limb appears normal. Owners should therefore be warned to monitor the dog carefully for signs of angular deformity after such injuries.

Specific diagnostic techniques

Hip dysplasia

Hip dysplasia can be diagnosed using a combination of physical examination and radiography. The Ortolani test is useful to characterise the degree of hip dysplasia and to document the integrity of the dorsal acetabular rim. When learning this test, it is best performed in a heavily sedated/anaesthetised dog in lateral recumbency. The technique is performed as follows:

1. The stifle joint of the upper limb is grasped firmly and the hip is maintained with the femur perpendicular to the vertebral column. The thumb of the operator's other hand is gently applied to the greater trochanter.
2. Whilst applying a moderate compressive force proximally along the axis of the femur (simulating the force of weight bearing), the stifle is abducted slowly. In immature dogs with hip dysplasia and hip laxity, the proximally directed femoral force subluxates the hip joint. As the hip is *abducted*, a point is reached when the femoral head slips back into the acetabulum. This is palpably detected by the hand on the stifle and the thumb on the trochanter.
3. With axial force still applied to the stifle, the stifle is *adducted* and the hip is felt to subluxate. Whilst repeating this manoeuvre the clinician assesses the character of the transition between reduction and subluxation. A 'snap' indicates good integrity of the dorsal acetabular rim and a grating sensation indicates dorsal acetabular destruction.

Hip dysplasia can be diagnosed radiographically with ventrodorsal extended and 'frog leg' views (and where the service is offered, a PennHip© distraction view). Hip subluxation/luxation is visible on the ventrodorsal extended view and the distraction view (Figure 46.1). Secondary osteoarthritis occurs rapidly in dogs with hip dysplasia resulting in osteophyte formation most easily seen on the femoral head, neck and on the cranial acetabulum. In severe cases, the femoral head becomes flattened and the acetabulum becomes shallow and widened. The frog-leg view shows if the hip joint reduces when the femora are abducted, which can be useful for decision-making regarding surgical management.

Osteochondrosis

Osteochondrosis is diagnosed by radiological examination of the affected joint(s). Orthogonal views should be taken. Osteochondrosis lesions are identified as concavities within the articular surface due to failure of the subchondral bone to ossify normally, resulting in a thickened region of cartilaginous precursor that is radiolucent, unlike the normal surrounding subchondral bone (Figure 46.2). For the shoulder and stifle, mediolateral projections are most useful whilst hock osteochondrosis is more obvious on a dorsoplantar projection. When there is a mineralised osteochondrosis dissecans lesion, the mineralised cartilaginous fragment is visible as a small/thin and faintly radio-opaque structure lying at the level of the expected articular subchondral bone contour. For the shoulder joint an arthrogram is extremely useful to investigate for the presence of an osteochondrosis dissecans flap since its presence is a determinant for recommending surgical management. If the flap detaches, the mineralised cartilage is visible in the joint cavity (known as a joint mouse).

Elbow dysplasia

Elbow dysplasia is best identified radiologically in a mediolateral projection of a fully flexed elbow joint and a craniocaudal view of the extended joint (Figures 46.3 and 46.4). The disease is associated with rapid development of secondary osteoarthritic signs and osteophytes can be seen on the anconeal process on the fully flexed elbow projection. If an ununited anconeal process is present, this is clearly identified by a radiolucent line on the anconeal process (dogs must be over five months of age in order to make this diagnosis, since fusion does not occur in some dogs until this age). Lesions of the medial humeral condyle are detected on the craniocaudal projection. In affected dogs, a subchondral lucency (see above) is visible and it is often observed with a blunting of the ulnar coronoid region. Some dogs with 'medial com-partment disease elbow dysplasia' have no radiological signs at the time of examination and a diagnosis may require nuclear scintigraphy, MRI, CT or arthroscopic investigation.

Patellar luxation

Patellar luxation is most readily diagnosed by physical examination, not by radiological investigation. Furthermore, confirmation is best in the conscious animal, since tension in the quadriceps mechanism assists luxation and reduction of the patella. It is best to examine the stifle with the dog in a standing position, supporting the caudal abdomen to prevent the dog sitting down. The stifle is held in a standing position, with the foot lifted slightly from the ground. The hind paw is internally rotated and with the operator's other hand, pressure is applied to the lateral aspect of the patella, pushing it medially, whilst the stifle is slowly flexed. This will displace the patella medially in cases of medial patellar luxation. Once the stifle is flexed, lateral pressure is applied to the patella and the stifle is extended, with the foot externally rotated. This will reduce a reducible medially luxated patella (a severe patella luxation will not reduce on physical examination, but remain luxated throughout). Some crepitation may be detected during manipulation, indicating articular cartilage loss and osteoarthritic change. Lateral patellar luxation is detected by applying lateral pressure to the patella with external rotation of the hind paw during flexion of the stifle.

Aseptic necrosis of the femoral head

Aseptic necrosis of the femoral head is best diagnosed radiologically. Ventrodorsal extended and frog-leg views are useful. Heavy sedation or anaesthesia is required for positioning. Radiographs show mottled lucency and increased bony density of the femoral head with apparent widening of the hip joint space (Figure 46.5). Sometimes, the lesions are more obvious on one view than the other, although only a single view is required if a diagnosis is made on the first projection.

Panosteitis

Panosteitis can be difficult to diagnose radiologically at first presentation because radiological signs lag behind the clinical signs and are often subtle, manifesting as only subtle increases in trabecular density in some cases. A characteristic radiological appearance of panosteitis is an increase in bony density in the middle of a long bone, almost like a thumb print (Figure 46.6). Several such lesions may be present, either in a single bone or in several bones. If panosteitis is suspected, it is useful to perform a skeletal survey to try and find a bone with radiological signs. It is also helpful to take radiographs two weeks after first clinical presentation because radiological signs of disease are not present during the initial phase of inflammation and pain. In some cases, a definitive radiological diagnosis is never achieved because the clinical signs disappear before further radiographs are taken.

Physeal fractures

Physeal fractures and angular limb deformities are readily diagnosed on radiological investigation using standard orthogonal views. It is helpful to radiograph both limbs using identical settings and positioning. Physeal fractures are characterised by displacement and/or widening of the lucent physis and there may be limb deformity.

Angular limb deformity secondary to physeal injury is characterised by mineralisation of the normally lucent growth plate and by abnormal limb alignment, by length discrepancy between the paired bones of the affected limb and by length discrepancy between contralateral bones (affected bone shorter and curved). In severe cases, subluxation of a joint (e.g. the elbow joint) may be apparent.

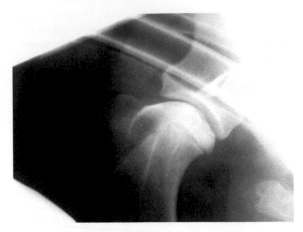

Figure 46.2 **Lateral view of the shoulder showing irregular lucent appearance to the caudal humeral head subchondral bone typical of osteochondrosis**

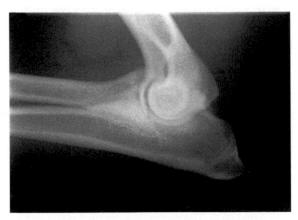

Figure 46.3 **The flexed mediolateral view of the elbow is the most sensitive radiograph for detecting osteophytes and hence osteoarthritic change. This radiograph shows osteophyte formation on the anconeal process and osteophyte remodelling of the radial head. In a young Labrador, these changes are most likely secondary to elbow dysplasia (coronoid disease)**

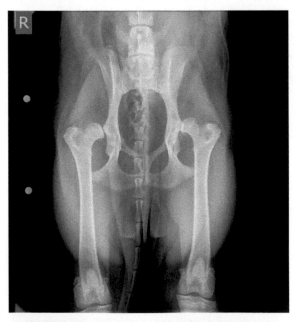

Figure 46.1 **Ventrodorsal view radiograph showing severe hip dyplasia in a dog. Both hips are luxated due to marked soft tissue laxity**

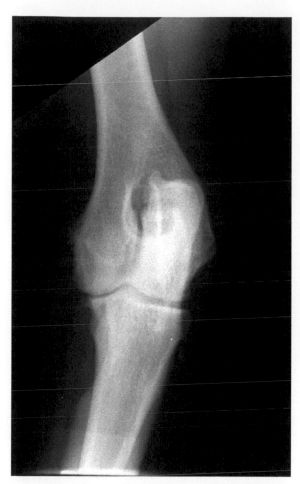

Figure 46.4 **Craniocaudal view radiograph of the elbow showing osteophyte formation on the proximal medial ulna in the region of the coronoid process. The osteophyte indicates osteoarthritis and in a young Labrador, the most likely cause is elbow dysplasia**

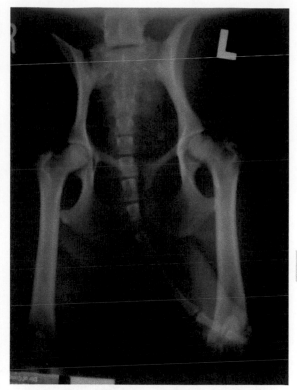

Figure 46.5 **Ventrodorsal projection of the hips of a Jack Russell Terrier showing mottling of the left femoral head and widening of the hip joint space. These are typical radiological features of aseptic necrosis of the femoral head**

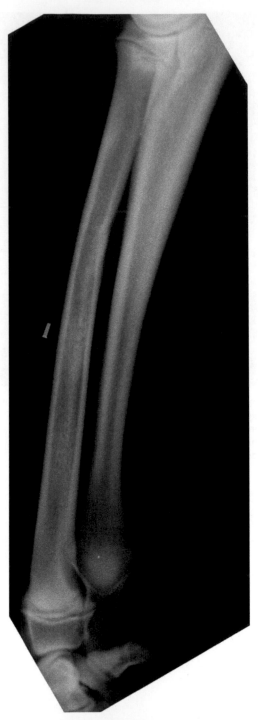

Figure 46.6 **Mediolateral view of the radius and ulna of a young large-breed dog showing irregular mottled radiopacity of the diaphysis of the radius. In a young male large-breed dog, this appearance is typical of panosteitis**

Treatment

Hip dysplasia

Some dogs with hip dysplasia can be effectively managed conservatively and, as they become skeletally mature, their clinical signs diminish and normal levels of activity are possible. Dogs affected with hip dysplasia should be treated for their discomfort. A four-week course of NSAIDs should be given to control pain and a controlled, restricted exercise programme initiated, designed to reduce activity-induced joint pain which occurs with high repetitive impact during play. Frequent, short, lead walks are recommended. Dogs that will respond to conservative management will be markedly improved within two weeks. Dogs that do not respond to conservative management but have good dorsal acetabular integrity (see above) should be promptly referred for surgical management (pelvic osteotomy surgery) if debilitating hip osteoarthritis of the hips is to be prevented. If surgical management is not under consideration due to clinical or financial constraints, conservative management that aims to reduce pain can be continued whilst the puppy matures, at which point the acute pain of hip dysplasia tends to subside. Once clinical signs are controlled, the duration of the slow lead walks can be gradually increased. Controlled activity (and, if necessary, NSAIDs) should be continued until skeletal maturity. If a particular NSAID appears ineffective and pain is marked, a switch to an alternative NSAID can be helpful in some cases (see Chapter 50) and additional analgesia can be provided with non-licensed products such as tramadol and/or amantadine.

Surgical options for management of hip dysplasia include:

* Acetabular rotation pelvic osteotomy – useful for young dogs with an intact dorsal acetabular rim and mild laxity. A grating sensation on Ortolani testing precludes this surgery
* Total hip replacement – useful for dogs nearing or at skeletal maturity that are still painful despite medical management
* Femoral head and neck excision – a cheaper option which is useful for dogs that do not respond to conservative management when financial limitations preclude referral for total hip replacement.

Shoulder osteochondrosis

Shoulder osteochondrosis in which no dissecans flap is apparent should be treated conservatively with restricted activity and a four-week course of NSAIDs. When a dissecans flap is present, removal of the flap (arthroscopically or via arthrotomy) produces a much quicker resolution of pain and lameness (2–4 weeks) than conservative management (6–12 months). When there are bilateral flaps, unilateral staged treatments are recommended. Arthroscopic removal of dissecans flaps reportedly gives faster recoveries than the traditional open surgical approach.

Elbow dysplasia

Elbow dysplasia is most painful for growing dogs and tends to improve with skeletal maturity. At initial presentation and diagnosis, affected dogs should be treated with strictly controlled restricted activity and a four-week course of NSAIDs. The NSAID should be changed if there is not a satisfactory response within two weeks (see Chapter 50). Failure to respond to four weeks of conservative management suggests that one of the following surgical options may provide a more rapid improvement in comfort and lameness:

- Endoscopic investigation and fragment arthroscopic retrieval treatment (FART) – preferred for coronoid and medial humeral condylar disease. Following arthroscopic treatment, up to 70% of dogs treated become NSAID-independent as they reach skeletal maturity
- Proximal ulnar osteotomy and lag screw fixation of the anconeal process – for dogs with united anconeal process that do not respond to conservative management, provided radiological evidence of associated osteoarthritic change is not severe enough to limit the postoperative outcome
- Coronoid debridement
- Coronoidectomy
- Proximal ulnar osteotomy
- Sliding humeral osteotomy
- Biceps ulnar release procedure.

These latter techniques are reserved for dogs with severe disease and for dogs not responding to FART, but no consensus supports any one of these treatments. It should be noted that progressive osteoarthritis is a common sequel to elbow dysplasia, irrespective of whether it is treated surgically or medically.

Aseptic necrosis of the femoral head

Aseptic necrosis of the femoral head (Legg–Calvé–Perthes disease) is best treated surgically by femoral head and neck excision. Approximately 10% of affected dogs are thought to respond to conservative management. Occasionally, small dogs can be reluctant to use their limb after surgery which is a poor prognostic indicator for long-term function. Following surgical treatment, early limb use and physiotherapy are to be encouraged.

Patellar luxation

Patellar luxation in immature dogs is best managed surgically. Surgical techniques include tibial tuberosity transposition, femoral trochlear sulcoplasty, and femoral and tibial osteotomies. Patellar luxation is primarily a mechanical problem and medical treatment is not corrective.

Panosteitis

Panosteitis is treated conservatively using NSAIDs during episodes of pain and lameness, with strict restriction of activity. Often a seven-day course is sufficient but the disease appears to be episodic and further episodes of lameness can be expected. Clients owning affected dogs may learn to recognise the signs of discomfort and administer a short course of NSAIDs on an 'as needed' basis.

Hypertrophic osteodystrophy

Hypertrophic osteodystrophy (metaphyseal osteopathy) is a severe disease and affected dogs usually require hospitalisation, supportive IV fluid therapy, effective analgesia and supplementary feeding. There is currently no known specific treatment for hypertrophic osteodystrophy but generally, supportive therapy is sufficient for recovery in most affected dogs.

Physeal fractures

Physeal fractures are treated on an individual basis and specialist veterinary orthopaedic advice is recommended for interpretation of radiographs and management. Some fractures with limited displacement which are still stable can be managed with a support dressing and appropriate analgesia. Other physeal fractures require surgical fixation using implants, which may require elective removal shortly after placement, to avoid iatrogenic physeal growth arrest. Angular limb deformities are best treated by veterinary orthopaedic specialists, as surgical management can be technically challenging and a good long-term prognosis requires specialist knowledge and experience.

What if it doesn't get better?

Patients that do not respond to initial management should be re-examined within 2–4 weeks, in order to re-evaluate the diagnosis. Re-examination of radiographs should also be performed in the light of the findings of the most recent physical re-examination. Sometimes, some of the painful, developmental joint diseases (e.g. hip dysplasia) do not improve rapidly with NSAIDs alone. With hip dysplasia, one component of the lameness is joint laxity and not simply the pain, so even when comfortable the gait of such dogs is not normal. For cases in which pain is not controlled, additional analgesia may be helpful, using the agents described above. It is also useful to re-interrogate the dog's owner and check that the patient's activity is strictly restricted, as previously instructed. If conservative management proves to be unsuccessful, consideration should be given to the surgical options mentioned above.

The low-cost option

For most of the common differentials listed, a diagnosis can be made with a high level of certainty based on the history and a thorough orthopaedic examination, in association with the breed and signalment. However, whenever possible, a radiological diagnosis should be obtained and in most cases, such an examination should be possible using sedation, rather than anaesthesia. For some of the differential diagnoses discussed above, if the orthopaedic problem responds to conservative management, this approach can be continued in the longer term, since many developmental joint diseases appear to become less painful as puppies mature.

When should I refer?

Conservative management of the above conditions is well within the scope of general practice. Advice regarding referral should be sought when a problem eludes a diagnosis after the second or third consultation. Referral should also be offered when challenging orthopaedic surgery is one of the treatment options, since surgical intervention is generally preferred early in the course of disease, when there is still the potential to modify the course of disease.

Martin Owen

Forelimb lameness is common in both young and adult dogs. It is uncommon in cats once infections and trauma have been excluded. It can be acute or chronic, and occur due to trauma or an atraumatic disease process. Severe lameness may result in the animal carrying the limb, whereas less severe lameness can be noticed by the animal 'nodding' on the sound limb when it is walking or trotting. In most cases, forelimb lameness is due to pain.

Common differential diagnoses

Traumatic

- Digital pad or interdigital prick injury
- Foreign bodies – grass seeds, glass
- Nail (claw) injuries
- Ligament sprain of carpus or phalangeal joint
- Cat bite infection (mainly seen in cats)
- Fracture
- Joint luxation.

Atraumatic

- Foot problems – nail bed infections, pododermatitis, plasma cell infiltration of the pads in cats
- Developmental elbow problems – young, medium and large breed dogs (see Chapter 46)
- Shoulder osteochondrosis – young, medium and large breed dogs (see Chapter 46)
- Osteoarthritis – often follows developmental disorders that occurred when young. Most common in the elbow, followed by the shoulder/carpus and the foot
- Tumours – most commonly osteosarcoma (seen most often in the distal radius and proximal humerus; very rarely soft tissue sarcomas)
- Inflammatory arthritis – either septic arthritis, usually affecting a single joint, or immune-mediated polyarthropathy, usually affecting multiple joints
- Soft tissue shoulder problems – bicipital tendonopathy and bursitis, infraspinatus and supraspinatus tendonopathy, glenohumeral ligament insufficiency
- Bone diseases – panosteitis, hypertrophic osteodystrophy.

100 Top Consultations in Small Animal General Practice, First Edition
By Peter Hill, Sheena Warman and Geoff Shawcross
© 2011 Blackwell Publishing Ltd

Diagnostic approach

Some of the traumatic disorders mentioned above may be immediately apparent from the owner's history and a cursory examination. Some diseases are specific to young growing dogs. However, for most of the conditions, clinicians should question the owner to determine if the lameness was the result of trauma or if it had an insidious onset, and to establish the duration, progression and severity of the condition. It should be determined if the lameness varies following rest or activity, or is related to the nature of the ground on which the animal walks (foot problems are often worse on hard ground). In mature dogs, inflammatory and degenerative disorders of joints are often characterised by 'stiffness after rest/exercise', whilst tumours and chronic degeneration of ligaments are characterised by lameness that is unaffected by exercise or rest.

It is important to examine all the limbs of a lame patient as many cases of atraumatic lameness have more than one limb/joint affected, even though the lameness may only be obvious (to the owner) in one limb. Identification of the affected limb(s) is best achieved by observing the pet moving (preferably trotting, though this is not possible for cats or for dogs with severe or multiple limb lameness). A thorough orthopaedic examination of all limbs should be conducted, initially checking topographical anatomy for limb symmetry, muscle atrophy (which indicates a chronic problem or neurological deficit) and swelling. Most clinicians start the examination at the foot and work upwards. Each limb is checked using a combination of visual examination, palpation and physical manipulation. Abnormal anatomical features and any sources of pain should be identified and localised. Comparison with the opposite limb is useful, especially when assessing a pain response. As a general rule, the farther down the limb the lameness is localised, the more severe the lameness appears. As a corollary to this, severe lameness originating high up the limb invariably has a serious cause.

It should also be determined if the pet is in good general health since the diagnostic investigation will be influenced by the presence of concurrent problems.

The most useful ancillary aid for investigating severe or chronic lameness cases is radiography. Many of the conditions listed above can be diagnosed on good quality radiographs (Figure 47.1). Clinicians should choose the sites to be radiographed based on the anatomical/functional abnormalities detected on physical examination. In many cases, it is valuable to radiograph the opposite limb to allow comparison.

Other tests that may be required to investigate forelimb lameness include:

- Cytological (and in some cases bacteriological) analysis of samples of joint fluid from painful or swollen joints (Figure 47.2)
- Cytology of needle aspirates, which is useful for soft tissue swellings
- Suspected tumours should be biopsied, using a Jamshidi needle for bony lesions
- If a neoplastic limb lesion is suspected, radiographs of the inflated thorax should be examined to check for metastatic disease. In these cases, haematological and serum biochemical tests are also indicated.

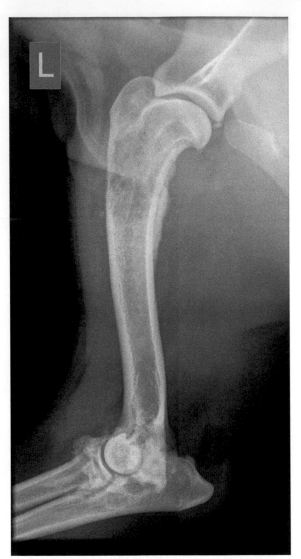

Figure 47.1 Mediolateral radiograph of the humerus showing mottled radiopacity and lucency typical of an osteosarcoma

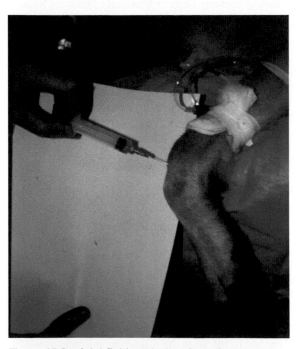

Figure 47.2 Joint fluid aspiration from the carpus

Section 5

Treatment

Minor traumatic injuries are usually treated by removal of any foreign bodies, treatment or prevention of secondary infection and the use of protective/supportive dressings. Nail injuries are best treated by cutting the nail short, application of a protective dressing and use of a broad-spectrum antibiotic to treat/prevent infection. Mild sprains of the distal limb should be supported by a padded dressing for five days. Cat bites or other infections of the limb require systemic antibiotics. More severe traumatic injuries such as fractures or joint luxations require in-patient treatment.

Painful lameness should be treated with appropriate analgesia. For a mild lameness of recent onset, when physical examination shows no evidence of severe disease, the pet's activity should be markedly restricted and a 5-day course of NSAID prescribed. Failure to respond is an indication that further investigation is required. More severe or persistent lameness should be investigated further before prescribing empirical analgesic therapy. Chronic osteoarthritis is managed with an initial 4-week course of NSAIDs and strict rest, followed by gradual increase in controlled activity appropriate to an observed improvement. Following withdrawal of NSAID medication, osteoarthritic pain and lameness may return in some cases and under such circumstances, long-term use of NSAIDs is indicated (see Chapter 50).

Bone tumours or soft tissue sarcomas can be treated by amputation, but the prognosis is poor due to the likelihood of metastatic spread. The welfare of the animal should be considered paramount and advice should be sought from an orthopaedic specialist or oncologist. Inflammatory arthritis can be challenging to diagnose and treat and clinicians should consider referring such cases to appropriate specialists. Developmental conditions of the elbow and shoulder may require surgical intervention (see Chapter 46).

What if it doesn't get better?

The prognosis for forelimb lameness depends on the diagnosis. Many of the traumatic conditions will respond to appropriate conservative management with appropriate analgesia. If the lameness is not responding to what is considered rational treatment,

the animal should be re-examined prior to prescribing further medication. The clinician needs to determine if the diagnosis is correct, or if there an alternative diagnosis which may explain the lack of response.

Soft tissue injuries (sprains, strains and shoulder soft tissue problems) often take more than four weeks to resolve. Distal limb injuries should be continually supported with a padded dressing (checked and/or changed every five to seven days) during the recovery period to prevent further injury through mechanical over-loading of healing tissues.

Refractory lameness due to chronic osteoarthritis may respond to a switch in NSAID, an increase in dose, or adjunctive therapies (see Chapter 50).

Some conditions (such as neoplasia) inherently carry a poor prognosis and a full recovery is very unlikely.

The low-cost option

Costs can be minimised by performing ancillary tests based on a carefully performed physical examination. Radiography of the whole limb in an attempt to find the cause of lameness is not a cost-effective strategy. Most lameness is caused by benign disease and so a 'response to treatment' approach can be taken initially with reasonably low risk of missing a serious disease such as neoplasia. If such an approach is taken, use of the most cost-effective NSAID would be prudent.

When should I refer?

Referral should be discussed if there is no diagnosis and the lameness persists after four weeks of investigation/treatment. Conditions which would benefit from the expertise of a specialist include developmental diseases, difficult fractures, limb tumours (especially if post-amputation chemotherapy is considered), inflammatory arthritis and soft tissue shoulder problems. If referral of the case is not an option, many referral centres provide a radiograph reading service which can enhance the chance of making a definitive diagnosis. Chronic osteoarthritis is usually managed in general practice but surgical options such as total elbow replacement are available at certain referral centres.

Martin Owen

Hindlimb lameness is common in both young and adult dogs. Like forelimb lameness, it can be acute or chronic, and occur due to trauma or an atraumatic disease process. Severe lameness may result in the dog carrying the limb, whereas less severe lameness can be detected by increased vertical displacement of the hindquarter on the affected side, or a shortened stride length. Mild hindlimb lameness and bilateral hindlimb lameness can be difficult to detect and historical findings can be helpful in identifying the problem limb(s), such as obvious stiffness on rising on the affected side. In most cases, hindlimb lameness is due to pain, or pain in combination with a mechanical problem such as joint instability. Hindlimb lameness may be unilateral or bilateral but clinicians should remember that unilateral lameness commonly occurs due to a bilateral disease in which the clinical signs are worse, or more advanced in the lame limb.

Common differential diagnoses

Traumatic

- Digital pad or interdigital penetrating injury
- Foreign bodies – grass seeds, glass
- Nail (claw) injuries
- Cat bite infection (mainly seen in cats)
- Fractures
- Hip luxation
- Stifle ligament rupture, traumatic patellar luxation, stifle luxation
- Hock luxation/shear injury
- Achilles tendon laceration/rupture
- Ligament sprains.

Atraumatic

- Foot problems – nail bed infections, pododermatitis
- Cranial cruciate ligament insufficiency – young large-breed dogs, middle-aged medium-sized dogs and old-aged small-breed dogs (see Chapter 49)
- Patellar luxation – medial in small, medium and large breeds; lateral in giant breeds
- Hip dysplasia
- Osteochondrosis (stifle and hock)

- Osteoarthritis – often follows developmental disorders that occurred when young, e.g. hip dysplasia/osteochondrosis or cranial cruciate ligament disease
- Tumours – osteosarcoma seen most often in the distal femur and tibia; soft tissue sarcoma more commonly affects the stifle and hock
- Inflammatory arthritis – either septic arthritis, usually affecting a single joint and generally osteoarthritic as such joints are prone to developing sepsis from haematogenous spread, or immune-mediated polyarthropathy, usually affecting multiple joints, especially the hocks and carpi
- Soft tissue problems – Achilles tendon injury, gastrocnemius tendonopathy, gracilis contracture (mainly seen in German Shepherd dogs)
- Neurological problems – lumbar and lumbosacral intervertebral disc prolapse, fibrocartilaginous embolus, nerve tissue tumours
- Bone diseases – panosteitis, hypertrophic osteodystrophy (also called metaphyseal osteopathy).

Diagnostic approach

Some of the traumatic disorders mentioned above may be immediately apparent from the owner's history and a cursory examination. However, for most of the conditions, a detailed history should be obtained, establishing whether the lameness was due to trauma or had an insidious onset, and its duration, progression and severity. The presence or absence of lameness or stiffness in other limbs in addition to the limb of primary concern should be determined. In mature dogs, inflammatory and degenerative disorders of joints are often characterised by 'stiffness after rest/exercise'.

It is important to examine all the limbs of a lame patient as many cases of atraumatic lameness have more than one limb/joint affected, even though the lameness may only be obvious (to the owner) in one limb. The lame limb(s) should be determined by observing the pet moving (preferably trotting, though this is not possible for cats or for dogs with severe or

100 Top Consultations in Small Animal General Practice, First Edition
By Peter Hill, Sheena Warman and Geoff Shawcross
© 2011 Blackwell Publishing Ltd

multiple lameness). A thorough orthopaedic examination of all limbs should be conducted, working from distal to proximal. Each limb is examined using a combination of visual examination, palpation and physical manipulation in order to check for pain, limb symmetry, muscle atrophy or swelling. Joints should be flexed and extended to detect pain, laxity or crepitus. Specific manipulations used to assess hip dysplasia and cruciate ligament insufficiency are described in Chapters 46 and 49. The pet's general health should also be assessed as diagnostic investigations are influenced by the presence of concurrent problems.

For severe or chronic lameness, the sites of anatomical/functional abnormality identified on orthopaedic examination should be radiographed under heavy sedation or general anaesthesia (Figure 48.1). Further physical examination under sedation/anaesthesia often reveals additional findings not detected in the conscious animal.

Other tests that may be required to investigate hindlimb lameness include:

- Cytological (and in some cases bacteriological) analysis of samples of joint fluid from painful or swollen joints
- Cytology of needle aspirates from soft tissue swellings
- Biopsy of suspected tumours, using a Jamshidi needle for bony lesions
- Radiographs of the inflated thorax to check for metastatic disease if a neoplastic limb lesion is suspected
- Haematological and serum biochemical tests if neoplastic or immune-mediated disease is suspected.

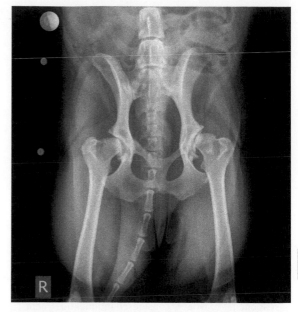

Figure 48.1   Ventrodorsal view of a dog's hips showing severe changes of osteoarthritis

Treatment

Minor traumatic injuries are usually treated by removal of any foreign bodies, treatment or prevention of secondary infection and the use of protective/supportive dressings. Nail injuries are best treated by cutting the nail short, application of a protective dressing and use of a broad-spectrum antibiotic to treat/prevent infection. Mild sprains of the distal limb should be supported by a padded dressing for five days. Cat bites or other infections of the limb require systemic antibiotics. More severe traumatic injuries such as fractures or joint luxations require

in-patient treatment. Cases requiring surgical intervention should be identified and treated as soon as possible.

Non-surgical, painful lameness should be treated with appropriate analgesia. For mild, short-duration lameness, when orthopaedic examination does not reveal a diagnosis for which there is a specific treatment, the pet's activity should be strictly restricted and a five-day course of NSAIDs prescribed. Failure to respond is an indicator for further investigation. Suspected sprains of the distal limb should be supported by a padded dressing for five days and NSAIDs should be given. If clinical findings, radiology and/or needle aspiration suggest a neoplasm is present, prompt staging of the tumour and appropriate treatment are indicated. Clinicians should seek specialist advice to identify the most current treatment options.

Specific surgical treatment options generally give the best outcomes for the management of severe hip dysplasia, cruciate ligament rupture, patella luxation and osteochondrosis (see Chapters 46 and 49). These procedures should be performed by clinicians with expertise in orthopaedic surgery. If surgical management is not pursued, medical treatment with NSAIDs is beneficial for affected patients but ongoing lameness and progressive osteoarthritis is inevitable.

Osteoarthritis affecting joints in the hindlimb can be managed with NSAIDs, rest and body weight reduction as described in Chapter 50. Suspected septic arthritis should be investigated by analysis of a joint fluid sample taken from the affected joint and treated with antimicrobial agents selected on the basis of culture and sensitivity testing. Broad-spectrum therapy, e.g. amoxicillin/clavulanic acid, should be administered pending bacterial sensitivity results.

The low-cost option

Costs can be minimised by directing ancillary tests based on carefully performed physical examination, avoiding unnecessary imaging or tests on normal structures. Most lameness is caused by benign disease and so a 'response to treatment' approach can be taken initially with reasonably low risk of missing a serious disease such as neoplasia.

What if it doesn't get better?

The prognosis for hindlimb lameness depends on the diagnosis. Many of the traumatic conditions will respond to appropriate conservative management with appropriate analgesia. If the lameness is not responding to what is considered rational treatment, the animal should be re-examined prior to prescribing further medication. The clinician needs to determine if the diagnosis is correct, or if there is an alternative diagnosis which may explain the lack of response. Any new findings should be investigated.

Some conditions that might have been managed medically initially (e.g. cruciate ligament disease, hip dysplasia or patellar luxation) may require surgical intervention in order to resolve the lameness. Once osteoarthritis is present, long-term intermittent lameness can be expected and various strategies may need to be employed to keep the animal comfortable (see Chapter 50). Some chronic hindlimb lamenesses, in which a diagnosis has been made but for which there is no useful surgical intervention, may be assisted by aquatic exercise.

Some conditions (such as neoplasia) inherently carry a poor prognosis and a full recovery is very unlikely.

When should I refer?

Referral should be discussed if there is no diagnosis and the lameness persists after four weeks of investigation/treatment. Conditions which would benefit from the expertise of a specialist include developmental diseases, difficult fractures, limb tumours (especially if post-amputation chemotherapy is considered), inflammatory arthritis and soft tissue problems. If referral of the case is not an option, many referral centres provide a radiograph reading service which can enhance the chance of making a definitive diagnosis. Chronic osteoarthritis is usually managed in general practice but surgical options such as total hip and stifle replacement are available at certain referral centres.

Martin Owen

Aetiology and pathogenesis

Cranial cruciate ligament insufficiency (CCLI) is the most common cause of spontaneous unilateral hindleg lameness in the dog. It occurs due to degeneration and stretching or progressive rupture of the CCL. The cause of the ligamentous degeneration is unknown but disease is most common in medium- and large-breed dogs, from four years of age onward. Prevalence is increased in females and with obesity. In giant breeds, CCL degeneration may occur more rapidly, resulting in clinical signs at a younger age. In contrast, in small breeds, CCL degeneration occurs more slowly so clinical signs generally occur in older dogs. Minor trauma to the degenerate ligament often leads to tearing, or complete rupture. Occasionally, a healthy CCL ligament can be ruptured by trauma (this may be the most common cause in cats), and rarely, it occurs secondary to immune-mediated polyarthritis (but this usually affects multiple joints). In all cases, CCLI is associated with joint inflammation, effusion and the development of secondary osteoarthritis. Most cases of CCLI develop cranio-caudal laxity of the stifle joint which can lead to meniscal tearing, especially in medium and large dogs.

History and clinical signs

CCLI can present in one of two ways. The first is a history of stiffness and mild lameness, which initially responds to rest and analgesia. Progressively, the lameness worsens and becomes refractory to medical management. The second presentation is a sudden onset severe lameness. Sudden worsening of a mild chronic lameness is likely to indicate progression of a partially torn ligament to a full tear, and/or a meniscal injury. Physical examination reveals lameness varying from 1/10 to 10/10 and various anatomical changes around the stifle joint that can be detected by careful palpation (see below). Examination often reveals bilateral disease in dogs with unilateral lameness. With degenerative disease, once one CCL ruptures there is a 30–50% chance of subsequent contralateral CCL rupture.

100 Top Consultations in Small Animal General Practice, First Edition
By Peter Hill, Sheena Warman and Geoff Shawcross
© 2011 Blackwell Publishing Ltd

Specific diagnostic techniques

Careful palpation of the affected limb identifies pain on full flexion and extension of the stifle. There may be atrophy of the thigh muscles. On the cranial aspect of the joint the palpable definition of the patellar ligament is obscured by joint swelling and joint effusion. In most cases, palpation of the medial aspect of the stifle and proximal tibia reveals a smooth fibrous swelling (known as medial buttress) that is characteristic of the chronic joint pathology of CCL disease. This finding alone has high diagnostic accuracy.

In advanced cases, cranio-caudal laxity is detectable. Two specific techniques can be performed to evaluate cranio-caudal stifle instability. In conscious animals, the 'tibial thrust test' is the preferred method because it is relatively painless (Figure 49.1). The femur is restrained in one hand with the index finger aligned on and passing distally over the patella, the patellar ligament and onto the tibial tuberosity. The hock and foot are held in the other hand and the hock is flexed whilst resisting the resultant reciprocal flexion of the stifle. CCLI allows cranial translation of the proximal tibia and the tibial tuberosity displaces the index finger. The 'cranial drawer test' is best performed in sedated/anaesthetised patients, or only in stoical conscious patients (Figure 49.2). The distal femur is held with the fingers on the patella and the thumb on the lateral fabella. The second hand grasps the proximal tibia with the fingers on the tibial tuberosity and thumb on the fibula head. Cranially directed force is applied to the proximal crus, avoiding twisting or flexing/extending the stifle. CCLI allows cranial translation ('draw') of the tibia. The test should be performed both with the stifle flexed and extended to avoid missing a partial CCL rupture. There is a degree of skill required in both of these manipulations and new graduates should first perform them under the guidance of an experienced clinician in order to ensure that correct results are obtained.

Radiography is valuable to characterise secondary changes in the stifle joint, and to ensure that no other disease process is causing the stifle lameness (such as a fractured patella, an osteosarcoma of the tibia or femur, or osteoarthritis secondary to stifle osteochondrosis). The radiographic signs are those of joint effusion and degenerative joint disease. The mediolateral view will show increased soft tissue density of the cranial joint space due to effusion and loss of the infrapatellar fat pad. Osteophytes (on the trochlear ridges and fabellae) and patellar ligament enthesiophytes (present at the tibial and patellar insertions) are usually present. Joint fluid analysis is only useful if immune-mediated disease is suspected.

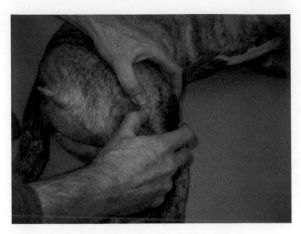

Figure 49.2 **Cranial drawer test. The stifle is carefully grasped with both hands, on the recognised bony landmarks. With cranial cruciate ligament rupture, the tibia can be drawn cranially in a direction that is parallel with the tibial plateau**

Treatment

In the majority of small dogs (less than 15 kg) and cats, medical management gives a satisfactory outcome. Restoration of function may be achieved more rapidly following surgical intervention, though there is no supportive evidence for this from controlled clinical studies. In these small patients, CCL disease often presents with an acute episode of painful lameness and complete rupture of the CCL. Conservative management requires strict restriction of activity for four weeks. The discomfort is treated with NSAIDs as long as obvious pain is present. A light support dressing placed from the proximal thigh, distally to include the toes applied for five days may further improve patient comfort. Such dressings are only practicable in long-legged lean dogs, otherwise they do not remain in place. As the lameness gradually improves, and as the stifle restabilises with fibrosis, limited incremental lead exercise is permitted. The lameness should resolve after approximately 12 weeks.

In larger dogs (more than 15 kg) the choice of treatment is influenced by the stage of the disease process and the severity. Early in the course of the degenerative form of CCLI, the milder signs of stiffness and lameness can be controlled using NSAIDs and restriction of activity. Such recommendations

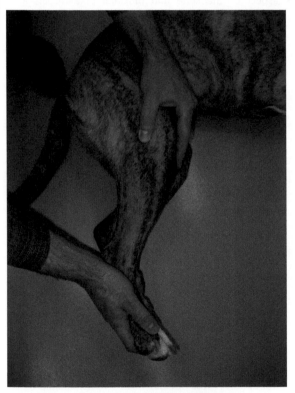

Figure 49.1 **Tibial thrust test. The stifle is maintained at a fixed angle, simulating weight bearing. The hock is slowly and progressively flexed firmly whilst the tendency for reciprocal flexion of the stifle is resisted. The index finger of the hand grasping the stifle is placed on the tibial tuberosity. With cranial cruciate ligament rupture, tibial thrust is detected by displacement of the index finger on the tibial tuberosity**

may control the clinical signs but they do not affect the progression of the disease. Eventually the problem becomes refractory to NSAID treatment. At this stage, there may be no instability, mild instability or complete ligament rupture.

Surgical intervention is recommended for severe, acute cases, or those that have progressed from a less severe form but now have intractable lameness. Further rest and NSAIDs are unlikely to give a satisfactory outcome in these cases. A number of surgical techniques are currently recommended for the management of CCLI, but they all involve a mechanism to address cranio-caudal instability. The two most commonly used procedures are:

- Extracapsular stabilising techniques, e.g. lateral fabellotibial suture
- Tibial osteotomy techniques, e.g. tibial plateau levelling osteotomy, tibial tuberosity advancement, triple tibial osteotomy.

Surgical techniques that were previously used, but are no longer recommended, include the 'over the top' technique, the intracapsular skin graft technique and fibular head advancement. Regardless of the technique used, an arthrotomy should be performed to check for, and treat, medial meniscal tears.

Analgesia and strict rest are essential following surgery. After suture removal at 10 days, a programme of gradual return to activity is recommended, with exercise level dictated by rate of resolution, post-surgical discomfort and lameness. Provided progress is satisfactory, the following approach is recommended, although the degree of commitment by the owner will determine how much of the advice is followed.

Weeks 1 and 2

- Strict house confinement apart from 5 minutes of slow walking on the leash three times a day
- Physiotherapy comprising gently flexing and extending all the joints in the leg, ten times, three times a day.
- Aquatic exercise (swimming/treadmill) may be introduced if available following healing of the skin incision. Evidence suggests that the greatest benefits are achieved following intensive early postoperative aquatic exercise.

Weeks 3 and 4

- 10–15 minutes of slow leash walk three to five times a day
- Physiotherapy as above. Encouraging 'sit to stand' transitions may improve stifle joint flexion at this stage.
- Aquatic exercise as above.

Weeks 5 and 6

- 20–25 minutes of leash walks three to five times a day
- Aquatic exercise as above.

Weeks 7 and 8

Leash walks of 30-minute duration three to five times per day.

Brisk walks and gentle off-leash exercise can be introduced after eight weeks, and thereafter, gradual return to normal activity should be pursued, in accordance with the patient's previous function and exercise behaviour. A full return to normal activity levels may not be possible for 4–6 months.

The longer term problems associated with osteoarthritis can be managed as described in Chapter 50.

What if it doesn't get better?

The recovery from CCLI is generally slow, taking 3–6 months with either conservative management or surgery. Clients must be warned about this in advance so that they have realistic expectations. If there is no improvement with conservative management, the possibility of meniscal injury should be evaluated either by arthrotomy or arthroscopic surgery. Owners should also be aware that even with successful surgery, it may not be possible for the dog to return to full athletic activity without there being a degree of lameness. Also, the development of degenerative joint disease is almost inevitable and will lead to some lameness in the future. The presence of inflammatory joint disease will also result in failure to improve with medical management. This can be diagnosed by joint fluid analysis.

The low-cost option

Costs can be minimised in the diagnostic phase by a skilful and careful physical examination to identify medial buttress and/or a positive thrust test. In a patient with the appropriate history and signalment, this is almost pathognomonic for CCLI. This can prevent the need for further tests such as radiography of other joints. To reduce costs, it is possible to take a conservative management approach in all sizes of patients, in the knowledge that it will be effective in most small animals but fewer large dogs. In the latter group, surgery is recommended if the lameness is not showing signs of resolution after six weeks. If this is still not possible, clients must be warned that long-term lameness is likely to be the outcome.

When should I refer?

Conservative management of CCLI is readily performed in the general practice setting. Surgical management of this disease is best performed by clinicians with the necessary expertise to offer a range of surgical options (including dynamic stabilising techniques), and the ability to deal with meniscal injuries. This may require referral to a specialist. If referral is not an option, clinicians may have to offer the surgical technique with which they are most familiar, although clients should be advised that this may not be the optimal approach.

Martin Owen

Aetiology and pathogenesis

The development of osteoarthritis is a complex process involving the interaction between degradative and repair processes in cartilage, bone and synovium, with a secondary component of inflammation. The disease mainly affects articular cartilage but changes also occur in the subchondral bone, the synovium and the synovial fluid. The process is irreversible and progressive, despite any current medical interventions. Most osteoarthritis in dogs and cats is secondary, resulting from problems such as developmental abnormalities, joint instability, joint incongruity or trauma. Osteoarthritis typically follows such conditions as osteochondrosis, hip dysplasia, patellar luxation, CCL disease or fractures involving the joint. Primary osteoarthritis (where there is no known predisposing cause) is uncommon in animals but it can occur in the elbow joint of cats.

History and clinical signs

Osteoarthritis in dogs most commonly presents as lameness or reluctance to walk. Usually, the disease has been present for some considerable time before clinical signs are evident. Owners' observations include stiffness, reluctance to exercise and reluctance to jump/play/climb stairs. In early or mild cases, the lameness may be most noticeable after rest but can disappear during exercise. In more severe cases, the lameness may be exacerbated after exercise. Acute presentations are often associated with minor trauma or with excessive exercise. Exacerbation of signs may occur with cold, damp weather. Cats with osteoarthritis may just appear to be less active than normal.

Specific diagnostic techniques

Osteoarthritis is best evaluated using a combination of physical examination and radiography. Palpation of

the joints and testing for range of motion will reveal some of the following findings:

- Joint swelling (effusion, peri-articular fibrosis, osteophytes)
- Reduced range of motion (detected by passive flexion and extension to extremes of joint motion)
- Joint pain (evident at extremes of joint range of motion)
- Crepitus
- Heat and swelling (only in cases with active inflammation).

The osteoarthritic stifle joint should be examined for craniocaudal instability using the cranial drawer test or the tibial thrust test to check for CCL disease (see Chapter 49) and the patella should be checked for luxation since these underlying diseases may be responsible for osteoarthritis.

Diseased joints should be radiographed, taking two orthogonal views, but clinicians should remember that the severity of any radiographic signs of osteoarthritis do not necessarily correlate with the severity of clinical signs. Typical radiological features of osteoarthritis include:

- Osteophytosis (new bone formation at the margins of the joint)
- Bone remodelling (evident as a change in contour of the articular bone, e.g. flattening of the femoral head, shallowing and widening of the acetabulum)
- Soft tissue swelling
- Joint effusion (only visible in the stifle joint)
- Intra-articular and peri-articular mineralisation (particularly in cats)
- Subluxation (partial separation of articular surfaces)
- Subchondral sclerosis (visible as increased radiopacity of subchondral bone adjacent to the articular surface).

If the joint pain is marked or the diagnosis is uncertain, a joint fluid sample should be taken for cytological examination to investigate for inflammatory joint disease.

Treatment

The medical treatment of osteoarthritis is palliative and not curative. It is unlikely that a dog or cat with osteoarthritis will be able to achieve sustained athletic performance, but a reasonable level of normal pet activity should be the goal of effective treatment. There are three components to the treatment regime:

Lifestyle adjustment

Initially, the activity of lame/stiff pets should be strictly restricted for 4 weeks. High impact activity, such as jumping and rapid acceleration/deceleration should be avoided. Once clinical signs are controlled, gradual re-introduction to gentle activity is permitted. Activity levels are gradually increased to a satisfactory level that does not induce lameness. If, at any stage, lameness recurs, a short period of rest of up to four weeks is necessary to achieve resolution, before resuming exercise. Activity/exercise should be regular and controlled each day since irregular levels or types of activity predispose to joint pain. Exercise levels need not be unnecessarily restricted provided that activity-induced lameness/stiffness does not occur.

Treatment of pain and inflammation

A 7-day course of NSAID is recommended initially (see Appendix 3 for drugs and dosages). If there is a satisfactory response to treatment, continued therapy for 2–4 weeks is recommended to prevent early recurrence of lameness/stiffness. Once clinical signs have been controlled for 4 weeks, trial withdrawal of medication is recommended to establish if long-term medication is necessary.

If clinical signs are not controlled after four weeks of treatment, a change to a different NSAID is indicated. Rapid switching from one NSAID to another has resulted in severe gastrointestinal problems in some animals. In order to avoid this, a 5–7-day 'wash out' period is recommended before introducing the new drug. During this time, pain relief can be provided with paracetamol (acetaminophen, 10 mg/kg q12 hours, but not in cats), codeine (0.5–2 mg/kg q12 hours) or tramadol (2–4 mg/kg q12 hours).

In many dogs and cats, the discomfort associated with osteoarthritis becomes so chronic that they become NSAID-dependent. These animals should be given the long-term medication that is most effective at relieving their clinical signs. It is prudent to con-

sider the implications of long-term NSAID medication and to perform regular checks (clinical and laboratory) to ensure continued safety (see Appendix 3 for further details).

Nutraceuticals such as glucosamine and essential fatty acids have proven clinical efficacy in the management of osteoarthritis, both in humans and in dogs. These can be given either as dietary supplements, or in diets specially formulated for the management of osteoarthritis. In mild cases, these products may be able to control the pain of osteoarthritis as sole agents. In more severe cases, they can be used as adjunctive treatments or to facilitate lower doses of NSAIDs. They may also slow the clinical progression of disease. If effective, they should be given on a long-term basis.

Other products that are available as aids in the management of osteoarthritis due to their putative chondroprotective effects include pentosan polysulphate, chondroitin sulphate and hyaluronic acid. Although some clinicians perceive a benefit from using these products, there is currently no strong scientific evidence to support their use in osteoarthritic dogs and cats. Likewise, although acupuncture has been described as a treatment for osteoarthritis, to the author's knowledge, there is as yet no published evidence of its efficacy. In some cases, physiotherapy and hydrotherapy appear to be beneficial.

Weight control

Obesity is a major contributor to the progression and signs of osteoarthritis. Obesity is to be avoided and lean body mass should be achieved by ensuring that osteoarthritic patients follow a calorie-controlled diet.

What if it doesn't get better?

Failure of osteoarthritis to respond to the above treatment recommendations can occur for the following reasons:

- There is an undetected underlying condition such as CCL disease, patellar luxation, fragmented coronoid disease, hip dysplasia, or lumbosacral disc disease
- There is an additional undetected orthopaedic problem such as stifle disease in a dog with osteoarthritis of the hips

- There could be septic arthritis (a joint fluid sample should be taken to investigate)
- The osteoarthritis may be too severe to control with medical management.

Intra-articular injection of methylprednisolone may be helpful when there is a single painful osteoarthritic joint that is refractory to systemic medication. Prior to injection, joint fluid should be examined and the possibility of joint sepsis must be excluded. Strictly aseptic precautions must be used to avoid introduction of potential pathogens since intra-articular steroids compromise local immune mechanisms.

For some of the above problems, surgical options are available that can resolve the chronic pain of osteoarthritis. These include total hip replacement, excision arthroplasty, total stifle replacement, total elbow replacement, and arthrodesis of the hock and carpus.

The low-cost option

A presumptive diagnosis of osteoarthritis can be made on the basis of a careful history and physical examination. Empirical treatment can be prescribed in such cases, even if financial limitations preclude radiography. However, failure of the condition to respond to a one-week trial of NSAID therapy is an indication for further investigation. Prednoleucotropin, an older anti-inflammatory drug combination, is less costly than some of the newer NSAIDs and it can be effective in managing the pain of chronic osteoarthritis. The prednisolone component of this drug may not be desirable in a long-term treatment plan, but the potential for side-effects may have to be accepted if financial restrictions dictate.

When should I refer?

Most cases of osteoarthritis are manageable in the general practice setting. Referral should be considered if the stiffness/lameness has not been satisfactorily controlled after three consultations, in case additional problems have gone undetected. The surgical management of arthritic joints by total replacement or arthrodesis should only be undertaken by specialist orthopaedic surgeons.

Section 5

Martin Owen

Aetiology and pathogenesis

Fractures occur when bones are subjected to forces that exceed their ability to resist deformation. Most fractures occur as a result of trauma, in which a substantial force is applied to a bone of normal strength. Pathological fractures occur when smaller forces are applied to abnormal bone, which has reduced strength secondary to a disease such as neoplasia or nutritional secondary hyperparathyroidism.

History and clinical signs

Generally, a traumatic event has occurred, though this may not have been observed. A fracture to a single limb usually results in non-weight-bearing lameness, but patients suffering major trauma may be non-ambulatory, because of multiple injuries or perhaps due to spinal trauma. In such cases, compromise to other body systems (e.g. the thorax or abdomen) may be obvious. If a long bone fracture occurs in an adult large-breed dog without any history of trauma, the clinician should be suspicious of a pathological fracture, since bone tumours are prevalent in such dogs.

Specific diagnostic techniques

Prior to examination, owners may need to be given advice about moving an animal with a suspected fracture, or an injured animal may need to be carried into the hospital from a car. Although the use of blankets or stretchers can be helpful, this method of moving injured animals can result in the animal struggling which may induce further injury to a fractured limb or an injured spine. Hence if the animal is small enough, it is preferable to carry it with one arm under its neck and another under its abdomen, letting its

legs hang down. Dogs usually accept this position without struggling and limb fractures will not be further damaged. Cats should be carefully lifted into a basket in order to be transported.

Animals that cannot walk should be investigated carefully for evidence of spinal damage. Spinal fractures are generally associated with vertebral column pain and signs of neurological dysfunction (rigidity or flaccidity) of the forelimbs, hindlimbs and/or the tail/anal sphincter. Care should be taken to avoid twisting and bending the vertebral column until the possibility of a spinal injury is eliminated by physical and neurological examination.

Patients with fractures should be initially assessed for more serious problems such as internal injuries or shock. For suspected road traffic accident patients (see Chapter 77), thoracic radiographs are indicated, checking for signs of serious injury such as rib fractures, pneumothorax or free pleural fluid. In many cases, especially those with hindlimb trauma, abdominal radiographs should also be performed and particular care should be paid to checking the integrity of the urinary system. The circulatory function of trauma cases must be carefully monitored, with attention paid to peripheral pulse quality, mucous membrane colour and capillary refill. Haematological and serum biochemical analyses can also provide useful information, although changes in such variables can lag behind pathological changes occurring in organs and body systems.

Examination of a suspected fracture requires careful physical examination including gentle palpation and manipulation. This usually reveals pain and swelling. Instability and crepitus may be evident when the limb is moved, depending on the bone involved. Limb injuries should be carefully examined for penetration of the skin and soft tissues (an open fracture). These require urgent treatment and carry a more guarded prognosis than closed fractures. Pinching the toes should elicit conscious pain perception and withdrawal, indicating that neuronal function is intact. Sometimes, it is necessary to squeeze the entire digit (bone and soft tissues together) firmly with a haemostat to elicit a response. Absence of withdrawal may indicate a nerve injury.

100 Top Consultations in Small Animal General Practice, First Edition
By Peter Hill, Sheena Warman and Geoff Shawcross
© 2011 Blackwell Publishing Ltd

Painful and/or unstable limb segments and/or joints should be radiographed. Often a single mediolateral projection radiograph is adequate to identify a fracture (Figure 51.1). For thorough evaluation of the injury, two orthogonal views of the fractured region should be taken. If repair of a limb fracture is intended, radiographs of the contralateral limb region are also useful, since the shape of the normal bone is a good template for planning fracture repair. When spinal injuries are investigated, only lateral projection radiographs are required, avoiding unnecessary repositioning of the patient. These radiographs should be evaluated carefully because fractures and subluxations can self-reduce because of the splinting effect of the axial musculature, minimising the displacement visible radiographically.

Treatment

Patients showing signs of circulatory system failure should receive appropriate rates of IV fluid therapy in order to support and maintain circulatory function. Treatment should be given for life-threatening problems and analgesia should be provided with judicious use of opiates and NSAIDs, once management of the circulatory function compromise is under way.

Prior to the definitive repair of fractures, 'first aid' treatment can be provided with support dressings (Figure 51.2). These improve patient comfort and avoid further damage occurring at the fracture site through displacement. Modified Robert Jones dressings are most appropriate, incorporating splinting material, if possible, to increase rigidity of the dressing. However, splinting needs to be carried out with care and circumspection in conscious animals. Splinting a fracture in a conscious patient can be an extremely painful process, especially if the fracture is not reduced and/or if a joint is involved. Successful splinting of the proximal limb (above the elbow or stifle) requires incorporation of the trunk into the limb bandage. This can be particularly challenging and is not possible in all cases. Splinting is most effective in the anaesthetised/sedated patient, but such sedation/anaesthesia should only be carried out once the patient's physiological status indicates that it is reasonable to do so.

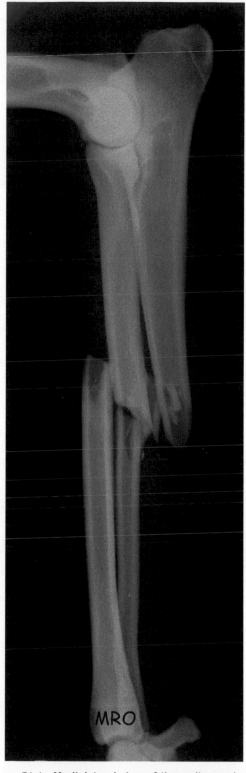

Figure 51.1 **Mediolateral view of the radius and ulna of a dog showing a closed, mildly comminuted fracture of the mid shafts of the radius and ulna**

Open fractures are orthopaedic emergencies and additional care is indicated. In the short term, the wound should be covered with sterile dressings and a support bandage as necessary. As soon as practicable, the patient should be anaesthetised and the contaminated wound should be cleaned, using surgical principles of asepsis. The hair should be clipped in a wide zone surrounding the wound. The wound should be covered with a hydrogel so that clipped hair that enters the wound will stick to the gel and can be subsequently flushed away. The surrounding skin should then be aseptically cleaned. Exposed bone is lavaged with isotonic sterile saline and all contamination and dead tissue is carefully removed (Figure 51.3). Any protruding bone fragments that are still attached to soft tissues should be replaced within the soft tissue envelope. Small bone fragments without soft tissue attachments should be discarded because they risk becoming sequestra as the healing process progresses. Once thoroughly lavaged, a bacterial culture swab should be taken from the fracture site for culture and sensitivity testing. The wound should then be covered with hydrogel and a sterile dressing, and the fracture should be support dressed/splinted. Following emergency first-aid treatment, definitive fracture stabilisation should be planned and performed, generally within the next 48 hours.

Patients with vertebral column fractures should ideally be restrained in lateral recumbency, on a flat, firm surface in order to prevent them from moving and further displacing the fracture fragments, risking spinal cord injury. If necessary, chemical restraint can be carefully administered, avoiding compromise to cardiorespiratory function. However, some patients become very anxious if physically restrained in lateral recumbency and struggle to assume sternal recumbency with a risk of making matters worse. Clinicians therefore need to assess the situation on a case-by-case basis in order to provide an optimal level of movement restriction. In some cases it is preferable to maintain the patient in a quiet and comfortable rested/mildly sedated state in a kennel whilst maintaining appropriate analgesia.

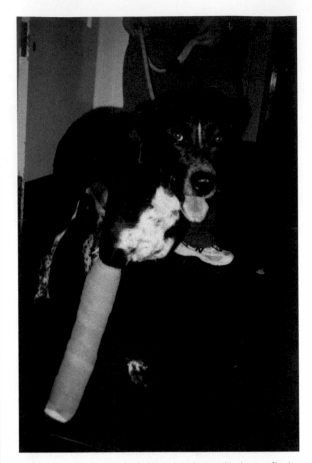

Figure 51.2 **A splinted dressing is applied as a first aid measure to stabilise a radius and ulnar fracture**

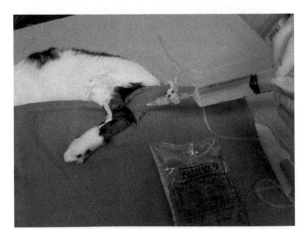

Figure 51.3 **An open fracture of the hock is lavaged using sterile saline. The surrounding hair has been clipped and the skin has been aseptically prepared and gross debris and necrotic tissue has been removed using sterile surgical instruments**

What if it doesn't get better?

Following reduction and stabilisation of a limb bone fracture, weight-bearing is expected within one to five days. Failure to use the limb, or worsening lameness following initially satisfactory progress, are indicators for re-investigation including repeat radiological evaluation. Conservatively managed patients with fractures that are not stabilised (e.g. pelvic fractures) should start to be ambulatory, with assistance, within five days of injury; failure to achieve this warrants re-evaluation and consideration of prompt surgical management.

For vertebral column fractures, the prognosis depends on the degree of spinal cord damage. If deep pain perception is present the prognosis is fair-to-good for recovery. If deep pain perception is absent, the prognosis for recovery is negligible and euthanasia is recommended.

stable/unlikely to displace further with conservative treatment.

Fractures suited to conservative management are identified following radiographic examination of the anaesthetised patient. For suitable long-bone fractures, reduction is achieved by manipulation under general anaesthesia. Stabilisation is then achieved using a cast. The cast should be longitudinally split once applied, to facilitate planned removal and rechecking of the limb at a later date. The cast can then be replaced without the requirement for anaesthesia.

For patients with severe fractures, multiple fractures or spinal fractures, euthanasia may have to be considered if there are insufficient funds to cover the costs of repair.

The low-cost option

Unfortunately, only a few selected fractures in dogs and cats can be managed satisfactorily with conservative management. These include:

- Some pelvic fractures
- Some small-bone fractures such as metatarsal and metacarpal bones
- Some long-bone fractures that are inherently stable once they are reduced by external manipulation (e.g. diaphyseal/metaphyseal tibial/radial fractures with intact fibula/ulna, respectively)
- Some physeal fractures in immature animals that are minimally displaced and which are

When should I refer?

Many fractures require specialist veterinary orthopaedic treatment for an optimal outcome. Clinicians should carefully assess each fracture patient on an individual basis in order to determine if satisfactory fracture repair can be performed in their own clinic. If radiological interpretation of the fracture indicates that repair will be challenging or that there is a significant risk of a poor outcome using the practice facilities, then expert advice and/or referral should be sought. It is preferable that specialist orthopaedic treatment is sought at initial presentation rather than making an initial attempt at fracture repair in the primary clinic which is likely to have an unsatisfactory outcome.

Martin Owen

Spinal pain can be one of the most severe forms of pain that dogs experience. It is one of the few occasions in which dogs may scream in pain in anticipation of being touched. Intervertebral disc disease is the most common cause of spinal pain and/or paresis/paralysis in dogs (Figure 52.1). It is most prevalent in chondrodystrophoid dogs (e.g. Dachshunds) but it also occurs in non-chondrodystrophoid dogs and in cats. It occurs due to degeneration of the nucleus pulposus which loses its 'shock-absorbing' properties. The hardened nucleus of the disc may subsequently tear through the annulus fibrosus and herniate into the vertebral canal. This pathology results in perineural inflammation resulting in spinal pain. Severe herniation into the vertebral canal crushes the spinal cord leading to cord ischaemia and disturbance of neuronal transmission. Disc protrusions can be acute (Type I, most common in chondrodystrophoid breeds) or slowly progressive (Type II, most common in large breed, non-chondrodystrophoid dogs, such as the German Shepherd dog).

Spinal pain also occurs less commonly with developmental problems, inflammatory diseases, neoplasia or secondary to musculoskeletal trauma. Spondylosis of the spine is a common finding in radiographs of older dogs but it is rarely a cause of spinal pain.

Common differential diagnoses

- Intervertebral disc disease
- Developmental abnormality (e.g. atlanto-axial subluxation, cervical spondylopathy)
- Spinal trauma
- Meningitis/granulomatous meningoencephalitis
- Discospondylitis
- Immune-mediated polyarthropathy
- Spinal neoplasia, affecting a vertebral body or nervous tissue
- Fibrocartilaginous embolism.

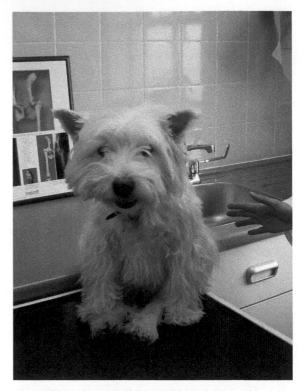

Figure 52.1 Paraplegic dog sitting abnormally because of loss of motor function in the pelvic limbs

100 Top Consultations in Small Animal General Practice, First Edition
By Peter Hill, Sheena Warman and Geoff Shawcross
© 2011 Blackwell Publishing Ltd

Diagnostic approach

A detailed history should be obtained since spinal disease can be accompanied by other organ system disease (e.g. bacterial infection of the urinary tract, which occurs commonly with discospondylitis). A full clinical examination should be performed to check for signs of disease in other body systems prior to investigating neurological function and spinal pain. Pyrexia in particular may heighten suspicion of an inflammatory or infectious process, although in some cases, severely painful lesions alone can result in mild pyrexia.

Making a specific diagnosis in a dog or cat with spinal pain requires a careful spinal and neurological examination. If the animal can still walk, its gait should be observed to see if there is any weakness or ataxia (see Chapter 85). A methodical neurological examination should then be performed to localise any neurological deficits to a region(s) of the spinal cord. The severity of any compromise to spinal cord function should be determined by careful interpretation of the neurological tests. Milder spinal cord injuries are characterised by increased reflexivity when the extensor muscles/tendons are percussed. The loss of conscious pain sensation is consistent with a severe spinal cord injury. Conscious pain sensation can be assessed by firmly pinching the bony part of the toes with haemostats. If present, the patient will show a behavioural response to the painful stimulus (e.g. cry, attempt to move away, look at or try to bite the clinician). If absent, there will be either no movement of the limb, or a reflex movement of the limb with no behavioural response.

Localisation of the spinal pain is the last part of the examination and is achieved by careful palpation, manipulation and application of pressure to the spine. Clinicians should be aware that this can lead to sudden extreme pain and the dog/cat may scream, especially when the cervical spine is involved.

In view of the possibility of spinal pain occurring in the presence of systemic disease (e.g. inflammatory spinal disease or neoplasia), and as a pre-anaesthetic check, routine haematological and serum biochemistry analysis is prudent before considering undertaking further investigations.

Patients without evidence of additional body system disease should be anaesthetised in order to perform a radiological examination of the abnormal region of spine. A carefully positioned, well-collimated series of images taken using appropriate radiographic settings is essential and careful interpretation is necessary to identify relevant spinal pathology. The radiographic technique is critical. The spine must be absolutely parallel to the table or the intervertebral disc spaces will look smaller than they actually are, leading to a potential misdiagnosis of a diseased intervertebral disc.

Radiological changes commonly associated with disc disease include mineralisation of the intervertebral disc, narrowing of the disc space, and/or presence of mineralised disc material superimposed upon the vertebral canal (Figure 52.2). The width of the disc space is more important than disc calcification because narrowing of the disc space suggests loss of nuclear material (i.e. disc herniation). Radiological changes are not normally seen with polyarthropathies or with meningitis. Radiological changes associated with discospondylitis may not be apparent early in the course of the disease. Typically, dogs affected with discospondylitis have marked vertebral column pain and sometimes, neurological deficits are evident. When radiological signs are evident, they are characterised by destruction of the end plates of the vertebral bodies adjacent to the affected disc. The intervertebral disc space appears irregular in width. Later in the disease, the disc space appears narrowed due to collapse. Chronic discospondylitis is associated with ventral spondylosis.

If plain radiographs do not yield a diagnosis, further advice should be sought prior to performing additional tests, which might include CSF analysis, myelography or advanced imaging using computed tomography (CT) or MRI. Ideally, such tests should be performed by a specialist, since expertise is required to perform them and interpret the results.

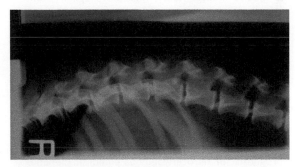

Figure 52.2 Lateral view of thoracic spine of a dog with intervertebral disc disease. The radiograph shows a mineralised disc at T13/L1 and a narrowed intervertebral disc space at L1/2

Treatment

The main objectives when approaching the management of these cases is to rapidly determine if the case requires medical or surgical management, and to determine the prognosis. Emergency surgical management is generally indicated if there are acute onset neurological deficits that prevent ambulatory function, and for most spinal fractures, where sensory function remains. The prognosis in these cases is dependent on the severity of the neurological injury. For intervertebral disc herniations, the prognosis is good, provided there is conscious pain sensation. The prognosis is guarded if there is loss of deep pain sensation, although if cases are treated surgically within 48 hours, up to 70% of affected dogs will recover ambulatory function. Most dogs with sensory function following a spinal fracture will recover ambulatory function. The prognosis is generally inversely related to body weight.

Elective surgical management may be beneficial for dogs with recalcitrant vertebral column pain due to intervertebral disc disease, even if there are no signs of spinal cord compromise. It may also be beneficial for large-breed dogs with Type II protrusions. The prognosis for control of pain by intervertebral disc fenestration is good, though some cases take several weeks of strict rest for resolution of pain. The prognosis for dogs affected by Type II disc protrusions is uncertain but generally guarded since surgery can result, in some cases, in a calamitous deterioration in neurological function for several weeks.

Medical management is indicated for spinal lesions characterised by milder pain and for cases with no or only mild neurological deficits (fibrocartilaginous emboli, granulomatous meningoencephalitis, polyarthritis). The prognosis for dogs with mild forms of intervertebral disc extrusion is generally good. Several weeks of strict rest (in a cage) is required to reduce the chance of exacerbation of disease that occurs with progressive disc extrusion with excessive activity. Recurrence is not uncommon following initially successful conservative management. The prognosis for fibrocartilaginous embolism depends on the region of the spinal cord affected. Dogs/cats showing signs of lower motor neuron compromise have a poor prognosis. Upper motor neuron lesions have a good prognosis but, in all cases, several weeks are required for recovery and most patients will have residual neurological deficits.

Due to the severity of spinal pain, medical management is best achieved with a combination of NSAIDs and opioids. Patients in marked pain should be hospitalised so that activity is severely restricted pending test results and further investigations. Periods of hospitalisation from five to 14 days are typically required whilst the dog is becoming comfortable and eight weeks of strict (cage) rest is generally advised, especially if a herniated disc is managed conservatively, rather than surgically.

Corticosteroids are rarely indicated for intervertebral disc herniations. Glucocorticoids are very effective analgesics for dogs with discogenic pain, but following their administration, dogs are often excessively active and such activity can result in massive disc hernation and severe spinal cord injury. Furthermore, dogs with intervertebral disc disease are predisposed to gastrointestinal ulceration and administration of steroids increases the chance of severe gastrointestinal disease. Occasionally, an anti-inflammatory dose of glucocorticoid can be helpful for large-breed dogs with Type II disc herniation.

What if it doesn't get better?

The prognosis for the various causes of spinal pain varies dramatically depending on the cause and it is important that the owner has a realistic expectation from the outset. Some conditions (e.g. severe traumatic spinal injuries) carry a hopeless prognosis and a recovery cannot be expected. In other conditions, the prognosis may be variable and the dog may only achieve a partial recovery (e.g. post-surgery for a severe disc herniation with severe neurological deficits). Conservatively managed patients recovering from spinal compression due to disc herniation have generally predictable rates of recovery according to the severity and location of the lesion and in indirect relation to body mass (see neurological texts for further guidance). If a patient does not show the predicted pattern of recovery, or if there is deterioration in neurological function, specialist advice should be sought promptly.

If the dog does not respond to the initial treatment as expected, the diagnosis should be re-evaluated. In cases of confirmed intervertebral disc herniation, failure to control spinal pain may be due to inadequate restriction of activity and it may be useful to hospitalise such patients, during which time potent analgesics should be administered. If failure of management is manifest as worsening of neurological deficits, specialist advice should be sought promptly.

The low-cost option

Intervertebral disc disease is common in chondrodystrophoid dogs aged 4–8 years, so if the signalment, history and clinical signs are consistent with the disease, a presumptive diagnosis can be made with reasonable certainty. Confirmation requires radiological examination and for especially placid dogs, lateral spinal radiographs may sometimes be obtained without sedation/anaesthesia. For cases of intervertebral disc disease causing spinal pain but without marked neurological deficits, recovery is possible using strict confinement to prevent further disc herniation and analgesia to control discomfort. However, owners should be made aware that where there is significant neurological compromise, recovery rates are generally lower and recovery times are generally longer than following surgical intervention.

When should I refer?

Spinal problems are challenging to diagnose, often unpredictable in their progression and they can be challenging to treat. Furthermore, a definitive diagnosis often requires advanced imaging techniques and skills that are not readily available in general practice. Consequently, specialist advice should be sought promptly in any case showing neurological deficits in which there is uncertainty regarding the diagnosis, prognosis or treatment. Referral should be discussed with the owner for cases with spinal pain in which the pain is not controlled within 24 hours of hospitalised treatment. Cases requiring spinal surgery are best dealt with by specialists.

Section 5

Section 6
Cardio-respiratory problems

Paul Smith

Coughing is a protective mechanism that helps to remove material (secretions or inhaled particles) from the bronchial tree or pharynx. It can be elicited by particulate matter, pulmonary congestion, intra- or extra-luminal compression of the airways, extremes of air temperature, irritant fumes, various inflammatory mediators and excessive production of mucus. Coughing is more common in dogs than in cats. When a cough persists for two months or more, it is referred to as chronic. Coughing needs to be distinguished from gagging/retching, which normally indicates a pharyngeal or gastrointestinal problem.

Common differential diagnoses

Dog

Upper airway disorders

- Acute tracheobronchitis ('kennel cough')
- Laryngeal paralysis
- Tracheal collapse
- Lungworm (*Oslerus osleri*)

Lower airway disorders

- Chronic bronchitis
- Airway foreign body
- Eosinophilic bronchopneumonopathy

Lung parenchymal diseases

- Pneumonia (inhalational or infectious)
- Intra-pulmonary haemorrhage (consider trauma or bleeding diathesis secondary to *Angiostrongylus vasorum*)
- Pulmonary neoplasia (primary or metastatic)
- Idiopathic pulmonary fibrosis

Cardiac disease

- Left-sided congestive heart failure (see Chapter 57)
- Left-atrial dilation causing airway compression

Mediastinal disease

- Neoplasia (e.g. thymoma, lymphoma)

100 Top Consultations in Small Animal General Practice, First Edition
By Peter Hill, Sheena Warman and Geoff Shawcross
© 2011 Blackwell Publishing Ltd

Cat

Lower airway disorders

- Acute bronchitis (e.g. infection with *Bordetella bronchiseptica*)
- Chronic bronchitis
- Feline asthma syndrome
- Bronchial/pulmonary neoplasia
- Airway foreign body
- Lungworm (*Aelurostrongylus abstrusus*)

Lung parenchymal diseases

- Pneumonia (bacterial or mycoplasmal)

Mediastinal disease

- Mediastinal neoplasia (e.g. thymoma, lymphoma)

Diagnostic approach

The first step in determining the cause of a cough is to ascertain if the cough results from a cardiac or respiratory disorder. Diagnosing cardiac disease is usually relatively straightforward. In contrast to dogs, cats with heart disease rarely cough, so a respiratory disorder is usually present in this species.

Although it is important to keep an open mind regarding possible differential diagnoses, age and breed predispositions to many cardiorespiratory disorders do exist (Table 53.1). It is also useful to have information regarding the vaccination and worming status of the animal, knowledge of any exposure to other dogs/cats or wild animals (e.g. foxes), any history of foreign travel, and details of the animal's environment.

Many clues to the cause of coughing can be obtained from the history. Acute tracheobronchitis causes a characteristic cough that may occur following a period in kennels or other exposure to dogs (see Chapter 54). Sudden onset, acute coughing is often associated with inhalation of foreign bodies. Chronic bronchitis typically results in a cough that is worse after a period of lying down/sleeping (e.g. in the morning), whereas laryngeal paralysis typically results in a cough and respiratory stridor that occurs during excitement or activity. Tracheal collapse often leads to a type of cough described as 'honking'. Signs that may indicate a more severe or widespread problem include dyspnoea, syncope, exercise intolerance, lethargy, inappetence or weight loss.

Auscultation of the thorax forms an important part of the examination of animals with a cough because it can help to differentiate between cardiac or respiratory disorders.

Physical examination findings that support a diagnosis of a cardiac disorder include:

- Identification of a heart murmur and/or gallop sounds.
- Disappearance of sinus arrhythmia (dog).
- An elevation of the heart rate – typically greater than 140 bpm (dog) or 200 bpm (cat).

The femoral pulse quality may or may not be abnormal in an animal with heart failure. It should also be noted that the presence of a heart murmur alone does not necessarily mean that a cough is caused by cardiac disease. Mitral valve disease resulting in an audible murmur is common in dogs but many of these patients will not develop congestive heart failure for many years.

Auscultation of the upper airways and lung fields is performed to evaluate the intensity of the normal breath sounds and to identify adventitial (abnormal) sounds. In most cases, the presence of an abnormal sound is not specific enough to confirm a diagnosis, but some findings can be suggestive of particular disorders. For example, an audible expiratory wheeze in a cat is highly suggestive of lower airway disease (chronic bronchitis or asthma), and the presence of severe diffuse crackles in a small breed dog without evidence of heart failure is suggestive of pulmonary fibrosis. However, further investigations are still required to confirm these diagnoses. Thoracic auscultation is a relatively insensitive technique for the detection of pulmonary changes such as mild oedema, and over-reliance on its diagnostic potential should be avoided.

With the exception of kennel cough, most cases of coughing will require further investigation in order to distinguish definitively between cardiac and respiratory causes, and to assess their severity. The nature and type of investigation will depend on whether or not a heart or respiratory disease is suspected, the severity of the signs, the index of suspicion of the differential diagnoses, and the presence or absence of concurrent clinical signs. The most useful initial diagnostic test is thoracic radiography. A full evaluation would include a dorso-ventral or ventro-dorsal view plus right lateral ± left lateral views. Left-sided congestive heart failure is nearly always accompanied by an enlargement of the cardiac silhouette, and is also characterised by the presence of pulmonary venous congestion and pulmonary oedema.

Further evaluation of suspected cardiac problems would include a standard 6-lead ECG (particularly if an arrhythmia is detected on physical examination) and echocardiography (to assess heart function, chamber sizes, and to determine the aetiology of the heart disease present). Performing and interpreting ECGs is within the scope of many general practitioners, but echocardiography is a specialist investigation that will require referral. Whether or not these tests are recommended will depend on various factors including the severity of the case, the confidence of the clinician in their diagnosis, and the wishes of the client.

Further evaluation of the respiratory tract might include any or all of the following:

- Examination of the upper airway and laryngeal function under light general anaesthesia.
- Radiographic evaluation of the trachea. This should be made after extubation, at peak inspiration and expiration if tracheal collapse is suspected.
- Faecal parasitology (faecal samples obtained over three separate days) and/or trial treatment with parasiticides effective against lungworm and *Angiostrongylus vasorum*.
- Bronchoscopy, broncho-alveolar lavage cytology ± microbial culture and sensitivity testing. These are advanced techniques that should only be undertaken by clinicians who have received specific training.
- A PCR panel for respiratory pathogens
- Full haematology and serum biochemistry, which can be valuable in providing a baseline prior to starting certain drugs.

Occasionally, it is difficult to determine the origin of a cough in dogs with concurrent respiratory and cardiac disease, especially if the former is responsible for the cough. In such cases, response to trial treatment, an echocardiogram (mainly to assess left atrial size) and/or measurement of canine N-terminal pro-B-type natriuretic peptide (NT pro-BNP) may be employed (see Chapter 57).

Table 53.1 Recognised age/breed predispositions to diseases resulting in coughing in the dog and cat.

Disorder	Age/Breed predisposed
Tracheal collapse	Toy breed dogs (e.g. Yorkshire terrier)
Chronic bronchitis	Middle-to-old aged dogs, Siamese cats
Pulmonary neoplasia	Middle-to-old aged dogs
Airway foreign body	Active / working / farm dogs
Angiostrongylus vasorum	Young dogs
Oslerus osleri	Young dogs, Greyhounds
Pneumocystosis	Young Cavalier King Charles Spaniels
Laryngeal paralysis	Elderly, large-breed dogs (e.g. Labrador Retriever)
Idiopathic pulmonary fibrosis	West Highland White Terrier
Mitral valve disease	Cavalier King Charles Spaniels, but all dogs susceptible

Treatment

Successful treatment of coughing requires identification and management of the underlying cause. In some cases, the history and physical examination may provide sufficient information to allow initiation of empirical treatment (e.g. kennel cough – see Chapter 54). However, in most cases, further investigation is required before specific treatment can be recommended. The following treatment regimes are commonly used to treat coughing:

* Management of congestive heart failure – see Chapter 57
* Antiparasitic drugs – indicated for treatment of lungworm and *Angiostrongylus vasorum* infections
* Antibiotics – indicated for upper and lower airway bacterial infections, and bacterial pneumonia
* Antitussive therapy (e.g. butorphanol) – this can be useful in cases of kennel cough and refractory chronic bronchitis but should be avoided if there is active inflammation or severe infection (e.g. pneumonia)
* Corticosteroids – these are useful for treating non-septic inflammatory disease such as chronic bronchitis, but should be used cautiously when there is an infection
* Bronchodilators – these can be useful for treating diseases such as feline asthma, tracheal collapse or refractory chronic bronchitis.

Management changes such as weight loss in obese pets, use of a harness rather than a collar, and avoidance of airway irritants, may also help to reduce the severity of a cough.

What if it doesn't get better?

Most mild viral/bacterial infections will resolve or improve markedly after one or two weeks of appropriate antimicrobial therapy. Left-sided congestive heart failure usually improves after one or two days' treatment. If a cough persists beyond this time, despite appropriate treatment, both the diagnosis and therapeutic strategy should be re-evaluated. Further investigation may be required to obtain a more specific diagnosis. For example, clinicians should note that concurrent heart and respiratory disease is common, and, even in dogs with obvious signs of cardiac disease, it cannot always be assumed that the cough is of cardiac origin. If the diagnosis is certain, a change in drug or drug dosage may be indicated. For example, chronic bronchitis does not usually respond to antibiotics but may improve markedly with glucocorticoid treatment to alleviate the airway inflammation. Clients should also be warned that some conditions cannot be cured and a successful outcome requires lifelong therapy. In other situations, such as pulmonary metastatic disease, the prognosis for recovery is hopeless.

The low-cost option

Costs can be kept to a minimum by obtaining a diagnosis and establishing an effective treatment strategy as quickly and efficiently as possible. This may be possible from the history and physical examination alone, but carefully chosen diagnostic tests, if performed at an early stage, may be the most cost-effective approach in the long term. In situations where finances are limited, and owners decline further evaluation, clinicians may have to initiate one or more of the treatment strategies listed above based on a limited investigation and their index of suspicion. For example, owners of older dogs with suspected congestive heart failure may favour a trial course of therapy rather than pursuing thoracic radiography. However, owners should be warned that the prognosis in these circumstances is not as certain as it would be if a definitive diagnosis had been made. Despite this, it may still be possible to achieve a successful outcome in various cardio-respiratory disorders when clinicians initiate treatment based on clinical findings alone, including cases of congestive heart failure, bacterial infection of the upper and lower respiratory tract, bacterial pneumonia, mycoplasmal pneumonia, chronic bronchitis, lungworm infestation, *Angiostrongylus* infestation and feline asthma.

Although many causes of coughing in dogs and cats require long-term management, some of the drugs commonly used for treatment are relatively inexpensive, including furosemide, digoxin, potentiated sulphonamides, oxytetracycline, prednisolone and codeine.

When should I refer?

Many common causes of coughing can be managed in general practice. However, referral should be discussed if a diagnosis cannot be reached using investigations that can be performed within the practice, or if a condition is not responding to treatment as the clinician would expect. Echocardiography and bronchoscopy are advanced procedures and should only be carried out by clinicians with the appropriate expertise. Medical management of some cases of congestive heart failure and chronic respiratory disorders may benefit from the expertise of a specialist. The surgical management of laryngeal paralysis and tracheal collapse also usually requires referral to a specialist surgical centre.

Paul Smith

Aetiology and pathogenesis

Kennel cough, or acute tracheobronchitis, is a common, highly contagious, respiratory disorder of dogs. Although one or more of a number of different infectious agents may be implicated (Table 54.1), kennel cough is usually attributable to a concurrent bacterial and viral infection. The disease is usually transmitted between dogs in close contact by aerosolized respiratory secretions (i.e. during coughing or sneezing).

History and clinical signs

Kennel cough is characterised by a paroxysmal, high-pitched cough that may be worse during periods of excitement or activity. The bout of coughing often ends with a gag, resulting in the production of a small amount of frothy phlegm. A history of recent (typically within 2–10 days) exposure to other dogs (e.g. attendance at boarding kennels, dog shows or training classes) is commonly reported. Most dogs are afebrile at presentation although a transient pyrexia may be identified in some cases. Although most affected dogs remain bright and have a normal appetite, some may be lethargic and inappetent. Some affected dogs may also develop a concurrent nasal or ocular discharge. Rarely, kennel cough may progress to pneumonia.

Table 54.1 **Infectious agents that may cause kennel cough.**

Agents commonly implicated	Agents less commonly implicated
Canine parainfluenza virus	CAV 2
Bordetella bronchiseptica	Reoviruses
Canine adenovirus (CAV) 1	Canine herpesvirus
	Canine distemper virus
	Mycoplasma species

100 Top Consultations in Small Animal General Practice, First Edition
By Peter Hill, Sheena Warman and Geoff Shawcross
© 2011 Blackwell Publishing Ltd

Specific diagnostic techniques

A diagnosis of kennel cough is usually made from the history and physical examination alone. Light tracheal palpation often elicits a bout of coughing, confirming tracheal sensitivity. Auscultation of the chest usually reveals no abnormal sounds, unless pneumonia has developed.

Treatment

Although most infections tend to be self-limiting, treatment with antibiotics against *Bordetella bronchiseptica* and other opportunistic bacterial infections is recommended. Although they will not affect the viral component of the condition, they should prevent the development of secondary bacterial pneumonia. The first choice antibiotic is doxycycline, but suitable alternatives include oxytetracycline, potentiated sulphonamides or amoxicillin/clavulanic acid. A 7–10 day course is typically employed, but longer courses may occasionally be necessary as *Bordetella bronchiseptica* can persist in the airways for up to 3 months. Concurrent treatment with an antitussive such as butorphanol may help to provide some relief from the cough but should be avoided in dogs with pneumonia. Paradoxically, although glucocorticoids should normally be avoided in the face of active infection, anecdotal reports suggest that a five-day course of prednisolone given at a dose of 0.5–1 mg/kg/day may help to ameliorate the cough more quickly than when antimicrobials are used alone. However, this approach should only be taken in adult dogs that are non-febrile, have a severe cough, appear systemically well and have a clear chest on auscultation.

Prevention and control of kennel cough is best achieved by vaccination and strict segregation of dogs at risk. Dogs are unlikely to be contagious once they have stopped coughing. Minimizing population density and maximising ventilation can also reduce the incidence within boarding kennels and veterinary premises. In addition to the yearly parenterally administered vaccinations, intranasal vaccines against *Bordetella bronchiseptica* plus canine parainfluenza virus (Nobivac KC, Intervet UK Ltd) are available. Immunity to *Bordetella bronchiseptica* takes 72 hours to develop whereas protection against parainfluenza is not achieved for three weeks. Although immunity is considered to be good, lasting up to 12 months, owners should be made aware that the use of these vaccines does not provide guaranteed protection against kennel cough, and dogs may still become symptomatic after receiving them.

The low-cost option

As kennel cough is a self-limiting disease, most dogs will recover without treatment. In mildly affected dogs, conscientious monitoring by the owner may be all that is necessary, as long as the affected dog is not putting other dogs at risk. If treatment is deemed necessary, drugs such as oxytetracycline or potentiated sulphonamides would represent the cheapest options.

What if it doesn't get better?

Owners should be advised that most dogs with kennel cough usually recover after one to two weeks, but rarely, some dogs will continue to cough for up to six weeks. Viral infections may cause a chronic cough associated with increased bronchial reactivity, a syndrome referred to as 'chronic tracheobronchial syndrome'. Chronicity may also occur due to concurrent airway collapse or the development of secondary bacterial infection/pneumonia.

If the cough persists for longer than anticipated (i.e. 2–6 weeks) further investigations (e.g. full haematology, thoracic radiography and bronchoscopy) should be performed to rule out other differential diagnoses or concurrent disease(s). Chronic tracheobronchial syndrome is a diagnosis of exclusion and, if present, is usually treated with an antitussive such as butorphanol. Concurrent non-septic inflammation of the lower airways may require a course of glucocorticoids. Pneumonia is potentially a life-threatening disease and should be treated with broad-spectrum antibiotics (initially administered intravenously), intravenous fluid therapy, supplemental humidified oxygen (as necessary) and supportive care.

When should I refer?

Kennel cough is a disease that is readily managed on an out-patient basis in general practice. In rare cases where the cough persists for longer than anticipated and the necessary equipment and expertise to investigate for other possible causes is not available, a referral may be offered. Dogs with pneumonia may initially require intensive 24-hour therapy and observation, and referral to a specialist practice should be considered if appropriate facilities are unavailable at the primary practice. It may also be advisable to seek expert advice in situations where substantial economic losses could occur (e.g. boarding or Greyhound kennels).

Andrea Harvey

Sneezing and nasal discharge are common presenting clinical signs in both dogs and cats, usually indicating disease within the nasal cavity or nasopharynx. They are more common in cats because of the relatively frequent occurrence of 'cat flu'.

Common differential diagnoses

- 'Cat flu' – a feline upper respiratory tract infection caused by herpes virus (FHV), calici virus (FCV) or *Chlamydophila*, either alone or in combination (although the latter organism rarely causes significant nasal disease on its own). Secondary bacterial infection is common.
- Dental disease with oronasal fistula/tooth root abscess
- Foreign body – e.g. blade of grass
- Neoplasia (lymphoma most common in cats, carcinoma most common in dogs)
- Nasopharyngeal polyp – cats
- Nasopharyngeal stenosis – cats
- Fungal infection (*Aspergillus* in dogs, *Cryptococcus* in cats but rare in UK).

In some cases, the underlying cause of the nasal discharge cannot be identified and a diagnosis of idiopathic chronic rhinitis has to be made, following investigations to rule out other causes. Cats that have previously suffered from 'cat flu' are predisposed to chronic rhinitis, but it is much less common in dogs, usually affecting large breeds.

Diagnostic approach

Important historical features that allow the differential diagnoses to be prioritised include the age and breed of the animal, the speed of onset, the duration of clinical signs, the presence of additional clinical signs, the nature of the discharge, and whether it is unilateral or bilateral. It is also important to find out if any in-contact animals have had similar clinical signs, and if the animal is vaccinated.

100 Top Consultations in Small Animal General Practice, First Edition
By Peter Hill, Sheena Warman and Geoff Shawcross
© 2011 Blackwell Publishing Ltd

Physical examination should focus on assessing the nature of any discharge (serous, purulent, haemorrhagic), determining if it is worse or predominant on one side, listening for stertor, checking the symmetry of the nose and examining it for pain or discomfort, examination of the mouth and teeth, and evaluating the animal's general systemic health. A microscope slide, a few hairs, or a wisp of cotton wool can be held against each nostril in turn to help assess airflow.

'Cat flu' is typically acute in onset resulting in bilateral serous or purulent nasal discharge, with or without an ocular discharge (Figure 55.1). It is most common in young cats, but can occur at any age, and in vaccinated cats. The cat may also be systemically unwell and may have other signs of upper respiratory tract viral infection such as ulcers on the tongue (FCV) or corneal ulcers (FHV). Foreign bodies are typically associated with acute onset severe sneezing, often accompanied by pawing or rubbing the face. The nasal discharge usually starts a day or two later and is typically purulent, pungent smelling, and most often unilateral, but can be bilateral (see Chapter 79). Neoplasia occurs most commonly in older animals and is more likely to be associated with dyspnoea and a haemorrhagic and/or unilateral nasal discharge compared with animals with chronic rhinitis, which often show sneezing and bilateral nasal discharge. Neoplasia, nasopharyngeal polyps and nasopharyngeal stenosis in particular are likely to be associated with easily audible stertor. Cats with nasopharyngeal polyps are usually younger and they may also have signs of middle ear disease. Nasal aspergillosis most commonly occurs in dolicocephalic, large breeds of dog.

In cats with sneezing or nasal discharges, a diagnosis of 'cat flu' or chronic rhinitis can usually be made on the basis of clinical signs alone. Further investigation should be performed in recurrent or severe cases, or if the signalment, history and clinical findings suggest that any of the other differential diagnoses are more likely. A plain swab can be submitted for a PCR panel of feline respiratory pathogens (FHV, FCV, *Chlamydophila* and *Mycoplasma*). FCV can also be isolated from an oropharyngeal swab (submitted in viral chlamydial transport medium). Ideally, complete haematology, biochemistry, FIV and FeLV tests should be performed to assess systemic health, particularly in older animals.

Nasal radiographs are helpful to look for abnormalities such as soft tissue densities, turbinate destruction, or radiopaque foreign bodies in the nose. Intra-oral views of the nasal cavity are most useful, but radiographs of the lateral pharynx and bullae can also be helpful. Dental radiography can be used to evaluate disease of the tooth roots, and thoracic radiographs are indicated if pulmonary complications are suspected. If endoscopy is available, anteriograde and retrograde rhinoscopy is useful for visualising masses, fungal plagues or foreign bodies. Foreign bodies extending into the pharynx may also be seen without endoscopy, by pulling the soft palate forward and/or using a dental mirror. A useful technique for detecting and removing blades of grass from the nasal cavity of cats is to gently insert a piece of monofilament suture material into the nose to push the blade back into the nasopharynx. Nasal biopsies can be taken to confirm or rule out neoplasia. Cytology of nasal flushes can sometimes be useful, particularly when nasal lymphoma is a differential diagnosis. Bacterial culture of nasal discharges is rarely helpful.

In dogs, chronic rhinitis is much less common and therefore further investigations should be performed much earlier in any dog presenting with a nasal discharge. A blood test for *Aspergillus* antibody should be performed if this is considered likely. A positive result would be highly suggestive of *Aspergillus* infection, but it should not be excluded on the basis of a negative result as the antibody tests are not highly sensitive. Assessment of general health and for the presence of additional clinical signs involving other body systems is important. If no differential diagnoses can be prioritized, a complete nasal investigation would include haematology/biochemistry, radiographs, rhinoscopy and biopsies.

Treatment

Appropriate treatment is based on establishing a diagnosis. In cats with nasal discharge due to 'cat flu' or chronic rhinitis, a 7–14 day course of antibiotics is indicated as a first-line treatment. Broad-spectrum antibiotics such as amoxicillin/clavulanic acid, cefalexin or doxycycline are good first-line choices. Supportive care, good nursing and encouragement to

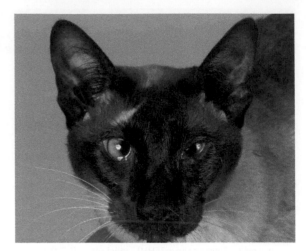

Figure 55.1   A cat with upper respiratory tract disease ('flu')

eat are important. Saline nebulisation or steam inhalation (10–15 minutes twice to three times daily initially) is useful to reduce viscosity of secretions and encourage productive sneezing. A nebuliser can be purchased from most pharmacies and the water vapour directed into a small area that is contained and covered (e.g. a cat basket or igloo type bed covered with a plastic bag or cloth). An alternative is to place the cat in a steamy room (e.g. bathroom). The mucolytic bromhexine hydrochloride (Bisolvon, Boehringer Ingelheim) can also be used as an aid to loosening viscous discharges (a pinch in the food twice daily), but this is unlikely to have much benefit used on its own, and is not as effective as nebulisation.

In dogs, nasal discharge is rarely due to primary bacterial disease and empirical use of antibiotics is unlikely to be of lasting benefit, although bacterial infection may occur secondary to dental disease, foreign bodies or neoplasia. Further investigations should therefore be performed earlier in the course of disease. Nasal discharges due to dental disease or foreign bodies should respond to appropriate dental care (see Chapter 36) or removal of the responsible object. Nasopharyngeal polyps require surgical removal. Nasal lymphoma is usually very responsive to chemotherapy (e.g. cyclophosphamide, vincristine, and prednisone protocol), whilst other nasal tumours (e.g. carcinomas) can be palliatively treated with radiotherapy. The treatment of choice for nasal aspergillosis is trephination of the frontal sinus and infusion of clotrimazole, which may require referral.

What if it doesn't get better?

If there is no response to initial treatment, or if signs recur, then further investigations should be carried out as discussed above. In some cases, advanced imaging (MRI or CT) can yield useful additional information. In cats with chronic rhinitis, prolonged courses (6–8 weeks) of antibiotics may be required, and some cases need ongoing continuous or pulse antibiotic therapy. Continuation of saline nebulisation or steam inhalation is important. Intermittent nasal cavity flushing under general anaesthesia can sometimes be helpful to remove inspissated secretions. Some cases will improve with meloxicam treatment. Alternatively, topical glucocorticoids (inhaled or drops) may be appropriate. Corticosteroids should be avoided if acute viral infections are present, and they should not be given concurrently with NSAIDs.

Idiopathic chronic rhinitis in dogs is a diagnosis of exclusion, although it is more common in certain breeds such as Irish Wolfhounds. Potential treatment strategies include intermittent antibiotics, antihistamines, oral and inhalational steroids and NSAIDs. Some dogs may respond partially to doxycycline or azithromycin, although it is unclear whether the response is related to the antimicrobial or anti-inflammatory properties of these drugs. Hydration of the nasal cavity with nasal drops or aerosols may limit nasal discharge, and some animals may improve with inhalant glucocorticoids.

Although nasal neoplasia may respond to appropriate treatment, owners should be warned that relapse, at some point, is likely.

The low-cost option

Most common causes of sneezing or nasal discharge in cats can be managed without incurring high costs. For cats with flu, providing antibiotics, advising steam nebulisation and allowing the owner to nurse the cat at home will minimise costs. If the rhinitis becomes chronic, periodic use of antibiotics is the most appropriate option. In dogs, trial treatment with antibiotics is unlikely to be cost-effective and will probably add unnecessarily to the overall cost of treatment. Narrowing down the differential diagnoses as much as possible using history and clinical signs, and then targeting the investigation most likely to yield a diagnosis, will save costs. For example, if neoplasia appears very likely, nasal biopsies would be essential; if a foreign body is suspected it may be possible to visualise and remove it from the nasopharynx with forceps; in large-breed dolicocephalic dogs, an *Aspergillus* antibody test would be a sensible first step in investigation. Conditions such as nasal neoplasia in dogs cannot be managed at low cost and euthanasia should be considered when the dog's quality of life is affected.

When should I refer?

Most cases of sneezing and nasal discharge can be managed in general practice but some of the conditions require investigations that may not be routinely undertaken in the practice (e.g. nasal biopsies, advanced imaging), or require protocols that are best performed by specialists (e.g. treatment of nasal aspergillosis, radiotherapy). Referral could also be considered in cases that relapse frequently despite appropriate investigation and treatment, or if there are systemic complications that cannot be adequately managed within the practice (e.g. concurrent pneumonia and 'cat flu', anorexic patients requiring assisted feeding).

Paul Smith

Aetiology and pathogenesis

A heart murmur is a heart sound produced by turbulent blood flow, or less commonly, by vibrations of a cardiac structure such as chordae tendineae. Turbulent blood flow may be caused by an increase in blood velocity, a change in blood viscosity (e.g. anaemia) or by the passage of blood from a narrow region into a much larger one.

Common differential diagnoses

Apart from innocent puppy/kitten murmurs (thought to be caused by an increased stroke volume relative to aortic size), the following differential diagnoses should be considered:

- Aortic stenosis
- Pulmonary stenosis
- Hypertrophic cardiomyopathy
- Patent ductus arteriosus (PDA)
- Congenital mitral valve disease
- Congenital tricuspid valve disease
- Ventricular septal defect
- Aortic insufficiency (i.e. aortic valve regurgitation; produces a diastolic heart murmur)
- Anaemia (haemic murmurs).

Diagnostic approach

Murmurs are detected on auscultation of the thorax. Auscultation should be performed in a quiet room with the dog or cat standing, if possible. Panting may be prevented in dogs by holding the mouth closed, and purring may be prevented in cats by waving an alcohol-soaked swab in front of the nose. Most stethoscopes have a bell and diaphragm (Figure 56.1). The diaphragm is used to detect high frequency sounds (e.g. most heart murmurs and lung sounds) and should be applied firmly to the chest wall, whereas the bell is best used to detect low frequency sounds

100 Top Consultations in Small Animal General Practice, First Edition
By Peter Hill, Sheena Warman and Geoff Shawcross
© 2011 Blackwell Publishing Ltd

(e.g. gallop sounds) and should be held lightly against the chest wall. The clinician should move the chest piece slowly from apex to base as well as high up in the axilla on each side of the chest (a murmur associated with PDA may only be audible in this region). Auscultation of the sternal area is also important, particularly in cats that often have loud murmurs in this region.

Murmurs can be characterised by their intensity (which can be graded from 1 to 6, see Table 56.1), point of maximal intensity (PMI), and timing (i.e. systolic, diastolic or continuous). In addition, the area of the chest wall overlying the heart (precordium) should be palpated to identify the location of the heart within the chest and to determine if a precordial thrill (palpable vibration) is present. If present, this signifies a murmur intensity of at least 5. Palpation of the femoral pulse should also be performed as this may help to narrow the differential diagnoses. For example, a weak pulse may be felt in severe aortic stenosis whereas a stronger than normal pulse may be felt with PDA.

The characteristics of murmurs found in various disorders of puppies and kittens are shown in Table 56.2. Puppies and kittens with a heart murmur often have no clinical signs; consequently a heart murmur may be detected as an incidental finding. If clinical signs are absent, either a heart murmur is present in the absence of cardiac disease (e.g. 'innocent murmurs') or cardiac disease is present but is not severe enough to result in clinical signs (i.e. the cardiovascular system is able to compensate for the defect present). Most puppies and kittens with cardiac disease have either innocent murmurs or a congenital malformation. However, hypertrophic cardiomyopathy (an acquired heart disease) has been observed in cats as young as six months of age. Puppies and kittens with severe cardiac disease may develop congestive heart failure (CHF; see Chapter 57).

Innocent murmurs in puppies and kittens usually disappear by 16 weeks of age. Therefore, if a low intensity systolic murmur (i.e. grade 3 or less) is detected at the left heart base in a puppy or kitten without clinical signs, it might be prudent to wait until the animal is over 16 weeks of age before recommending a diagnostic investigation. However, this has to be balanced against the possibility that the owner may wish to return the puppy or kitten to the breeder if a more serious disorder is present. Which approach is taken can only be decided following discussions between the owner and breeder. If the murmur persists, precise diagnosis of cardiac disease in puppies and kittens requires echocardiography. As this is a specialist investigation, referral to a cardiologist is recommended. Additional tests usually employed in a typical cardiac investigation also include a standard 6-lead ECG, and thoracic radiography to confirm the presence or absence of CHF.

Table 56.1 Murmur intensity scale.

Murmur grade	Description
1	A very quiet murmur over a localised area, audible only in a quiet room after a period of concentrated listening. Some vets and new graduates are unable to detect grade 1 murmurs.
2	A quiet murmur that is easily heard over the PMI but has minimal-to-no radiation to other areas.
3	Moderately loud, easily heard over a moderate area of radiation but unlikely to radiate to the opposite side of the chest.
4	A loud murmur with a wide area of radiation (i.e. to the opposite side of the chest) but no palpable precordial thrill.
5	A very loud murmur with extensive radiation and a palpable precordial thrill.
6	As in 5, but murmur audible with the chest piece held just off the chest wall.

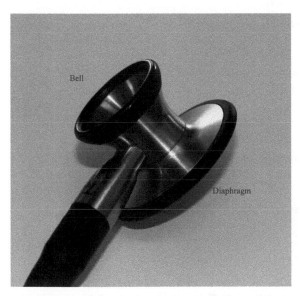

Figure 56.1 Stethoscope chest piece to show the diaphragm and bell

Treatment

The requirement for treatment depends on the underlying cause of the heart murmur, and whether or not heart failure is present. Many animals with heart murmurs do not (and may never) require treatment and regular monitoring is all that is required. If a PDA or pulmonary stenosis is suspected, early diagnosis and intervention can be curative. A PDA with left-to-right shunting can be treated by transcatheter embolisation (a minimally invasive technique that obviates the need for thoracotomy) or surgical ligation. Pulmonary stenosis can be treated with balloon valvuloplasty (also minimally invasive). These are specialist interventions that can only be performed by cardiologists and experienced surgeons. If heart failure develops, treatment with standard protocols can be instituted (see Chapter 57), but euthanasia may be warranted in animals with severe, symptomatic, congenital cardiac disease in which the long-term outlook is poor.

Table 56.2 Characteristics of murmurs seen in puppies and kittens.

Cause	PMI	Grade	Timing	Femoral pulse	Predisposed breeds
Innocent murmur	Left heart base	3 or less	Systolic	Normal	Any
PDA	Axilla on left side of chest	Usually ≥5	Continuous	Hyperdynamic	Toy and Miniature Poodles, Border Collie, English Springer Spaniel
MVD	Left heart apex	1–5	Systolic	Normal-to-weak	Large, pure-bred dogs
TVD	Right heart apex	1–5	Systolic	Normal-to-weak	Large, pure-bred dogs including Labrador Retriever
VSD	Usually right sternal border but possibly left heart base	The higher the intensity, often the smaller the defect	Systolic (concurrent AI may lead to an additional diastolic murmur)	Usually normal	Any
AS	Left or right heart base	Intensity often correlates with the severity of the stenosis	Systolic	Normal-to-weak	Boxer Golden Retriever Newfoundland
PS	Left heart base	Intensity often correlates with the severity of the stenosis	Systolic	Normal	English Bulldog, West Highland White & Border Terriers, Cocker Spaniel
HCM	Often over the left or right sternal border	Murmur may or may not be present (0–6)	Systolic	Normal-to-weak	Cats
Anaemia	Usually left heart base but the hypoviscosity may elicit murmurs at other locations	3 or less	Systolic	Variable: may be bounding or weak if hypovolaemic	Any

Abbreviations: PMI = point of maximal intensity; PDA = patent ductus arteriosus; MVD = mitral valve disease; TVD = tricuspid valve disease; VSD = ventricular septal defect; AI = aortic insufficiency; AS = aortic stenosis; PS = pulmonary stenosis; HCM = hypertrophic cardiomyopathy.

Section 6

What if it doesn't get better?

With the exception of innocent murmurs, haemic murmurs, or following successful treatment of PDA, it is unlikely that the murmur will disappear. The owner should be made aware of the clinical signs that may occur in the future and would require treatment, such as the development of heart failure.

The low-cost option

The lowest cost option in a puppy or kitten with a heart murmur but no clinical signs is to withhold therapy until such time as clinical signs develop, if indeed they do. Where there are financial constraints, diagnosis and treatment of heart failure, if this ensues, is possible without obtaining a specific diagnosis of the underlying cardiac disease, but the owner should be made aware that the diagnosis is uncertain and thus optimal treatment may not be achieved. If there are severe clinical signs, and insufficient funds for treatment, euthanasia may have to be considered.

When should I refer?

Referral to a cardiologist should be offered if a murmur persists beyond 16 weeks of age and a precise diagnosis is required. This might be the case if the owner is particularly worried, if the clinician feels that a precise diagnosis would be helpful, or in animals with breeding potential. If a left-to-right shunting PDA, or pulmonary stenosis, is suspected, a referral should be offered as soon as possible to allow prompt treatment.

Section 6

Paul Smith

Aetiology and pathogenesis

Heart failure is a syndrome that occurs when a cardiac or pericardial disease becomes so severe that either: (1) the heart cannot pump enough blood into the aorta or pulmonary artery to maintain a normal arterial blood pressure or perfusion to all tissues – forward heart failure, or (2) can do so, but only with elevated atrial pressures – backward, or congestive heart failure (CHF). Depending on the side of the heart affected, CHF may be either right- or left-sided.

Common differential diagnoses

CHF

- Severe mitral valve regurgitation
- Severe tricuspid valve regurgitation
- Patent ductus arteriosus (PDA)
- Dilated cardiomyopathy (DCM)
- Slowly developing pericardial effusion (e.g. idiopathic haemorrhagic pericardial effusion)
- Cardiac arrhythmia – depends on heart rate and presence or absence of structural disease

Forward heart failure

- Aortic stenosis (AS)
- Pulmonic stenosis (PS)
- Rapidly developing pericardial effusion (e.g. haemorrhage due to haemangiosarcoma).

All the causes of CHF listed above can also cause forward failure if they become advanced or are left untreated.

History and clinical signs

In left-sided CHF, increased left atrial pressure results in increased pulmonary capillary hydrostatic pressure. This causes transudation of fluid from the pulmonary capillaries into the pulmonary interstitium, causing pulmonary oedema (Figure 57.1). Typical clinical signs include a cough, tachypnoea and dyspnoea. It is important to note that dogs with heart disease may also cough in the absence of pulmonary oedema due to compression of the left mainstem bronchus by the enlarged heart. In right-sided CHF, increased right atrial pressure tends to cause ascites. A pleural effusion may also be present but this occurs less frequently.

Forward heart failure produces clinical signs of weakness, exercise intolerance, syncope and peripheral vasoconstriction (e.g. cold extremities, pale mucous membranes, sluggish CRT and hypothermia), irrespective of the side of the heart affected. Clinical signs associated with forward heart failure are often exacerbated during exercise.

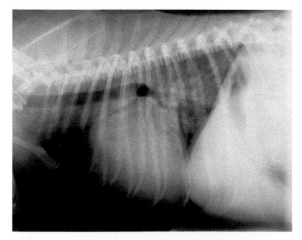

Figure 57.1 **Right lateral thoracic radiograph obtained from a crossbreed dog with left-sided congestive heart failure (pulmonary oedema) caused by chronic degenerative mitral valve disease. The cardiac silhouette appears enlarged and a diffuse mixed lung pattern is present in the dorsocaudal lung fields. Pulmonary venous congestion (i.e. enlargement of the pulmonary veins) can also be seen**

100 Top Consultations in Small Animal General Practice, First Edition
By Peter Hill, Sheena Warman and Geoff Shawcross
© 2011 Blackwell Publishing Ltd

Specific diagnostic techniques

Careful evaluation of the cardiovascular system is required before making a diagnosis of heart failure. A combination of a cough and a heart murmur do not necessarily mean that the dog has left-sided CHF (see Chapter 53). Additional clinical features that support a diagnosis of CHF include an elevated heart rate (typically >140 bpm) and disappearance of sinus arrhythmia (although this can also disappear in dogs that are excited or anxious). The presence of sinus arrhythmia and a low-to-normal heart rate virtually rules out CHF.

A right lateral thoracic radiograph is often sufficient to be able to confirm a diagnosis of left-sided CHF (Figure 57.1). However, a dorsoventral view will help in evaluating the cardiac silhouette and lung fields more thoroughly. Where left-sided CHF is present, the left side of the heart is usually enlarged. An exception to this is acute onset, severe mitral regurgitation caused by a ruptured chordae, in which left-sided CHF may ensue without left atrial dilation.

Occasionally, in a dog with both respiratory and cardiac disease, it remains very difficult to determine whether or not left-sided CHF is present. A useful adjunctive diagnostic test in such circumstances is the assessment of serum canine NT pro BNP. This peptide is released from the ventricular wall in response to myocardial 'stress'. An elevated concentration, therefore, supports a diagnosis of cardiac, rather than respiratory disease. It is important to note that dogs with reduced renal function may also have high levels of NT pro BNP.

Right-sided CHF is usually suspected from the physical examination. Typical findings include ascites, an elevated heart rate and either muffled heart sounds ± a weak/paradoxical femoral pulse (seen with pericardial effusion) or a right-sided heart murmur (seen with tricuspid valve regurgitation). Confirmation of the diagnosis may require echocardiography, and other causes of ascites need to be ruled out (e.g. peritonitis, abdominal neoplasia).

Forward heart failure may produce intermittent signs (such as episodic weakness as seen with subaortic stenosis), or persistent weakness and regular collapse (as seen with severe dilated cardiomyopathy or acute cardiac tamponade). The diagnostic approach will, therefore, vary accordingly. Echocardiography is required to determine if there is a pericardial effusion, severe myocardial failure or valvular obstruction. The investigation of episodic weakness may also require referral to a specialist for further tests (e.g. 24-hour ambulatory ECG).

Conventional echocardiography cannot be used to diagnose heart failure *per se* but is extremely useful in determining the precise aetiology and severity of cardiac or pericardial disease. Echocardiography can also elucidate the diagnosis where a distinction between cardiac and respiratory disease cannot be made from thoracic radiographs. In uncomplicated cases showing classic clinical signs of mitral valve regurgitation, echocardiography is not essential, but it can help to verify the diagnosis, provide a more reliable prognosis and allow the clinician to select the most appropriate treatment. Detailed echocardiography should be regarded as a specialist procedure. However, it may be relatively easy in general practice to detect a pericardial effusion using cardiac ultrasound.

Treatment

CHF is often treated very successfully in general practice. However, a number of treatment options exist and knowledge of these, together with their potential side-effects, is necessary to maximise each dog's quality and longevity of life. With the exception of PDA, pulmonary stenosis, and some cases of pericardial effusion, most other causes of heart failure cannot be cured and usually require life-long management. Dogs with pericardial effusion require pericardiocentesis for effective management.

Drugs used to treat CHF include the following:

- Furosemide – Used to reduce the circulating fluid volume and thereby alleviate/prevent the recurrence of pulmonary oedema or ascites. The minimum effective dose must be used to minimise acid–base and electrolyte abnormalities. Increases in the dose are often required with progression of the disease and occurrence of diuretic resistance
- Pimobendan – Used to increase myocardial contractility and relaxation, and to cause veno- and arteriolar-dilation. May also decrease pro-inflammatory cytokine production

- Angiotensin-converting enzyme (ACE) inhibitors – By reducing the formation of angiotensin II, ACE inhibitors have several beneficial effects including veno- and arteriolar-dilation
- Spironolactone – Provides additional diuretic effect by acting at a different site within the nephron from furosemide
- Digoxin – Beneficial effects include a slowing of the heart rate (particularly useful in the treatment of atrial fibrillation) and diuretic properties. Digoxin toxicity is a common and quite debilitating side-effect. The optimum dose, therefore, needs to be established in each case, taking into account general condition, renal function, and serum protein and potassium concentrations. Some dogs appear to be very susceptible to digoxin toxicity and may not tolerate it
- Glyceryl trinitrate – A vasodilator, primarily used during the first 24 hours in dogs with acute left-sided CHF. The cream is usually applied to the inner aspect of the pinna (clip hair if necessary, and wear non-permeable gloves to apply).

The use of these drugs to manage heart failure is very much tailored to the individual dog, and depends largely on the aetiology and severity of the underlying heart disease. The most commonly treated condition in general practice is left-sided CHF. In severe cases, cage rest and treatment with furosemide (1–2 mg/kg SC q8–12 h) and pimobendan (0.1–0.3 mg/kg PO q12 h) is indicated initially. If very severe, the dose of furosemide can be increased (2–4 mg/kg IV q1–2 h for one to two doses, then given q6–8 h). Glyceryl trinitrate (¼ inch/5 kg q6–8 h topically) and oxygen supplementation can also be beneficial.

For maintenance treatment, current evidence suggests that concurrent treatment with furosemide (1–2 mg/kg PO q12–24 h), an ACE inhibitor (e.g. benazepril 0.25–0.5 mg/kg PO q24 h or ramipril 0.125 mg/kg PO q24 h), pimobendan (0.1–0.3 mg/kg PO q12 h) and spironolactone (2 mg/kg PO q12 h) provides the best outcome. However, the treatment regimen should be tailored to the individual dog and may vary according to specific findings, such as the presence/absence of concurrent disease or arrhythmias, owner compliance and finances, and response to treatment.

For right-sided CHF, similar strategies are usually employed, but periodic abdominocentesis may be required in some cases to treat refractory ascites. In such cases, it may also be beneficial to administer furosemide by subcutaneous injection because the intestinal oedema that accompanies ascites in right-sided CHF may impair gastrointestinal absorption.

Dogs being treated for CHF should be re-examined 1–2 weeks after initial presentation and then every 3–4 months. However, the exact timing of each re-evaluation depends on the response to treatment and the severity of the heart disease. At each visit, it is useful to assess serum electrolyte, urea and creatinine concentrations, and, if possible, systolic arterial blood pressure. Thoracic radiography may be employed to ensure adequate resolution of pulmonary oedema. Follow-up by a cardiologist will allow echocardiography to be employed to assess progression of the primary disease.

Cases of suspected forward heart failure are best referred to cardiologists for confirmation of the diagnosis and treatment recommendations.

What if it doesn't get better?

If a case is not responding to treatment as expected, it is critical to first ensure that the diagnosis is correct. If the clinician is uncertain, a second opinion would be valuable. If the diagnosis is correct, the treatment strategy should be re-evaluated. It should be remembered that, as the heart disease progresses, the therapeutic strategy may need to change, with intensification to be anticipated with advancing disease. Drugs that may be considered in refractory cases include digoxin and thiazide diuretics. The latter should be used cautiously since they can lead to severe acid–base and electrolyte abnormalities. Referral to a specialist may be appropriate before contemplating unfamiliar drug protocols.

Acute exacerbation of heart failure (known as decompensation) may also occur with chronic disease and may require modifications to the drug protocols and doses. Ultimately euthanasia may be necessary, which should not be considered a failure if all other avenues have been explored or are considered unlikely to be effective.

The low-cost option

Owners should be made aware at the outset that treatment of heart failure will result in ongoing expense. If financial limitations preclude an extensive diagnostic investigation, the clinician may have to initiate therapy based on the clinical findings alone. This can be a successful strategy in cases of left-sided CHF due to mitral valve disease, but the outcome is much less predictable with other cardiac disorders. Financial limitations may preclude the concurrent use of furosemide, pimobendan, ACE-inhibitors or spironolactone in dogs with CHF. In such cases, furosemide and pimobendan or an ACE-inhibitor represents a cheaper treatment protocol. In dogs with chronic degenerative MVD, furosemide plus pimobendan has been found to be more efficacious than furosemide plus an ACE-inhibitor. If this protocol is not possible, the cheapest option is to use furosemide plus digoxin, and if this is still not financially feasible, the long-term outlook is poor and euthanasia should be considered.

When should I refer?

Treating heart failure is to some extent 'more of an art than a science' and success rates depend on the clinician's experience. Although most dogs with CHF can be treated in general practice, referral to a specialist cardiologist may provide a better chance of improving both the quality of life and survival time. If cases are not responding well to routine treatment protocols, referral should definitely be discussed with the client. Dogs with more severe cardiac diseases (such as dilated cardiomyopathy or pericardial effusions), or those in which echocardiography is required for diagnosis (such as aortic or pulmonic stenosis) may also benefit from referral. The diagnosis and management of arrhythmias also requires considerable expertise. Treatment options such as implantation of artificial pacemakers and management of PDAs by transvenous embolisation or surgical ligation can only be carried out at specialist centres.

Paul Smith

Normal cats have a resting respiratory rate of 16–25 breaths per minute. Cats with breathing difficulty may have an increased respiratory effort (dyspnoea) and/or rate (tachypnoea). In the early stages, cats will adapt their lifestyle to accommodate thoracic disease and become less active. This may not be noticed by owners as quickly as it would be in dogs, often resulting in cats being presented with severe and critical signs. Severely dyspnoeic cats often crouch in a sternal or squatting position with their elbows abducted and neck extended.

Common differential diagnoses

- Trauma (e.g. diaphragmatic hernia, pneumothorax, pulmonary contusion, rib fracture)
- Pleural effusion (e.g. FIP, left-sided CHF, neoplasia)
- Pyothorax
- Chylothorax (e.g. mediastinal lymphoma, secondary to CHF, idiopathic)
- Asthma
- Pulmonary oedema (e.g. left-sided CHF due to hypertrophic cardiomyopathy)
- Cranial mediastinal mass (e.g. lymphoma, thymoma)
- Congenital diaphragmatic hernia
- Spontaneous pneumothorax
- Nasopharyngeal polyp
- Laryngeal disease
- Chronic bronchitis
- Pneumonia
- Pulmonary neoplasia
- Over-zealous fluid administration (hypervolaemia).

Diagnostic approach

Cats with respiratory distress are vulnerable to rapid decompensation and respiratory arrest. Consequently, *they should be handled with extreme care so as to prevent additional distress*. Immediate stabilisation prior to diagnostic testing (see below) is often required; however striking a balance between making an effective diagnosis and providing optimal treatment with minimal handling can be difficult.

100 Top Consultations in Small Animal General Practice, First Edition
By Peter Hill, Sheena Warman and Geoff Shawcross
© 2011 Blackwell Publishing Ltd

The differential diagnoses can often be narrowed significantly from the history, observation of the breathing rate and pattern, and a cursory physical examination. For example, where there is a history of coughing prior to the onset of dyspnoea, asthma is far more likely to be present than left-sided CHF (in contrast to dogs, cats with CHF rarely cough). A recent change in the meow, or presence of snoring, stridor or stertor is suggestive of nasopharyngeal or laryngeal disease.

A careful assessment of the breathing pattern can be helpful in differentiating the possible causes (Table 58.1). After a brief observation of the breathing rate and pattern, a cursory physical examination should be performed if possible, including observation of mucous membrane colour, assessment for visible signs of trauma, and cardiopulmonary auscultation. The presence of a heart murmur and/or gallop sounds in conjunction with a high heart rate (± an arrhythmia) support a diagnosis of left-sided CHF, in which case a pleural effusion and/or pulmonary oedema will be present. However, the absence of a heart murmur and/or gallop sounds does not completely discount the possibility that CHF is present. Chest percussion, to elicit areas of dullness, may also be employed to support a diagnosis of pleural effusion. Lack of compressibility may be detected in cats with a cranial thoracic mass.

After the initial evaluation, if a pleural effusion or pneumothorax is considered likely, thoracocentesis (usually under light sedation) may be employed without prior diagnostic imaging (see Figure 58.1 and below for technique). Samples of any fluid obtained should be placed in an EDTA tube (for cytology) and a plain tube (for assessment of protein levels and bacterial culture if appropriate). A fresh smear can be analysed in-house.

If it is unclear whether or not a pleural effusion or pneumothorax is present, a dorsoventral radiograph of the thorax may be obtained. Alternatively, thoracic ultrasound allows a more rapid diagnosis of pleural effusion, as long as clipping does not stress the cat. If a pleural effusion is not present, a more complete thoracic radiographic series would be valuable to investigate other possible causes.

Table 58.1 Differential diagnoses based on breathing pattern.

Restrictive breathing pattern	Obstructive breathing pattern	
Stiff lungs or pleural disease prevent full lung expansion and result in short, rapid and shallow breaths. Exhalation or both phases of respiration may appear laboured.	Airway narrowing results in increased respiratory effort. The location of narrowing determines which phase of respiration is more laboured (and often prolonged). Fixed upper airway obstructions may lead to increased difficulty throughout both phases of respiration.	
	↑ **Inspiratory effort** Abnormal inspiratory sounds may also be apparent (e.g. stridor or stertor).	↑ **Expiratory effort** Wheezing sounds may also be heard on exhalation.
• CHF • Pleural effusion • Pneumonia • Pulmonary neoplasia • Pneumothorax	• Laryngeal paralysis • Nasopharyngeal disease (e.g. polyp, neoplasia)	• Asthma

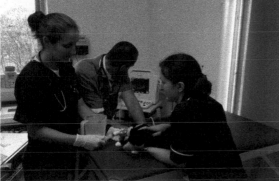

Figure 58.1 Thoracocentesis using a butterfly catheter attached to a 3-way tap. In most cases it is far safer and easier to have one or two people gently restraining the cat and one person holding the butterfly catheter in the chest. Ultrasound guidance is unnecessary but if available does help to optimise site for needle insertion. A third person actually drains the fluid

Treatment

In all cases, care must be taken not to increase patient distress. Consequently, oxygen supplementation, thoracocentesis, drugs or rarely, tracheostomy, may be required prior to diagnostic testing. Supplemental oxygen should be provided as soon as possible, initially by holding an oxygen tube near the nose or mouth at a flow rate of 5 L/min. An oxygen cage may then be employed to provide an oxygen-rich environment thereafter. Regardless of the underlying cause of the dyspnoea, sedation (e.g. butorphanol 0.2 mg/kg IM) often helps to alleviate anxiety and facilitate procedures such as thoracocentesis. Intramuscular administration of drugs is often less stressful in a dyspnoeic cat than restraint for intravenous injection.

Cats with pleural effusions or pneumothorax of unknown cause should receive supplemental oxygen and undergo thoracocentesis as soon as possible. Thoracocentesis is usually performed with the cat in sternal recumbency. An area over the chest wall should be clipped and aseptically prepared. Placement of the needle/catheter may be guided by thoracic ultrasound, thoracic radiography (or possibly even chest percussion). Otherwise the tap is usually made at the 7th to 8th rib space, usually at the level of the costochondral junction (slightly higher if a pneumothorax is present). A butterfly catheter, attached to a three-way tap and connected to a 20-ml syringe, is most often used.

Pyothorax may be treated with intravenous fluids, antibiotics and supportive care plus either intermittent thoracocentesis (using the aforementioned technique) or placement of one or two chest drains (which requires general anaesthesia). The latter may be preferable since this facilitates drainage and allows once or twice daily pleural lavage.

Cats with left-sided CHF will have pleural effusion and/or pulmonary oedema. If a pleural effusion is present, thoracocentesis should be employed as soon as possible, followed by low-dose furosemide to prevent recurrence and control any pulmonary oedema. Pulmonary oedema should be treated with furosemide (initially 2 mg/kg IV or IM) and glyceryl trinitrate (Percutol, Dominion Pharma), ¼ inch applied topically, usually to the medial aspect of the pinna. The respiratory rate and effort should be monitored, and the furosemide dose repeated after 1–2 h if the dyspnoea has not abated. Clinicians should note that cats are particularly sensitive to the dehydrating and potassium-depleting effects of diuretics; consequently the lowest effective dose of furosemide should always be used. Cats occasionally require administration of IV fluids (e.g. half maintenance rate) supplemented with potassium for 12–24 h after receiving IV furosemide. Hypokalaemia should be considered if the cat becomes inappetent, weak and lethargic after diuretic administration. Long-term management depends on the underlying cause and usually involves various combinations of furosemide, spironolactone, an ACE-inhibitor, antithrombotic therapy and antiarrhythmic agents. Pimobendan is also indicated in some cases. A referral to a veterinary cardiologist is recommended to establish a definitive diagnosis and optimal therapeutic regimen.

Cats with asthma should be treated initially with dexamethasone (0.25–0.5 mg/kg IV/IM) and the β_2-receptor agonist bronchodilator terbutaline (Bricanyl, AstraZeneca; 0.01 mg/kg IV/IM). Rapid improvement can be expected in most cases after 15–30 minutes. However, the terbutaline may be repeated after 30 minutes if insufficient response is noted.

If the underlying cause of the dyspnoea is unclear, treatment with furosemide (2 mg/kg IV/IM) plus dexamethasone (0.25–0.5 mg/kg IV/IM) may be employed together in the first instance. Terbutaline should be avoided if CHF cannot be discounted.

What if it doesn't get better?

When fluid or air is present in the pleural space, failure to adequately drain it will result in a poor response. Failure to respond may also be due to an incorrect provisional diagnosis or inappropriate treatment. Consequently, a change of treatment strategy with or without further diagnostic testing (if the patient is sufficiently stable) may allow progress to be made. If, however, there is such severe underlying pathology and/or respiratory fatigue that the patient is unable to adequately ventilate or oxygenate despite supplemental oxygen and initial stabilisation, it may be necessary to intubate and provide positive pressure ventilation. If this cannot be performed, euthanasia may be the kindest approach. Some causes of dyspnoea (e.g. lung tumours, FIP) carry an inherently poor prognosis.

The low-cost option

Empirical treatment based on the most likely diagnosis may be effective and could spare the cost of a diagnostic investigation. As long as a broad-spectrum approach is not undertaken, a favourable response to initial empirical therapy will then provide clues to the underlying cause of the dyspnoea, and may allow an on-going treatment plan to be established. However, given that dyspnoea is a life-threatening condition that may result in an extremely unpleasant and occasionally protracted death, cost-cutting should not be undertaken at the expense of patient welfare. If empirical treatment is ineffective, and the patient is suffering, euthanasia may be warranted.

When should I refer?

Most dyspnoeic cats can be stabilised in general practice. If the practice does not have the facilities or expertise to diagnose and manage some of the underlying conditions mentioned above, a referral should be offered. Referring a dyspnoeic patient is usually best done after an initial period of stabilisation, since the journey (usually done without supplemental oxygen) may endanger the life of the cat. Cats with CHF would benefit from an expert opinion to allow a precise diagnosis and optimal treatment regimen to be established.

Section 7
Eye problems

Jim Carter and Peter Hill

Aetiology and pathogenesis

Eyelid disease may be either hereditary (e.g. entropion, ectropion, nasal fold trichiasis, macropalpebral fissures) or acquired (e.g. trauma, neoplasia). Acquired eyelid disease becomes more common as the patient gets older.

Entropion is an inversion of one or both eyelid margins, normally with haired skin contacting the cornea or conjunctiva (Figure 59.1). It is extremely common in domestic species, but is more common in dogs than cats, and in certain breeds such as the Shar Pei, Mastiff, Rottweiler, Great Dane and Labrador Retriever. Although entropion is typically thought of as a disease of young patients (weeks to months), it may not be clinically present or noted by the owner of large-breed dogs until the dog is adolescent (12–24 months old).

Ectropion is an eversion of one or both eyelid margins with exposure of the bulbar and palpebral conjunctiva (Figure 59.2). It is known as diamond eye, and is common in giant breeds (especially St Bernards, Newfoundlands and Clumber Spaniels) but rare in cats.

Various disorders of the eyelashes are seen in dogs. Distichiasis is the presence of an abnormal row of eyelashes on the lid margin arising from the meibomian glands. It is common in Flat Coat Retrievers, Cocker Spaniels, Dachshunds and Cavalier King Charles Spaniels. Ectopic cilia are individual eyelashes that protrude via the palpebral conjunctival surface, having originated in the meibomian gland and are most common in Flat Coat Retrievers and Bull Dogs. Trichiasis refers to normal eyelashes or eyelid hairs that project towards the globe and contact the cornea or conjunctiva causing irritation. This is most common in toy breeds with excessive facial hair and Cocker Spaniels with a slipping facial mask. Eyelash disorders are rare in cats.

Blepharitis is inflammation of the eyelids. It is a multifactorial condition that can be seen in association with conjunctivitis, or with skin disease (allergies, demodicosis, pyoderma, fungal infections, autoimmune disease; Figure 59.3). The meibomian glands of the eyelid can also become inflamed or infected. Acute pyogenic infection produces a small abscess and is referred to as a

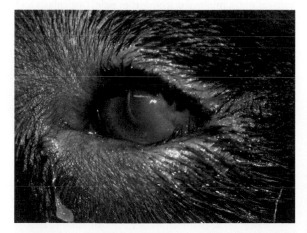

Figure 59.1 **Dog with entropion resulting in corneal ulceration**

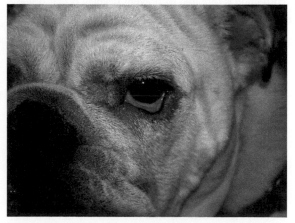

Figure 59.2 **Dog with ectropion showing eversion of the eyelid**

100 Top Consultations in Small Animal General Practice, First Edition
By Peter Hill, Sheena Warman and Geoff Shawcross
© 2011 Blackwell Publishing Ltd

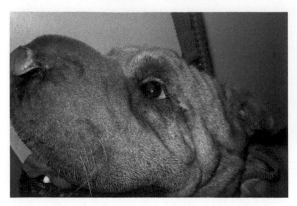

Figure 59.3 Blepharitis and periorbital dermatitis in a dog with allergic skin disease and secondary pyoderma

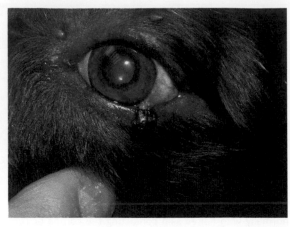

Figure 59.4 Meibomian gland adenoma on the eyelid

hordeolum (stye). Chronic inflammation produces a small nodule which is referred to as a chalazion.

Eyelid neoplasia is common in the older dog and is typically benign. The most common types of lid neoplasia in the dog are meibomian gland adenoma (Figure 59.4) or adenocarcinoma, papilloma or melanoma. Meibomian gland adenomas are associated with the meibomian gland epithelium and have a typical lobulated appearance at the lid margin, although papillomas may have a similar appearance and location. Eyelid neoplasia in cats is less common but more often malignant. Squamous cell carcinomas can also develop on the eyelids, especially when they are non-pigmented and following solar damage. Resection of eyelid masses may be curative, but restoration of the eyelid structure after excision is essential for maintaining long-term ocular surface health.

Traumatic damage to the lids often results in lacerations of the lid margin. An early diagnosis and accurate correction is required to prevent ongoing ocular disease. Misalignment of the lid margins due to previous surgery or trauma, or regions of lid margin that do not have the normal anatomical mucocutaneous smooth margin, can result in dramatic long-term and potentially sight-threatening corneal and intraocular disease.

History and clinical signs

Because of the visible nature of many of these conditions, many causes of eyelid disease can be diagnosed on the basis of the history and clinical examination alone. Additionally, in many cases, the duration of clinical signs will help with the location of the problem, as certain conditions, e.g. distichiasis, will not suddenly develop in an elderly patient. The owner should be asked which eye they feel is the problem, as many patients will arrive with multiple ocular lesions but not all will be an issue for the animal. The owner should be asked if they know of any obvious trauma or exposure to chemical irritants prior to the onset of the lid disease. Unless the diagnosis is immediately apparent, a full physical examination should also be carried out as some eyelid lesions can be a manifestation of a more widespread problem.

Most eyelid disorders present with blepharospasm and either an increase in lacrimation or a mucopurulent discharge. However, this is not the case for all patients, especially those with lid neoplasia as, at initial presentation, there may be little or no contact with the cornea and consequently, minimal discomfort or pain. Distichiasis and ectopic cilia can lead to cyclical symptoms at approximately 6–8 week intervals, as the hairs grow, contact the eye and then fall out.

Specific diagnostic techniques

A thorough ocular examination is vital in all cases of eyelid disease. It is important to assess the lid conformation without the aid of sedation as this will change the lid positions and also hinder neurological assessment. In many cases, lid conformation is best assessed from a distance without touching the patient as this may exacerbate blepharospasm or, in the case of some breeds such as the Shar Pei, preclude all examination due to excessive lid spasm. A Schirmer Tear Test should then be performed to ensure that there are no deficiencies in tear production.

Once this has been done, topical local anaesthesia can be applied if necessary to try to alleviate any spastic component of the lid deformity. It may also be used to confirm that the ocular discomfort is derived from the lids, conjunctiva or cornea, as pain from intraocular disease such as glaucoma or uveitis is not alleviated by topical anaesthesia.

Some lid disease such as distichiasis or ectopic cilia may not be clearly visible with the naked eye and so some form of magnification may be essential to obtain a diagnosis. This may take the form of an operating loupe, direct ophthalmoscope, slitlamp biomicroscope or even a magnifying glass. If these are not available within the practice then referral may be necessary for a more detailed examination.

In the case of lid neoplasia, cytological evaluation or histopathology may be required. Cytology can often be obtained either by fine needle aspiration or impression smears. Some lid neoplasms, such as squamous cell carcinoma, have a high exfoliation rate and cytology may be able to give an accurate diagnosis. However, in many cases biopsy will be required for definitive diagnosis. In such cases, the clinician needs to decide whether to take an excisional biopsy (for small tumours) or a partial, sectional, biopsy (for larger lesions). Advanced diagnostic imaging may be necessary for more invasive tumours to determine the full extent of the lesion. For example, a squamous cell carcinoma may already be invading the orbit at time of initial diagnosis.

Culture and sensitivity testing of ocular discharges may be beneficial but clinicians should remember that most eye infections are secondary to an underlying cause, so the results do not usually determine the primary treatment. Antibiotics should only be used if there is clinical evidence of infection, or secondary corneal injury has occurred due to the lid pathology. Initial medication may be either systemic or topical depending on the site of disease and extent of pathology.

Treatment

- Entropion and ectropion are best treated by surgical correction, but the operation is best left until the eyelids have reached a mature conformation (usually at least 6–12 months of age)

  However, young puppies with entropion may respond well to a simple lid-tacking procedure. If an operation is deemed necessary at this time, revisional surgery may be required at a later date. Entropion and ectropion surgery is best carried out by experienced clinicians or specialist ophthalmologists because over- and under-correction can both lead to a failed outcome. Also, the large number of surgical techniques available makes selection of the most appropriate procedure difficult. In complicated cases (such as Shar Peis or St Bernards), referral at initial diagnosis may be the best approach.

- Distichiasis and ectopic cilia may not always require treatment. Many dogs have abnormal lashes from a young age without having clinical signs. If required, surgical correction can be achieved by electrolysis, cryotherapy or several different resection techniques. The technique of choice varies between clinicians.

- The treatment of blepharitis requires an accurate diagnosis, which requires a consideration of both ocular and cutaneous differential diagnoses. Depending on the cause, treatment for bacterial infection, fungal infection, demodicosis or allergies may be required. Hordeolums and chalazions can be treated by incision, curettage and topical antibiotics.

- Eyelid tumours are best treated by surgical resection. Small eyelid tumours in geriatric patients can be carefully monitored without treatment, but once the tumour makes contact with the cornea, it will cause pain and inflammation. At this stage, surgical resection is required. In younger dogs, surgical resection is advised at an earlier stage because contact with the cornea is ultimately likely and the operation is easier when the tumour is small. Larger tumours may require more complicated blepharoplasty techniques, which are likely to require the expertise of a specialist.

- Traumatic lacerations are treated by careful suturing to reappose the cut edges.

Section 7

What if it doesn't get better?

Most of the above conditions can be cured or effectively managed. In most cases, failure to achieve a good outcome indicates a failure to make a correct diagnosis, or a sub-optimal outcome following surgical intervention. Some conditions, such as advanced lid neoplasia, inherently carry a poor prognosis and a long-term cure may not be possible.

The low-cost option

There are no ways of dramatically reducing the costs when dealing with eyelid disorders, which are usually diagnosed on the basis of history and clinical examination. In many cases, surgical intervention is required and there are no alternative medical options that might reduce the cost. Failure to achieve an optimal outcome initially may actually result in longer term problems, which incur additional costs. For this reason, referral to an ophthalmologist at an early stage can actually be the most cost-effective option.

When should I refer?

Many minor eyelid disorders can be managed in general practice. However, referral should always be discussed at an early stage for the more complex problems such as severe entropion, ectropion (diamond eye), lid trauma or extensive lid neoplasia. Referral should also be offered if particular skills, equipment or facilities are required, such as performing electrolysis for the treatment of distichiasis. Medical management of some eyelid disorders such as blepharitis can also be difficult, and referral should be offered if a good response to treatment has not been seen within the first week. Long-term inadequate management of such cases may result in scar formation within the lids causing further complications and disease progression. Some of these cases may benefit from collaborative input from both ophthalmologists and dermatologists.

Jim Carter

Conjunctivitis is inflammation of the conjunctiva, the mucous membrane that covers the sclera (bulbar conjunctiva), and inner aspect of the eyelids and third eyelid (palpebral conjunctiva). Conjunctivitis is the commonest cause of a 'red eye' and must be differentiated from corneal disease, anterior uveitis and glaucoma. The condition occurs in both dogs and cats, and has multiple aetiologies. It is worth remembering that some of the causes are not infectious, and certainly not bacterial, and therefore treatment with antibacterial agents may not always be appropriate.

Common differential diagnoses

Primary conjunctivitis

- Infectious
  - Dog – bacterial (mostly *Staphylococcus* spp.), Canine adenovirus-1, Canine distemper virus
  - Cat – *Chlamydophila*, *Mycoplasma* spp., FCV, FHV-1
- Allergic – atopic / allergic conjunctivitis
- Irritant/traumatic – foreign body, scratch, acid/alkali burns, smoke, wind, dust, sand.

Secondary conjunctivitis

- Tear film abnormalities – keratoconjunctivitis sicca (immune-mediated, neurogenic, congenital), meibomian gland disease
- Eyelid defects – entropion, ectropion, distichiasis, ectopic cilia
- Corneal disease – corneal ulceration, chronic superficial keratitis (pannus; only in dogs), eosinophilic keratitis (cats), corneal sequestrum (cats), herpetic keratitis (cats)
- Retrobulbar disease
- Periorbital disease
- Neoplastic infiltration (especially lymphoma)
- Intraocular disease (uveitis, glaucoma, lens luxation).

100 Top Consultations in Small Animal General Practice, First Edition
By Peter Hill, Sheena Warman and Geoff Shawcross
© 2011 Blackwell Publishing Ltd

Diagnostic approach

Although many cases of conjunctivitis are traumatic in origin (cat fights, foreign bodies, caustic agents), the initiating cause will often not have been witnessed by the owner. Patients typically present with a discharge that is unilateral or bilateral, and mucoid or mucopurulent. If severe, this may be adherent to the lid margins preventing opening of one or both eyes. Some causes (such as *Chlamydophila* infection in the cat) present with a serous discharge. Typically, conjunctivitis is sore and irritating but not acutely painful. If there is marked blepharospasm or ocular pain, it normally indicates an additional problem, such as corneal disease or glaucoma.

A full ocular examination should be performed in all cases of conjunctivitis. The eyelids and peri-ocular regions should be carefully checked, and the eyes examined for asymmetry or swellings. The conjunctiva will be hyperaemic. Prominent, tortuous blood vessels may be seen running across the sclera that are mobile with the conjunctiva, unlike those seen with episcleral involvement which are short, straight, perpendicular to the limbus and not mobile (Figure 60.1). In some instances, lymphoid follicles (small white nodules) can be seen within the ventral fornix and on, or under, the third eyelid.

In-house cytology of the discharge can be very valuable in characterising the role of bacterial infection and to help choose appropriate treatment, especially in recurrent cases. It is important to collect the sample before the discharge is cleaned away. A Schirmer Tear Test should then be performed as keratoconjunctivitis sicca is still largely under-diagnosed and is a major cause of recurrent conjunctival infections in dogs (Figure 60.2). In cats it is appropriate to submit dry swabs for PCR for FHV-1 and *Chlamydophila*, and swabs in virus transport medium for FCV.

The cornea should then be examined for evidence of corneal or intra-ocular disease, before and after application of fluorescein. With uncomplicated conjunctivitis, the cornea will be clear, whereas it can be cloudy or opaque with keratitis, uveitis or glaucoma. Positive staining with fluorescein indicates corneal ulceration as long as excess stain is flushed away immediately (see Chapter 61). The pupil appears normal with conjunctivitis and corneal disease, but it is typically small or irregular with uveitis and dilated with glaucoma.

Topical local anaesthetic can then be applied to the eye to allow the third eyelid to be gently lifted so that the bulbar aspect can be examined for foreign bodies or follicle formation.

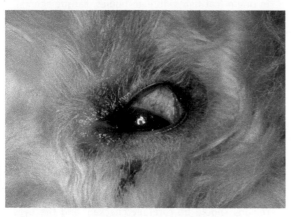

Figure 60.1   Conjunctivitis in a dog, showing tortuous scleral blood vessels (picture courtesy of Peter Hill)

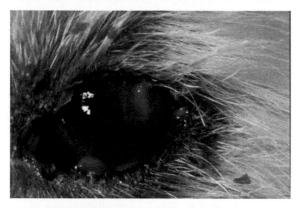

Figure 60.2   Keratoconjunctivitis sicca, causing a mucopurulent ocular discharge

Treatment

If the conjunctivitis is secondary to some other ocular problem, this will need to be treated specifically to allow resolution. For primary conjunctivitis, topical antibacterial agents are appropriate in most cases. The choice of antibiotic should be based on clinical signs, knowledge of the probable organism involved, and cytology ± culture and sensitivity testing. In most cases, the infection will have been triggered by foreign bodies, trauma or irritants and will respond to a limited selection of antibacterial agents such as fusidic acid or chloramphenicol. These antibiotics are readily available in eye ointments or drops and are typically applied three or four times daily in the case of chloramphenicol drops or once daily for fusidic acid, both for 5 days.

Chlamydophila infections require systemic treatment with doxycycline at 10 mg/kg for three weeks after the clinical resolution of signs (usually about 28 days in total). In cases caused by viral infection, the bacterial infection will be secondary, so antibacterial treatment will only result in a partial response. Therapy for viral-induced conjunctivitis will depend on the underlying cause. FHV in cats has shown good response to topical antiviral medications such as trifluorothymidine drops and may potentially respond to systemic famcyclovir, although evidence is mainly anecdotal at this time.

The use of topical corticosteroids or NSAIDs is indicated for follicular (allergic) conjunctivitis, but contraindicated if the cornea exhibits any indication of ulceration or erosion, as corticosteroids can potentiate the action of collagenases and elastases resulting in a 'melting cornea'. Patients with allergic conjunctivitis may require treatment with topical dexamethasone (Maxidex) or ketorolac trometamol (Acular), as well as appropriate management of any more-widespread cutaneous signs (see Chapter 20).

What if it doesn't get better?

In most cases, treatment failure arises because anti-biotics are being applied to the eye when the cause of the condition is not a bacterial infection. The initial diagnosis should be reviewed and more appropriate treatment instituted, rather than immediately trying an alternative antibiotic. For example, correction of diseases such as ectropion or KCS is paramount to treating the cause of conjunctivitis and repeated courses of antibiotics will be of no long-term benefit. It is also important to ensure that more sinister diagnoses such as uveitis or glaucoma have not been missed.

If a resistant bacterial infection is suspected, the choice of antibiotic should be made on the basis of bacterial culture and sensitivity testing. Empirical changes of antibiotic therapy are not appropriate. Antibiotics that can be beneficial when bacterial resistance is documented include un-licensed topical products such as ciprofloxacin (Ciloxan, Alcon) or ofloxacin (Exocin, Allergan).

Rarely, a conjunctival biopsy may be necessary in order to make a diagnosis (e.g. with lymphoma). This can usually be done under topical local anaesthesia and does not generally require sedation.

The low-cost option

Many cases of conjunctivitis can be managed at relatively low cost with appropriate topical treatment. The main way to prevent unnecessary costs is to get an accurate diagnosis from the outset to avoid unsuccessful treatments. Some of the causes of conjunctivitis are more serious conditions and treatment costs will inevitably be higher when this is the case.

When should I refer?

Most cases of primary conjunctivitis can be managed in general practice. Referral should be considered if the problem is secondary to a more serious ocular problem that cannot be dealt with within the practice, especially conditions such as uveitis or glaucoma. Also, if a case does not respond to initial therapy within 5–7 days, or there is progression to ulceration of the conjunctiva or cornea, an expert opinion from an ophthalmologist may be helpful.

Section 7

Jim Carter

Aetiology and pathogenesis

Corneal ulceration can be caused by trauma, cat scratches, foreign bodies, tear-film abnormalities such as keratoconjunctivitis sicca (KCS), abnormal eyelid conformation, contact of lashes with the cornea, FHV infection and neurological disorders such as facial nerve paralysis. In dogs, it is most common in brachycephalic breeds due to exposure of the central cornea. Most corneal ulcers are not due to primary infections, so antibiotic treatment is prophylactic rather than therapeutic.

History and clinical signs

Traumatic incidents are often not witnessed by the owner, although typically they will lead to a very acute onset of clinical signs. In brachycephalic dogs, owners will often not notice the start of the ulceration as the dogs normally have poor corneal sensitivity. Many of these dogs will have a history of recurrent corneal ulceration.

Corneal ulcers are painful and may lead to squinting or rubbing at the eye. The cornea may appear cloudy and there will often be an associated conjunctivitis with a serous discharge. The third eyelid may be prolapsed and the pupil may be small due to a reflex uveitis.

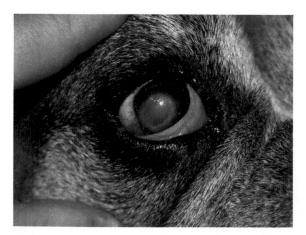

Figure 61.1   Large, indolent corneal ulcer

100 Top Consultations in Small Animal General Practice, First Edition
By Peter Hill, Sheena Warman and Geoff Shawcross
© 2011 Blackwell Publishing Ltd

Specific diagnostic techniques

The eye should be examined carefully for evidence of entropion, traumatic injury, distichiasis, ectopic cilia or KCS as these could all be potential causes of disease. There may be an obvious defect in the corneal epithelium when the eye is examined with an ophthalmoscope (Figure 61.1). With more severe ulcers, there may be a crater appearance to the central cornea. Corneal vascularisation may occur, appearing as small blood vessels that emanate from the limbus and traverse the cornea to the area of ulceration. These can give the cornea a reddish haze.

A mucopurulent discharge indicates the presence of secondary infection. If present, a sample should be examined cytologically to help establish the nature of the infection (gram-positive, gram-negative, cocci or bacilli). If resistant organisms are suspected, or if an infection has failed to respond to initial antibiotic therapy, a swab should also be submitted for culture and sensitivity.

The depth of ulceration can be ascertained with the help of fluorescein stain and a cobalt blue light source. Fluorescein does not adhere to the normal corneal surface, but does adhere to exposed corneal stroma. A positive result appears as a zone of green fluorescence under ultraviolet light. However, fluorescein does not adhere to Descemet's membrane (the basement membrane of the corneal endothelium). If the ulcer is deep enough to expose this membrane (causing what is known as a descemetocele), there will be a clear zone in the central area of the ulcer (Figure 61.2). When using fluorescein it is important to remember to flush the dye away almost immediately with sterile saline to help prevent false-positive results caused by pooling in healed stromal defects.

Tear film problems are a common cause of corneal ulceration, especially in dogs. It is vital to record Schirmer Tear Test values in all patients with ulceration. However, this procedure should not be performed in patients with full thickness perforation or an imminent chance of corneal perforation (descemetocele).

Treatment

The treatment protocol depends on the depth and location of the lesion and also on the underlying aetiology (Table 61.1). However all patients with corneal ulceration should receive:

- Appropriate analgesia during the course of treatment and healing phase with systemic NSAIDs
- Appropriate antibacterial therapy
- Appropriate treatment for any secondary uveitis, including systemic NSAIDs and mydriatics such as atropine sulphate or tropicamide.

It is becoming common to treat patients with topical NSAIDs rather than systemic medications but these will retard corneal epithelialisation (as will all topical medications). Prophylactic antibiosis is always recommended to prevent secondary corneal infection. For initial therapy, topical fusidic acid or chloramphenicol would be appropriate choices. If infection is already established, or occurs during treatment, the choice of antibiotic should be based on cytology ± culture and sensitivity testing (Table 61.2).

Superficial regions of ulceration should respond to treatment and be completely resolved within 7–10 days of injury. If not, clinicians should look for another underlying factor that is potentiating the ulceration and preventing resolution.

Deep ulcers (descemetocele) require surgical correction. This can only be achieved with correct surgical instruments, small suture materials (8/0 or smaller) and good magnification. The techniques are best performed by specialists (Figure 61.3).

The use of third eyelid flaps is a relatively simple procedure for covering corneal ulcers to assist with healing, but they are not the preferred choice of ophthalmologists because it is not possible to examine the cornea whilst they are in place.

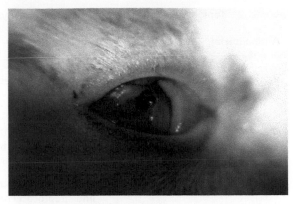

Figure 61.2 **A descemetocele**

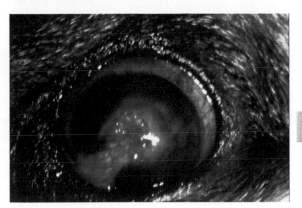

Figure 61.3 **Surgical repair of a deep corneal ulcer using a pedicle graft**

Table 61.1 **Depth of ulceration and treatment options.**

Depth	Medical treatment	Surgical treatment
Superficial	Topical antibiotics	Contact lens
<⅓ depth	Topical treatment	Contact lens or third eyelid flap
>⅓ depth	Topical treatment	Pedicle graft, corneoconjunctival transposition

Table 61.2 Topical antibiotics and spectrum of activity.

Antibacterial agent	Corneal penetration	Range of activity	Main indications
Bacitracin	Poor	Gram-positive infections, in particular streptococci	Often manufactured in combination with polymixin or with hydrocortisone
Chloramphenicol	Good	Broad spectrum but *Pseudomonas* may be resistant. Variably bacteriocidal, minimal corneal toxicity	Surface ocular infections, intraocular infections, prophylaxis following surgery
Ciprofloxacin	Good	Broad spectrum but some streptococci and streptococci resistant. Gram-negative coverage including *Pseudomonas*, gram-positive including some staphylococci and *Bacillus*	Gentamycin-resistant *Pseudomonas* infections
Fusidic acid	Good	Fusidic acid is only effective against gram-positive bacteria such as *Streptococcus*, *Staphylococcus* and *Corynebacterium*	Gram-positive ocular surface infections, bacterial lid infections and post-operative lid surgery
Gentamycin	Poor	Aminoglycosides are active against many gram-negative and some gram-positive bacteria. Not useful for anaerobic bacteria, or for intracellular bacteria, e.g. *Chlamydophila*	Gram-negative ocular surface infections
Polymixin B	Poor	Gram-negative bacteria including *Pseudomonas*	Often manufactured in combination with Neomycin or with steroids, e.g. Maxitrol

What if it doesn't get better?

If the ulceration fails to respond to appropriate treatment or continues to deteriorate despite treatment then referral should be discussed as a matter of urgency. Progression of an ulcer into the deeper layers of the cornea can lead to a descemetocele or even corneal rupture. Some corneal ulcers can become refractory (indolent). These are caused by failure of the epithelium to adhere to the underlying stroma and typically have a rim of loose epithelium around their edge. Indolent ulcers can be treated by debridement under local anaesthesia, grid keratotomy and application of bandage contact lenses (although these can be very difficult to retain in brachycephalic patients). These procedures are best performed by experienced clinicians and specialists.

Some ulcers undergo collagenolysis (melting ulcers). In such cases, application of topical plasma drops and EDTA preparations can help to prevent further progression. Plasma drops are prepared in-house from blood products, whereas EDTA drops can be obtained from specialist pharmacies.

In cats, the possible role of FHV should be considered, and a swab submitted for PCR. Another complication that can occur in cats is the development of a corneal sequestrum (Figure 61.4). This is a necrotic region of corneal stroma and generally is best treated by specialists with a superficial keratectomy and then some form of corneal repair, either with a pedicle graft or corneoconjunctival transposition.

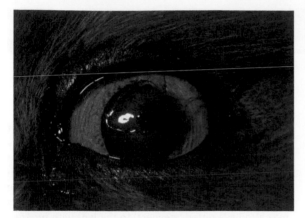

Figure 61.4 **Corneal sequestrum in a cat**

When should I refer?

Referral should always be discussed in cases of corneal perforation, deep regions of ulceration or marked uveitis, especially if the practice does not have suitable equipment for surgery or if the clinician is not experienced with the techniques. It should always be remembered that the cornea is not very forgiving of poor surgical technique and the best repair should be the first repair attempted.

The low-cost option

The cheapest and best way to get resolution in these cases is to obtain an accurate diagnosis at the first consultation by performing a detailed ocular examination. Money can be wasted by sequentially changing medications in the hope that one will work. In deep regions of ulceration associated with brachycephalic patients it may be expedient to discuss referral at an early stage and treat these cases as an emergency. Enucleation may also be considered as a therapeutic option as these patients often need combination procedures to correct the corneal defect and poor lid conformation which can prove to be expensive and not always effective.

Section 7

Jim Carter

Aetiology and pathogenesis

A cataract is an opacity that occurs within the lens or lens capsule. It results from a disruption in the water balance and protein content of the lens, or the normal arrangement of the lens fibres.

Cataracts can occur for a variety of reasons:

- Hereditary (most common in dogs; see Table 62.1)
- Intraocular disease such as uveitis, glaucoma, lens luxation, retinal detachment or retinal degeneration, e.g. progressive retinal atrophy (PRA), toxic insult, post inflammation
- Infectious diseases, especially in cats, in association with uveitis and lens epithelial damage
- Associated with metabolic disorders such as diabetes mellitus or hypocalcaemia in the dog
- Associated with milk replacer in young puppies (due to amino acid deficiency)
- Associated with traumatic injuries, e.g. foreign bodies or cat claws
- Idiopathic.

In the cat, most cataracts are secondary to trauma or infectious disease that causes uveitis and lens epithelial damage. Even if there is no obvious sign of uveitis, it should be ruled out, as subclinical disease may be present and can lead to development and progression of cataract. Hereditary forms of cataract are rarely seen in cats.

History and clinical signs

Owners may present their pet because they have noticed a change in the appearance of the eye(s) or suspect that vision is impaired. However, it is more common for cataracts to be detected incidentally at routine vaccination or geriatric check-ups, without the owner realising there is a problem with the pet's eyes. Most cataracts develop very gradually. However, those associated with diabetes mellitus can develop very rapidly, with marked swelling of the lens (intumescence) and lens-induced uveitis.

Owners may report some loss of vision in their pet, which may be apparent as difficulty in finding objects such as toys or biscuits (e.g. with cataract formation), or night blindness (associated with PRA and potentially secondary cataract formation). Difficulty locating objects may be noted more in bright sunlight as many hereditary cataracts are central in position; as the pupil constricts, there is a temporary marked visual impairment. The owners may also have noted 'greyness' to the lens with progression over time. Dogs that present with progressive visual impairment and alterations of the lens must have a full ophthalmic examination as there may be causes such as retinal degeneration, uveitis, glaucoma or diabetes driving the cataract progression.

Table 62.1 **Some canine breeds known to suffer from hereditary cataract. Ages indicate the mean age of onset.**

Golden Retriever	9 years
Labrador Retriever	9 years
Cavalier King Charles Spaniel	7 years
Standard Poodle	18 months
Staffordshire Bull Terrier	18 months
German Shepherd Dog	3 years
Old English Sheepdog	3 years
Welsh Springer Spaniel	3 years
Miniature Schnauzer	3 years
American Cocker Spaniel	6 years
Boston Terrier	Two forms: early 3 years; late 8 years
Irish Red and White Setter	9 years
Belgian Shepherd Dog	9 years
Siberian Husky	5 years
Chesapeake Bay Retriever	3 years
Leonburger	9 years
Norwegian Buhund	5 years
Large Munsterlander	9 years

100 Top Consultations in Small Animal General Practice, First Edition
By Peter Hill, Sheena Warman and Geoff Shawcross
© 2011 Blackwell Publishing Ltd

Specific diagnostic techniques

A thorough and complete ophthalmic examination must be performed with all cataract patients. Mydriasis is required to assess the lens equator for indications of cataract progression and also to enable the retina to be visualised around the cataract.

Cataracts appear on ophthalmoscopic examination as a visible opacity within the lens (Figure 62.1). This needs to be differentiated from nuclear sclerosis and age related thickening of the lens that occurs in all patients over the age of approximately seven years. With nuclear sclerosis, there is normally no detectable impairment of vision and no loss of tapetal reflectivity, as occurs with cataracts.

Cataracts can be classified by:

- Age at onset – congenital, juvenile (up to 6 years) or senile (over 6 years)
- Location – capsular, subcapsular, cortical or nuclear
- Severity
  - Incipient (<10% of retina obscured)
  - Immature (may be unable to examine the retina but will still have visible tapetal light reflection)
  - Mature (loss of tapetal light reflection)
  - Hypermature (the cataract is liquefying or reabsorbing and causing lens-induced uveitis. A tapetal light reflection can be visualised along with wrinkling of the lens capsule).

These classifications are of benefit in determining the origin and progression of the cataract. In combination with knowledge of the age and breed, they will help differentiate hereditary cataract from inflammatory, congenital or traumatic causes in many canine patients. Patients with rapid progression of cataract should be screened for diabetes mellitus.

To help differentiate retinal disease from lenticular disease causing visual impairment, patients may benefit from an obstacle course test in both light (photopic) and dark (scotopic) conditions. Those patients with hereditary retinal disease such as PRA often show clinical indications of night blindness not shown by patients with immature cataract.

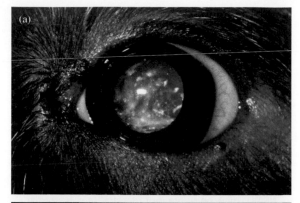

(a)

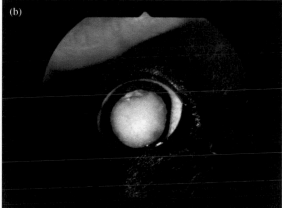

(b)

Figure 62.1 **Hypermature cataracts**

Treatment

Currently, there is no medical treatment that will resolve cataracts. The only therapeutic option is removal by phacoemulsification followed by intraocular prosthetic lens implantation. Phacoemulsification has the highest success rate in:

- Patients with immature cataracts (success rate approximately 94%)
- Patients with no other clinical systemic disease, e.g. diabetes mellitus (the presence of such diseases does not prevent phacoemulsification but it may increase the complication rate)
- Patients with no indication of concomitant ocular disease, e.g. chronic uveitis, progressive retinal atrophy.

Mature and hypermature cataracts can also be successfully treated with phacoemulsification but the long-term success rate is lower (85–90%) than in young patients with soft, immature cataracts.

If there is a secondary lens-induced uveitis (often associated with rapid cataract development), medical treatment is indicated to prevent the development of tertiary glaucoma. Appropriate medical treatment in this situation includes topical corticosteroids and a mydriatic (e.g. tropicamide or atropine sulphate). However, in some diabetics, even topical corticosteroids can contribute to insulin resistance so a topical NSAID may be more appropriate (e.g. ketorolac, trometamol or flubiprofen).

What if it doesn't get better?

Cataracts will not spontaneously resolve or reduce with medical management available at this time. Hence, without phacoemulsification, the disease will persist and possibly progress.

The low-cost option

If referral for full ophthalmologic assessment and possible phacoemulsification is not an option, owners should be advised on how to manage a visually impaired dog. Many dogs cope extremely well with blindness as long as there are minimal changes in their environment.

When should I refer?

Early referral for full ophthalmologic assessment is recommended in any patient with cataracts, to ensure that no underlying disease is present that would warrant specific treatment, and to discuss suitability for phacoemulsification. In diabetic patients, referral should be offered as soon as the cataracts become apparent; some ophthalmologists will recommend application of topical treatments (NSAIDs) until referral can be arranged. Referral is also advised in cases that have concurrent uveitis, glaucoma or lens luxations.

Jim Carter

Blindness is normally thought of as a lack or loss of the ability to see. This can range from being unable to negotiate around the house because of the loss of visual acuity, to complete absence of perception of light. Blindness is most commonly caused by lesions within the eye, but it can also be caused by central disease (due to optic nerve or brain disorders).

Common differential diagnoses

Conditions marked with an * are currently untreatable and lead to permanent blindness. All the others are potentially treatable if a correct diagnosis is made.

- Trauma
- Keratitis
- Cataract
- Intraocular haemorrhage (hyphaema)
- Uveitis (anterior, posterior)
- Glaucoma
- Chorioretinitis
- Retinal detachment*
- PRA*
- Sudden acquired retinal degeneration (SARD)*
- Optic neuritis
- Intracranial lesions
- Neoplasia
- Systemic hypertension
- Toxicity, e.g. ivermectin, enrofloxacin* (cats).

Diagnostic approach

When presented with a case of blindness, the clinician should rapidly try and determine:

- Can the condition be diagnosed within the practice (i.e. by a non-specialist)?
- Once diagnosed, can the condition be treated?

A detailed clinical history is very valuable when assessing blindness. Many of the conditions that cause blindness have breed or age predispositions. Blindness may occur suddenly (trauma, intraocular haemorrhage, SARD) or gradually (cataract, PRA). Some causes of blindness may be associated with pain (uveitis, glaucoma) whereas others are asymptomatic, apart from the visual loss.

A thorough physical examination is also essential as some causes may be due to more widespread systemic disease. In elderly cats, particular attention should be paid to the heart, thyroid gland and kidneys, as systemic hypertension is a common cause of blindness in this species. The patient should also be examined from a distance for signs of asymmetry (position of globe, deviations of nasal midline, etc), pain, neurological deficits, ocular discharge or behavioural changes.

Once the physical examination has been undertaken, a complete ophthalmic examination should be performed, including assessment of the cornea, lens, iris, anterior and posterior chambers, retina and optic nerve. The lens should be examined with a direct ophthalmoscope or pen light. Mydriasis is required to properly evaluate the retina and optic nerve. Mydriasis can be achieved with topical tropicamide for rapid onset (15–20 minutes) and short duration of action (2–3 hours). Atropine should not be used due to its long duration of action in most species (a matter of days in dogs and cats). Particular attention should be paid to the retinal vasculature and optic nerve head. Total retinal detachments should be easily visible, even without detailed ophthalmoscopic examination.

A neurological assessment is then indicated, including the following tests:

- Menace response – tested by hand movement in front of the globe
- Palpebral reflex – tested by touching the lid margins medially and laterally
- Vestibulo-ocular reflex – tested by gently moving the head up and down, left and right whilst observing globe movement
- Pupillary light reflex – tested by shining a pen torch into the eye and observing pupillary movement.

100 Top Consultations in Small Animal General Practice, First Edition
By Peter Hill, Sheena Warman and Geoff Shawcross
© 2011 Blackwell Publishing Ltd

- Dazzle reflex – tested by shining a bright light into the eye and observing the animal withdrawing from it.

A further evaluation often used by ophthalmologists to assess vision loss is an obstacle course (although this isn't practical in a typical general practice consultation). This can be done in both ambient and dim light conditions, as night blindness is a cardinal sign of PRA. It may be beneficial to cover one eye at a time to assess unilateral visual abnormalities.

Treatment

The management of blindness is totally dependent on achieving an accurate diagnosis as soon as possible. This will determine if any medical or surgical treatments are available to restore sight. It is important to ascertain if the disease is primarily ocular, neurological or systemic in origin, as this will help direct any medical or surgical management. Many causes of blindness have some systemic clinical disease or signs associated with them, e.g. cataract with diabetes mellitus; intraocular neoplasia with lymphoma; hyphaema with immune-mediated thrombocytopenia; chorioretinitis with toxoplasmosis.

Sudden-onset blindness can lead to anxiousness, confusion and possibly aggression and supportive care can be helpful initially. This normally takes the form of nursing care rather than medical management until a diagnosis is achieved. Some causes of acute blindness are also very painful (e.g. uveitis or glaucoma) and appropriate analgesia with opioids is indicated. Further details on the management of keratitis and cataracts can be found in Chapters 60 and 62.

What if it doesn't get better?

Some causes of blindness are not treatable (e.g. PRA, SARD) while others will only improve following specialist surgery. Some conditions may improve temporarily with treatment but relapse later (e.g. neoplasia). In general, the greater the period of time that the blindness persists, the less chance there is of recovery of any sight. Hence, the optimal outcome will be achieved with immediate diagnosis and aggressive early treatment. Unless the cause is immediately apparent to the clinician, early referral to a specialist is recommended.

The low-cost option

Costs can be minimised if the underlying cause of the disease can be identified on the basis of the history and clinical examination only. However, many of the causes need detailed and often expensive investigation in order to determine the exact cause. It must also be pointed out to clients that many of the long-term therapies for these patients can be expensive and their final expenditure may be reduced by initial capital outlay in investigation and obtaining a definitive diagnosis. If limited funds prevent a full investigation and/or treatment, the final decision about what to do will depend on whether or not the eye is painful. If it is painful, enucleation is a valid option. If it is non-painful, allowing the animal to adapt to life without vision remains the only option. This adaptation is aided by minimal changes to the pet's environment, i.e. not continually moving the furniture or washing the carpets; voice commands to help the patient and prevent injury; using a whistle when on walks to help the pet locate the owner.

When should I refer?

Unless the cause is immediately obvious, referral should be discussed with the client at the initial examination, as this will frequently offer the best prognosis for regaining or retaining vision. It is also sometimes more cost-effective to refer a case for specialist examination, because the diagnosis may be immediately apparent to a specialist when it was not to a less experienced clinician. The surgical treatment of cataracts and glaucoma should only be undertaken by specialists.

Section 8
Urinary tract problems

Sheena Warman

Clinical signs of lower urinary tract disease are common in dogs. Owners may notice increased frequency of urination (pollakiuria), difficulty urinating (dysuria), excessive straining (stranguria), inappropriate elimination, or abnormally coloured or strong-smelling urine. It is important to differentiate pollakiuria (associated with small volumes of urine) from true polyuria. In dogs (unlike cats), lower urinary tract inflammation is most commonly caused by bacterial infection. Infection is usually due to ascent of organisms via the urethra. It is more common in bitches and can be primary, or secondary to urolithiasis or neoplasia. Dogs with renal failure, diabetes mellitus and hyperadrenocorticism are at increased risk of urinary tract infections, although they may not always show clinical signs of lower urinary tract inflammation, despite the presence of a bacterial infection. Urethral obstruction is less common than in cats, and is very rare in bitches, but can occur as a result of urolithiasis.

Common differential diagnoses

Diseases of the bladder

- Bacterial infection
- Cystoliths
- Neoplasia (e.g. transitional cell carcinoma)
- Trauma
- Anatomical abnormalities (e.g. ectopic ureters)
- Sterile haemorrhagic cystitis due to cyclophosphamide administration.

Diseases of the urethra

- Uroliths
- Trauma (often due to prior attempts at catheterisation)
- Neoplasia (e.g. extension of transitional cell carcinoma).

It is also important to consider causes of haematuria that can arise from structures associated with the urinary tract e.g. the prostate, uterus, vagina or penis, or the signs associated with oestrus in the bitch. Disease in the upper urinary tract (kidneys, ureters) can cause haematuria, as can systemic bleeding disorders. Dysuria/stranguria can also be caused by prostatic or neuromuscular disorders.

Diagnostic approach

If urethral obstruction is suspected the patient should be admitted and treated as an emergency (for initial stabilisation refer to feline guidelines in Chapter 66). A thorough history should be taken from the owner, including information regarding previous signs of lower urinary tract disease, general demeanour, duration of clinical signs, whether or not urine is being produced during straining, and the appearance of the urine. Bleeding from the genital tract can be differentiated from urinary bleeding by comparing a voided sample to a cystocentesis sample.

Physical examination should be thorough. Most patients with lower urinary tract disease are systemically well. The abdomen should be palpated to assess bladder size. Palpation should be repeated following voiding to assess the presence of any large bladder masses, although this may be impossible in an overweight or very large dog. Rectal examination should be performed; in male dogs it is important to palpate the prostate, and in female dogs the urethra is usually palpable as it crosses the pelvis.

In all patients, a urine sample should be obtained for specific gravity, dipstick analysis, and sediment examination ± gram staining. If infection is suspected (inflammatory urine sediment with or without visible bacteria), then ideally a cystocentesis sample should be collected for bacterial culture and sensitivity prior to treatment. Commonly isolated bacteria include *E. coli*, *Staphylococcus* spp., and *Proteus* spp. If culture is not performed due to financial or practical limitations, some attempt at bacterial identification can be made based on results of pH and gram-staining. In acidic urine, gram-negative rods are most likely to be *E. coli*. In alkaline urine, gram-negative rods are most likely to be *Proteus* spp., whilst gram-positive cocci could be staphylococci, streptococci or enterococci.

100 Top Consultations in Small Animal General Practice, First Edition
By Peter Hill, Sheena Warman and Geoff Shawcross
© 2011 Blackwell Publishing Ltd

The presence of any type of crystals in urine is not necessarily abnormal. Crystalluria is influenced by urine concentration, pH and temperature, and does not necessarily reflect the presence of a urolith. Because not all uroliths will result in crystalluria, examination of urine sediment should not be relied upon for the diagnosis of urolithiasis; ultrasonography and/or radiography are much more reliable diagnostic tools. Identification of the type of uroliths is aided by knowledge of the breed, signalment, urinalysis results and radiographic findings (see Table 64.1). However, accurate identification often requires quantitative analysis of the stone. Patients with urolithiasis (particularly struvite) will frequently have a concurrent urinary tract infection. Surgery may be required for removal of uroliths or biopsy of suspected tumours.

If the dog is systemically unwell, or if a urethral obstruction is suspected, blood samples should be taken for a minimum of PCV, total solids, urea, creatinine and electrolytes. Ideally, a full haematological and biochemical profile should be obtained.

Table 64.1 Guide to predicting composition of uroliths.

Type of urolith	Breed predisposition	Gender predisposition	Age (years)	Urine pH	Radio-density	Associated abnormalities
Struvite	Miniature Schnauzer, Bichon Frise, Cocker Spaniel, Miniature Poodle	Female (>80%)	1–8	Neutral – alkali	++	Concurrent urinary tract infection common
Calcium oxalate	Miniature Schnauzer, Miniature Poodle, Yorkshire Terrier, Llasa Apso, Bichon Frise, Shih Tzu, Cairn Terrier	Male (>70%)	5–12	Acidic – neutral	+++	Occasionally hypercalcaemic
Urate	Dalmation, English Bulldog, breeds prone to portosystemic shunts	Male (>90%)	1–4	Acidic – neutral	+	Low urea, albumin and glucose and elevated bile acids in patients with portosystemic shunts
Cystine	Dachshund, Basset Hound, English Bulldog, Yorkshire Terrier, Irish Terrier, Rottweiler, Chihuahua, Mastiff, Tibetan Spaniel	Male (>95%)	1–7	Acidic	+	Usually none
Silicate	German Shepherd Dog, Golden Retriever, Labrador Retriever, Old English Sheepdog	Male (>95%)	4–9	Acidic – neutral	++	Usually none

Treatment

If a urinary tract infection is present, treatment with appropriate antibiotics should be instituted. Ideally, this should be based on culture and sensitivity results or at least following information provided by urine pH and gram-staining. If this information is not available, then amoxicillin, ampicillin or amoxicillin/clavulanic acid are appropriate first choices. A 7–10 day course is appropriate for uncomplicated infections.

If urolithiasis is suspected, based on clinical presentation of obstruction or following urinalysis and imaging, attempts should be made to identify the type of urolith, as outlined above. Specific specialised diets are available for the dissolution of struvite, urate and cystine uroliths. However, their use requires significant owner compliance as dissolution may take weeks to months, with monthly urinalyses and radiography or ultrasound to monitor progress. Diets should be continued for 4 weeks beyond radiographic dissolution of the uroliths. Concurrent urinary tract infections must be treated appropriately for the time that it takes for dissolution of the uroliths. Urine should be monitored to ensure pH is appropriate (depending on the type of urolith), that urine specific gravity is less than 1.020 (indicating adequate diuresis), and that there is no evidence of infection on sediment examination. If there is no reduction in the size of uroliths following 2 months of dietary treatment and treatment of any concurrent infection, then surgery should be considered.

Oxalate and silicate uroliths always require surgical removal as there is no diet currently available to aid in their dissolution. Surgery has the disadvantages of requirement for anaesthesia, possibility of complications, high initial costs, and possibility of failure to retrieve all uroliths. However, it allows retrieval of stones for definitive identification, and can provide an opportunity for correction of concurrent or predisposing problems such as bladder polyps. Appropriate textbooks should be consulted for further information on treatment and prevention of specific uroliths; recurrence is common unless underlying factors are addressed.

If there is no evidence of a urinary tract infection or urolithiasis, then the possibility of extra-urinary disease resulting in confusing clinical signs should be considered.

What if it doesn't get better?

If there is no response to treatment for a urinary tract infection, then the patient should be re-evaluated and the diagnosis reconsidered. If not already done, a cystocentesis urine sample should be obtained for culture and sensitivity. If infections recur then further investigations for underlying disease are appropriate. These should include ultrasound and/or contrast radiography of the urinary tract, haematology, and serum biochemistry. Underlying conditions such as uroliths, urinary tract tumours, prostatic disease, anatomical abnormalities or hyperadrenocorticism (if additional clinical signs are apparent) should be investigated and treated as necessary. Complicated or recurring urinary tract infections should be treated with antibiotics for a minimum of 4 weeks. Efficacy of antibacterial treatment can be confirmed by repeating urine culture after a few days of treatment and 1–2 weeks following the end of treatment.

In entire male dogs with a urinary tract infection, concurrent prostatic infection is extremely common. Whilst antibiotics such as ampicillin and amoxicillin may resolve the urinary tract infection, they do not penetrate the prostate effectively except in acute inflammation, and other antibiotics should be considered (see Chapter 69).

The low-cost option

Uncomplicated, occasional urinary tract infections can be diagnosed cheaply based on clinical signs and urinalysis (including culture when finances permit), and can often be treated with relatively inexpensive antibiotics such as ampicillin or amoxicillin. With recurrent infections, minimal investigations should include bacterial culture and sensitivity testing of a cystocentesis sample, and urinary tract ultrasound or contrast radiography. Ultrasound is usually cheaper as radiography is likely to require general anaesthesia, bladder catheterisation, and multiple exposures. Repeated courses of inappropriate antibiotics can delay diagnosis as well as encourage antibiotic resistance.

There are no cheap options for effective treatment of uroliths, as both surgical and medical treatments incur significant costs. Costs may be minimised following initial treatment by paying attention to prevention of recurrence by ensuring an appropriate diet is fed, diuresis maintained, and underlying conditions (e.g. infections, polyps) addressed. Urinary acidifiers (e.g. ammonium chloride) are not effective in treating urinary infections without concurrent use of antibiotics, but may be helpful in reducing the risk of recurrent struvite urolithiasis if financial limitations preclude the use of a specialised diet. Basic management changes such as increasing the dog's water intake, adding a quarter teaspoon of salt per day to the diet (contraindicated if the dog is receiving a struvite dissolution diet, or has hypertension, renal disease or congestive heart failure), and providing frequent opportunities for urination, may help reduce recurrence.

When should I refer?

Cases of cystitis are usually managed in general practice. Referral should be discussed if clinical signs persist despite appropriate treatment of any infection and investigation of any underlying diseases. It should also be considered if a urinary tract infection does not resolve or recurs more than twice despite appropriate antibiotic treatment, or if the practice does not have the facilities or expertise to investigate the possibility of underlying conditions. Surgery for prostatic disease requires specialist expertise.

Sheena Warman

Signs of lower urinary tract disease (LUTD) are common in cats. Owners may report pollakiuria (frequent urination), dysuria (pain or difficulty in urinating which is often manifested as vocalisation during voiding), stranguria (slow and painful discharge of urine), excessive licking of the genitalia, haematuria or inappropriate urination. Male cats in particular are prone to urethral obstruction. Particularly in cats that usually urinate outside, the problem may not be noted until the cat is systemically unwell due to post-renal azotaemia. Clinical signs include anorexia, vomiting, dehydration, abdominal pain, collapse or even death (blocked cats are discussed in more detail in Chapter 66).

Common differential diagnoses

- Feline idiopathic cystitis (FIC) – see below
- Urethral plugs
- Urethral spasm or strictures (often associated with inflammation following previous attempts at catheterisation)
- Uroliths/cystoliths
- Neoplasia (e.g. transitional cell carcinoma; uncommon in cats)
- Trauma
- Bacterial infection (rare as primary cause)
- Behavioural problem (inappropriate elimination)
- Constipation.

In many cases, the underlying cause of the signs remains uncertain and these cats are described as having feline idiopathic cystitis (FIC; previously known as idiopathic feline lower urinary tract disease). FIC is a diagnosis of exclusion. Cats which are overweight, live indoors, or eat dry diets are predisposed to FIC. The current theory is that neurogenic inflammation (release of substance P within the bladder due to stimulation of nerve endings by higher centres) leads to pain, swelling, bleeding, muscle contraction, inflammation and alterations in the glycosaminoglycan layer of the bladder, resulting in clinical signs of lower urinary tract disease. If both inflammatory proteins and urinary crystals (struvite or oxalate) are present, a urethral

plug forms and can cause obstruction, most commonly in male cats. In many cats, episodes are triggered by stress.

Extra-urinary problems such as neuromuscular disorders (particularly following trauma, e.g. tail avulsion injury), prostatic disease (rare in cats) and bleeding disorders should also be considered in appropriate cases.

Diagnostic approach

Any cat with signs consistent with LUTD should undergo immediate triage assessment, i.e. brief assessment of cardiovascular and respiratory status, and gentle palpation of the bladder, assessing size and turgidity. If the bladder is firm and painful, particularly in male cats (when it may be associated with visible swelling of the prepuce and penis), the cat may have an obstructed urethra and should be admitted and treated immediately (see Chapter 66).

Non-obstructed cats are usually systemically well, but can present with a similar history to obstructed cats due to persistent straining to urinate despite an empty bladder. A thorough history should be obtained, including information regarding any previous episodes of LUTD, trauma, and recent changes in the cat's environment or diet. Physical examination should be complete but with particular attention paid to palpation of the bladder and examination of the external genitalia. The bladder wall may be palpably thickened.

Urinalysis (specific gravity, dipstick and sediment evaluation) should be performed in all cats with lower urinary tract disease, ideally on a cystocentesis sample. Culture should be performed if bacterial infection is suspected (<5% of cats with LUTD). Gross or microscopic haematuria is common. If it is not present then urethral spasm, behavioural or neurologic causes of inappropriate urination should be considered. Crystalluria is influenced by pH, concentration and temperature of the sample, and samples should be examined as soon as possible after collection, ideally at 37°C. Crystalluria is usually a normal finding, particularly in samples with a high specific gravity. Care must be taken not to over-interpret the significance of any crystalluria; the presence of crystals does not necessarily indicate that a urolith is

100 Top Consultations in Small Animal General Practice, First Edition
By Peter Hill, Sheena Warman and Geoff Shawcross
© 2011 Blackwell Publishing Ltd

present. However, high numbers of struvite or oxalate crystals may contribute to signs of LUTD in cats and should be noted.

Further investigation in recurrent or severe cases focuses on identification of an underlying disease such as uroliths, infection, neoplasia or anatomical abnormalities such as urethral stricture. Full haematology and biochemistry, and testing for FIV and FeLV infection, should be performed particularly in older cats to assess general health. Ultrasound or contrast radiography is used to identify underlying urinary tract disease. Surgery may be required for definitive identification of uroliths or biopsy of suspected tumours identified with radiography or ultrasound. If no underlying disorder is identified, it is likely that the cat is suffering from FIC.

Treatment

For management of obstructed cats, refer to Chapter 66.

In non-obstructed cats, FIC usually resolves spontaneously within 3–5 days. NSAIDs (e.g. meloxicam) ± analgesia (e.g. buprenorphine) should be administered if signs are severe. Historically, antibiotics have often been given to these cats, despite the fact that less than 5% are likely to have a bacterial infection, and the apparent response is unlikely to be associated with the antibiotic treatment. However, bacterial infection is more likely if there is an underlying disease such as diabetes mellitus. Antibiotics should be reserved for cases with pyuria or bacteriuria on sediment examination, and ideally cases with confirmed infection (positive culture of a cystocentesis sample). The most important aspect of treatment is appropriate advice regarding maximising the cat's water intake (see below).

Wet diets are preferred, as they maximise water intake and reduce the risk of saturation of the urine with crystals. Acidifying diets are rarely required in cats with FIC; they may be considered if there is severe struvite crystalluria and confirmed alkaline urine. Inappropriate use of acidifying diets may cause further irritation to the bladder wall.

What if it doesn't get better?

If there is no response to initial treatment, or if signs recur, then further investigations should be carried out as discussed above. Underlying diseases

such as uroliths or neoplasia should be treated appropriately.

The ideal treatment for cats with recurring FIC is unknown, but various approaches may be useful in reducing the frequency and duration of episodes. The most important factor appears to be ensuring adequate water intake, to encourage the production of dilute urine. Wet food should be recommended, and multiple sources of fresh water should be available to the cat. Some cats prefer to drink from commercially available 'water fountains' designed for cats. Acidifying diets should only be used if there is severe struvite crystalluria and alkaline urine. Nutritional supplements that are thought to support the glycosamingoglycan lining of the bladder are available. Minimising stress is important and the use of pheromone sprays or plug-in devices (Feliway; Ceva) can be considered. Use of a NSAID such as meloxicam at the beginning of an episode (if obstruction has been ruled out) may be helpful. Urethral anti-spasmodic drugs (see Chapter 66) are helpful in some cats. It is important to note that most treatments remain anecdotal with little published information available regarding efficacy.

The low-cost option

Most non-obstructed cats with FIC will improve spontaneously over a few days, and will be managed as out-patients. A single dose of a NSAID such as meloxicam may help reduce signs and discomfort associated with the condition, and the owner should be encouraged to feed a wet diet. In cases that do not respond, or that recur frequently, urinalysis should be a priority. Ultrasound examination is likely to be the least expensive way of ruling out concurrent disorders, although retrograde contrast radiography will be required in some cases.

When should I refer?

Referral should be considered in cases that recur frequently despite appropriate investigation and treatment as outlined above, or if facilities/expertise are not available within the practice for further investigation. Referral to a veterinary-qualified behaviourist should be discussed if stress or behavioural issues appear to be part of the syndrome.

Sheena Warman

Aetiology and pathogenesis

The phrase 'blocked cat' refers to cats with urethral obstruction and is one of the most common emergencies encountered in small animal practice. Obstruction is far more common in male than female cats due to the length and shape of the penile urethra. Cats that are overweight, live indoors or are fed a dry diet are predisposed. The blockage is caused by the combined effects of inflammation (increased proteins and mucus) and urinary crystals (struvite or oxalate) that result in the formation of a urethral plug. In most cases, urethral obstruction is associated with feline idiopathic cystitis (FIC, see Chapter 65) but in some, primary urolithiasis may be more significant. Other causes include urethral spasm or strictures.

History and clinical signs

Urethral obstruction should be considered as a differential diagnosis in any unwell, male cat. The presenting signs depend on the duration of the obstruction. Early signs may not be apparent to the owner, particularly in cats that urinate outdoors. Initially, cats show frequent attempts at non-productive urination, often associated with pain and vocalisation. They often appear restless and lick their genitalia excessively. If the obstruction is not relieved within 36–48 hours, clinical signs of post-renal azotaemia and hyperkalaemia develop, including depression, anorexia, vomiting and dehydration, progressing to collapse, hypothermia and death. Hyperkalaemia can cause bradycardia or ventricular dysrhythmias.

Important differential diagnoses

- Non-obstructive lower urinary tract disease – see Chapter 65
  - FIC
  - Uroliths/cystoliths
  - Neoplasia
  - Trauma
  - Bacterial infection

100 Top Consultations in Small Animal General Practice, First Edition
By Peter Hill, Sheena Warman and Geoff Shawcross
© 2011 Blackwell Publishing Ltd

- Anatomical abnormalities
- Behavioural problems
- Any condition causing severe malaise in the (male) cat.

Specific diagnostic techniques

Suspected cases should undergo triage assessment, i.e. rapid assessment of respiratory and cardiovascular status, and bladder palpation. Critically ill cats may have signs of dehydration (reduced skin turgor and tacky mucous membranes), hypovolaemia (tachycardia, hypothermia, poor pulse quality, pale mucous membranes) and cardiac dysfunction (bradycardia or other dysrhythmias).

The presence of a blocked bladder is usually easy to determine by careful abdominal palpation; if there is any doubt whether or not the palpable structure is the bladder, then ultrasound can be used but is rarely necessary. Care should be taken as it is possible to rupture a blocked bladder. Bladder size varies, although the bladder is usually large, turgid and painful by the time the cat is presented. If the obstruction is not relieved, the bladder will become increasingly distended and eventually the bladder wall may lose some of its elasticity (detrusor atony). Rarely, the bladder ruptures spontaneously and may not be palpable. The external genitalia should be examined to see if a mucous plug is extruding from the penis.

A minimum of PCV, total solids, glucose, urea, sodium and potassium should be measured. Ionised calcium and blood gases are useful if available. If the cat has a fast, slow or irregular heart rate then an ECG should be taken. Changes associated with hyperkalaemia include spiking of T waves, loss of P waves and widening of the QRS complex, progressing to ventricular dysrhythmias, ventricular fibrillation and asystole. A urine sample should be collected for analysis either following successful catheterisation or by cystocentesis (see below).

Treatment

Blocked cats that are otherwise well and not azotaemic or hyperkalaemic should be sedated or anaesthetised for bladder catheterisation.

Cats that have cardiovascular compromise due to hypovolaemia, azotaemia or hyperkalaemia should be stabilised prior to sedation or anaesthesia.

- An IV catheter should be placed and fluid therapy started with 0.9% saline or Hartmann's solution (administering boluses of 5–10 ml/kg if hypovolaemia is present)
- Mild hyperkalaemia usually improves with fluid therapy and relief of the obstruction. Life-threatening hyperkalaemia (>7.5 mmol/L, or associated with a severe dysrhythmia) may require specific treatment:
    - Calcium gluconate (0.5–1 ml/kg of 10% solution given slowly IV over 10 min) helps protect the heart against the effects of hyperkalaemia
    - An IV bolus of glucose (0.25–0.5 g/kg) and glucose added to the IV fluids (to make a 2.5–5% solution) will help transport potassium into the cells (thus reducing serum potassium concentrations) and reduce the risk of hypoglycaemia if insulin is used
    - Neutral (regular) insulin will help lower potassium (0.1–0.25 IU/kg IV or IM) but can cause hypoglycaemia and is rarely used by the author
    - Sodium bicarbonate (1 mEq/kg IV) can also be administered, but is rarely required and can be associated with serious complications including hypocalcaemia, resulting in tetany or seizures.

Relief of the urethral obstruction usually requires sedation or general anaesthesia. Suitable sedative drug choices include ketamine/benzodiazepine combinations, or opioid/benzodiazepine combinations if cardiac abnormalities are present. Using sterile technique, the penis is extruded and a lubricated catheter (ideally an open-ended tom-cat catheter or lachrymal cannula) is gently fed into the tip of the urethra. It is useful to grip the prepuce around the penis to hold it in an extruded position whilst the catheter is being placed, to prevent the penis slipping back inside. Once the catheter is within the urethra, the penis is allowed to retract within the prepuce. The prepuce is then pulled dorsally and caudally towards the base of the tail to straighten the urethra as the catheter is advanced further. When resistance is felt, the catheter is flushed with pulses of sterile saline to help dislodge the plug. This may need to be done many times before the catheter can be advanced fully. Care is essential as the urethra is easily damaged by traumatic manipulation of the catheter. Once the obstruction has been relieved, the bladder is flushed repeatedly with saline until as much debris as possible has been removed. Occasionally, no physical obstruction is met; these cats are thought to suffer from urethral spasm and may respond to medication with anti-spasmodic drugs. They may require repeated or indwelling catheterisation whilst the drugs take effect. Anti-spasmodic drugs such as dantrolene (0.5–2 mg/kg PO q12 h) and prazosin (0.25–1 mg/cat PO q8–12 h) can also be useful to help prevent short-term recurrence of obstruction in cats with physical causes of obstruction.

If it is not possible to catheterise the urethra, then cystocentesis can be performed to provide short-term relief to the bladder. There is a small risk of causing uro-abdomen if an over-distended bladder wall with reduced elasticity tears or continues to leak urine through the cystocentesis site. If the urethral obstruction is still impossible to relieve on repeated attempts, a cystostomy tube may need to be placed as a temporary measure whilst urethral anti-spasmodic drugs are initiated.

Following successful catheterisation, it is usually recommended that a suitable catheter is sutured in place for at least 24–48 hours. This is particularly important if the cat is unwell, there is excessive haemorrhage or debris in the bladder, or detrusor atony is present. A soft, flexible catheter should be used as this will be less irritant to the inflamed bladder wall. The catheter should remain in place until the cat is alert and well, and the urine appears almost normal. Following removal of the catheter, the cat should be closely monitored to ensure it can urinate comfortably. If detrusor atony is present, the cat may be unable to fully empty the bladder, and the bladder will have reduced tone (i.e. a soft, non-turgid bladder will be palpable even immediately after observed urination). This can take days to weeks to improve, and may contribute to recurrence of clinical signs.

Following catheterisation of critically ill cats, monitoring of urine output and serum potassium concentrations is important. Post-obstructive diuresis is common, and dehydration can develop if adequate intravenous fluids are not administered to account for this. Hypokalaemia can develop in the post-catheterisation period, requiring supplementation of IV fluids with potassium chloride.

Opioid analgesia (e.g. buprenorphine) should be provided in all cases. In alert, non-azotaemic patients, following successful relief of the obstruction, NSAIDs may be useful to reduce inflammation. Ideally antibiotics should not be given whilst the urinary catheter is in place as this encourages development of resistant organisms. The catheter's tip should be cultured at the time of removal and antibiotics given if necessary. Patients suspected to have urethral spasm may benefit from treatment with dantrolene and prazosin. Further treatment and dietary/behavioural advice should be given as for management of FIC (see Chapter 65), and the owner warned of the possibility of recurrence.

The low-cost option

Cats that are presented early in an obstructive episode, whilst still alert and well, and when the obstruction is easy to remove, can be managed relatively inexpensively with minimal blood tests, sedation, and short-term catheterisation. Critically ill cats require intensive monitoring and treatment which will inevitably be more expensive. However, if well managed, the prognosis is usually good, even for critically ill cats, and attempts should be made to treat the cat and relieve the obstruction within the financial limitations imposed by the owner. Appropriate dietary and behavioural advice should be given to minimise the risk of recurrence, as some owners will opt for euthanasia if they are unable to meet the costs of repeated episodes.

What if it doesn't get better?

If the urethral obstruction cannot be relieved, an emergency perineal urethrostomy may be required, or a cystostomy tube placed until urethrostomy can be performed. If an individual cat suffers repeated obstructive episodes, further investigations (complete urinalysis, ultrasonography and/or contrast radiography) should be undertaken to evaluate any underlying disease, as for cats with repeated episodes of non-obstructive LUTD (Chapter 65). Cats with repeated episodes which do not respond to appropriate medical/behavioural management may benefit from perineal urethrostomy; however, this is potentially associated with complications such as stricture formation, urinary tract infection and ongoing cystitis.

When should I refer?

Most obstructed cats can be successfully managed in general practice. Referral should be considered if the urethral obstruction cannot be relieved. It should also be recommended if facilities/expertise are not available for further investigation or treatment (medical, behavioural or surgical) of cats with recurrent episodes of obstruction. Perineal urethrostomy should be performed by a surgeon experienced in the technique.

Section 8

Peter Holt

Aetiology and pathogenesis

Canine urinary incontinence is common, especially in bitches, and is as much a problem for the owners as it is for the dog. It can present as a congenital or acquired condition.

Eighty per cent of animals with urinary incontinence are suffering from urethral sphincter mechanism incompetence, a condition that can be congenital or acquired. It can affect both sexes but is much commoner in bitches. Factors that contribute to urethral sphincter mechanism incontinence include reduced urethral tone, a shorter urethral length, an intrapelvic bladder neck position, weak supporting mechanisms in the lower urinary tract, large body size, breed, ovariohysterectomy/ovariectomy, hormones and obesity. Large and giant breeds are particularly at risk, especially Dobermanns, Old English Sheepdogs, Rottweilers, Weimaraners, Springer Spaniels and Irish Setters.

The caudal movement of the bladder that occurs when a dog lies down is more pronounced in bitches with urethral sphincter mechanism incompetence. The importance of bladder neck position is thought to be due to the influence of abdominal pressure on the urethra which, if the bladder neck were intra-abdominal, would counteract increases in pressure on the bladder. This transference of pressure to the urethra is absent/reduced in dogs with an intrapelvic bladder neck.

There is an association between spaying and urinary incontinence, probably due to a lack of circulating oestrogens, although an excess of gonadotrophins may also be a factor. In general terms, spayed animals are nearly eight times more likely to develop this form of urinary incontinence than entire bitches. Thus, if 100 bitches were not spayed, by the age of 10, two of them would be incontinent. If 100 bitches were spayed, about 16 of them would be incontinent after 10 years. Spaying before the first season may increase the risk although this has yet to be proved conclusively.

Whilst not a cause of the condition, obesity may worsen the degree of incontinence.

Less common causes of urinary incontinence include:

- Congenital: ectopic ureters, bladder hypoplasia, pervious urachus, intersexuality and congenital neurological disorders
- Acquired: prostate disease, bladder neoplasia, ureterovaginal fistula, acquired neurological conditions, overflow incontinence associated with chronic retention, and detrusor hyperactivity/instability.

History and clinical signs

Urinary incontinence is normally noticed by the dog's owner. The dog itself rarely shows any clinical signs, other than attempts to clean itself. Incontinence is usually noticed where bitches have been lying down because sphincter mechanism incompetence is most pronounced when the animal is recumbent. Continuously dribbling urine is more likely to be due to ectopic ureters (especially in juveniles) or a ureterovaginal fistula. Haematuria, dysuria and/or pollakiuria may be present in dogs with prostatic disease, bladder neoplasia, neurogenic problems or detrusor hyperactivity/instability. Incontinence must be distinguished from behavioural problems associated with inappropriate urination such as loss of house training. In these cases there are usually large puddles of urine in inappropriate places, compared to typically frequent small patches of urine where an incontinent dog has been lying. Occasionally, urinary incontinence can become apparent when dogs become polydipsic due to disorders such as diabetes or hyperadrenocorticism.

Specific diagnostic techniques

In most cases, acquired incontinence in dogs can be attributed to sphincter mechanism incontinence on the basis of history and physical examination alone; no abnormalities can be detected on physical examination when dogs are suffering purely from this condition. As long as the dog is otherwise healthy, a trial treatment for this condition can be instituted without additional investigations.

100 Top Consultations in Small Animal General Practice, First Edition
By Peter Hill, Sheena Warman and Geoff Shawcross
© 2011 Blackwell Publishing Ltd

Treatment

Urethral sphincter mechanism incontinence can be treated medically or surgically. Medical treatment relies on sympathomimetic agents or hormone treatment. Sympathomimetic agents improve continence control by increasing urethral tone. Currently, the most popular medical treatment is the alpha-adrenergic drug phenylpropanolamine (Propalin, Vétoquinol; Urilin, Dechra). Affected spayed bitches may also respond to therapy with oestrogens such as oestriol (Incurin, Intervet). In some animals that respond initially to alpha-adrenergics or oestrogens, the response eventually ceases. In the case of oestrogens, this may be due to desensitisation of oestrogen receptors. Oestrogens sensitise the urethral smooth muscle to alpha-adrenergic stimulation so a combination of oestrogen and alpha-adrenergic therapy may be useful, reducing the dose required of each individual drug and lessening the chances of side effects. The reported long-term success rates of treatment with these drugs is approximately 50%. Androgens have been employed in castrated male dogs but, in the author's experience, the results are disappointing. In obese dogs, a weight reduction programme should be recommended. Incontinent juvenile animals should not be spayed, at least until they have had two seasons, since congenital urethral sphincter mechanism incompetence will sometimes resolve after the first or second oestrus.

The main surgical options for treatment are to:

- Increase urethral resistance by constructing peri-urethral surgical slings, using artificial sphincters, or by the intra-urethral injection of bulking agents
- Increase urethral length, using bladder neck reconstruction techniques
- Re-locate the bladder neck to an intra-abdominal position by means of colposuspension (bitches) or vas deferentopexy, urethropexy or prostatopexy (male dogs).

The typical success rate of surgical intervention is 50%. These techniques are best performed by specialist surgeons.

What if it doesn't get better?

If the incontinence does not respond to trial medical therapy as outlined above, further investigation is required to rule out alternative possibilities. Differentiation of the various causes of urinary incontinence may require contrast radiography, ultrasonography and, if available, urodynamic examinations. These techniques require considerable expertise and experience, and are best carried out by specialists.

If urethral sphincter mechanism incompetence is confirmed by subsequent investigations and there has been a poor response to medical treatment, then surgical management is recommended.

The low-cost option

As urethral sphincter mechanism incontinence is common, empirical medical treatment for this condition can be tried with little risk of the condition deteriorating should the diagnosis subsequently prove to be incorrect. The medical management of this condition should not incur large costs, although lifelong treatment is likely to be required. However, if the incontinence persists, higher costs will be inevitable as further investigations are required. Surgical management of the various conditions will incur initially higher costs, but in the long term can actually be cheaper than lifelong medical management, especially in a large dog. Weight reduction in obese animals should also be recommended as this can help to improve continence control.

When should I refer?

Medical management of sphincter mechanism incontinence is routinely undertaken in general practice. Referral to a specialist surgeon should be recommended if further investigation of urinary incontinence is required, or if surgical management is advised.

Sheena Warman

Aetiology and pathogenesis

Chronic renal disease is a common problem, particularly in elderly dogs and cats. In most cases the cause of the renal failure is unknown, as many different disease processes can result in irreversible glomerular and tubular damage. Potential causes include glomerulo-nephropathies, toxins, pyelonephritis, chronic interstitial nephritis, urolithiasis, congenital disorders, neoplasia and drugs (e.g. NSAIDs). Damage to nephrons results in a reduction in glomerular filtration rate and the accumulation of substances within the body which would usually be excreted in urine. The disease progresses over a period of time varying from weeks to years, depending on the severity and persistence of the renal insult. As the disease progresses and increasing numbers of nephrons are lost, the patient becomes azotaemic (a build-up of nitrogenous waste products within the circulation), and eventually uraemic (clinical signs as a consequence of azotaemia and associated abnormalities). Azotaemia generally occurs when 60% of nephrons are no longer functioning, and uraemia when 70% of nephrons are lost.

Abnormalities associated with renal failure include:

- A reduced ability to concentrate urine causing polyuria and polydipsia (PUPD)
- Hormonal changes – reduced erythropoietin production, increased parathyroid hormone production
- Gastrointestinal signs due to the effects of toxins on the vomiting centre and the development of uraemic gastritis and ulcers
- Hypertension, which can cause ocular damage and sudden blindness, particularly in cats
- Anaemia – due to reduced erythropoietin production, reduced red cell lifespan, gastrointestinal bleeding and anaemia of chronic disease.

History and clinical signs

Early in the course of renal disease, the patient may not show any clinical signs and should be described as having renal 'insufficiency' rather than 'failure'. In symptomatic patients, the owner may report that their pet has increased thirst and urination (which may be confused with incontinence), weight loss, inappetence and vomiting. On physical examination, the patient may be in poor bodily condition, with a dull unkempt hair coat. Halitosis and mouth ulcers due to uraemia may be evident (Figure 68.1). If the kidneys are palpable, they often feel small and irregular, depending on the underlying disease process. Dehydration can be extreme in patients that have been inappetent, vomiting, or denied access to sufficient water. Ocular examination may demonstrate changes consistent with hypertension (tortuous retinal vessels, hyphaema, retinal oedema, haemorrhage or detachment), especially in cats.

If pets with chronic renal insufficiency or failure suffer an additional insult to renal function (e.g. dehydration, hypotension, nephrotoxic drugs), they may suffer an 'acute-on-chronic' crisis, becoming very dehydrated with rapid worsening of clinical signs.

100 Top Consultations in Small Animal General Practice, First Edition
By Peter Hill, Sheena Warman and Geoff Shawcross
© 2011 Blackwell Publishing Ltd

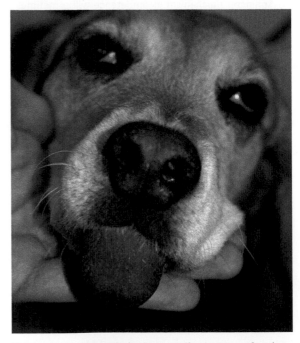

Figure 68.1 **Uraemic lesions on the tongue of a dog with severe renal failure**

Important differential diagnoses

- Hyperthyroidism (cats)
- Diabetes mellitus
- Neoplasia
- Dental disease
- Hepatic disease

See Chapters 4, 5, 6 and 38 for further differential diagnoses for inappetence, weight loss, PUPD and vomiting.

Specific diagnostic techniques

Renal disease is diagnosed on a combination of clinical and clinicopathological findings. Haematology may show a mild to moderate anaemia, which is usually non-regenerative. Serum biochemistry shows varying degrees of elevation of urea, creatinine ± phosphorus, depending on severity. Additional abnormalities can include hypo- or hypercalcaemia, hypoalbuminaemia (if there is significant urinary protein loss), and hypokalaemia due to reduced intake and increased loss. Urinalysis shows sub-optimally concentrated urine despite the presence of azotaemia, evidenced by urine specific gravity (USG) <1.030 in dogs or <1.035 in cats and there may be evidence of proteinuria which should be quantified by measuring the urine protein:creatinine ratio. Sediment analysis may show evidence of a concurrent urinary tract infection; in these cases a urine sample obtained by cystocentesis should be submitted for bacterial culture and sensitivity testing. Arterial blood pressure should be measured.

Pre-renal and post-renal causes of azotaemia must be excluded before a diagnosis of renal failure is made. Pre-renal azotaemia can be caused by a high protein diet, gastrointestinal bleeding, dehydration or hypovolaemia. Dehydrated or hypovolaemic patients without renal insufficiency will have concentrated urine (USG >1.030 in dogs and >1.035 in cats) unless there is another reason for an inability to concentrate urine (e.g. hypercalcaemia, or treatment with drugs such as furosemide or glucocorticoids). High protein diets or gastrointestinal bleeding can cause increased blood urea but creatinine concentrations should be normal. Post-renal azotaemia is caused by obstruction or rupture of the urinary tract and these cases will usually be identified on history and clinical examination.

Further investigations are not necessary in the majority of cases, but can be used to help rule out potentially treatable causes of chronic renal disease such as pyelonephritis or urolithiasis. Radiographs often show small, irregular kidneys, and ultrasound examination of the kidneys may demonstrate diffuse hyperechogenicity of the cortices, with reduced corticomedullary differentiation. In young patients, particularly if the kidneys appear normal on ultrasound, atypical hypoadrenocorticism (i.e. lack of cortisol but adequate mineralocorticoids) should be excluded by performing an ACTH-stimulation test, as these patients often present with vague signs of PUPD, weight loss, inappetence and vomiting. Renal biopsy is rarely performed unless the diagnosis is uncertain, or neoplasia is suspected.

Treatment

Animals that are dehydrated at the time of examination should be admitted for intravenous fluid therapy. A large component of the documented azotaemia could be pre-renal in origin, and the short-to-medium term prognosis may be good once they are rehydrated and managed as outlined below.

Treatment of chronic renal disease is focussed on slowing the progression of the disease, and reducing the severity and consequences of uraemia.

- Diet. Phosphate restriction is the most important reason for feeding a prescription renal diet, as this has been shown to slow disease progression. Serum phosphorus levels should be measured every few weeks initially to ensure adequate control. Protein restriction may help reduce the degree of azotaemia in uraemic patients. Sodium should be restricted to minimise hypertension. However, adequate caloric intake is essential to minimise weight loss, so if the patient will not eat a prescription diet then it is important that the pet is allowed to eat sufficient quantities of a favoured diet. Any food is better than no food
- Phosphate binders (e.g. lanthanum carbonate [Renalzin, Bayer], or chitosan with calcium carbonate [Ipakitine, Vetoquinol]) may be necessary if low dietary phosphate alone does not result in reduction of serum phosphate concentrations to within the normal range, or if the animal will not eat a low-phosphate diet

- Hypertension is usually treated with amlodipine (dogs 0.05–0.1 mg/kg q 12–24 h; cats 0.625–1.25 mg/cat q 24 h). ACE-inhibitors will also have some effect and can be tried initially but are not usually adequate as sole therapy for hypertension. Anti-hypertensive drugs must not be given to a dehydrated or hypovolaemic patient until the fluid deficit has been corrected, as they may cause a serious reduction in glomerular filtration rate
- Significant proteinuria (urine protein:creatinine ratio >0.5 in dogs or >0.4 in cats with no inflammatory sediment) justifies the use of ACE-inhibitors and regular monitoring of urine protein:creatinine ratio
- Water intake should be maximised by feeding wet food, adding water to food, and providing easy access to fresh water. Some owners can be taught to administer subcutaneous fluids to patients that are prone to recurring episodes of dehydration
- Oral potassium supplementation is advised if serum potassium concentrations are low, as hypokalaemia is a common cause of inappetence in renal failure patients
- Inappetence can also be a consequence of nausea which may respond to anti-emetic treatment (e.g. maropitant or metoclopramide). Nursing measures and appetite stimulants may be helpful (see Chapter 4). Assisted feeding, e.g. via a naso-oesophageal tube may be necessary in the short-term
- Vomiting and gastrointestinal ulceration can be minimised using anti-emetics (maropitant or metoclopramide) and gastroprotectants such as H_2-antagonists (cimetidine, ranitidine) and sucralfate (which will also have some activity as a phosphate binder)
- Any associated urinary tract infection should be treated appropriately (see Chapters 64 and 65)
- It is unusual for anaemia to be severe enough to cause clinical signs. Minimising gastrointestinal bleeding by minimising uraemia

is important. If anaemia is severe and causing clinical signs, then treatment with erythropoietin can be considered. This is administered by subcutaneous injection, in conjunction with iron supplementation. Currently, only recombinant human preparations are available, with an associated risk of development of antibodies which will cross-react with any endogenous erythropoietin, thus worsening the anaemia. Specialist advice should be sought before using this drug
- Owners may have questions about haemodialysis or renal transplantation as treatment options. Neither is widely available in the UK because of technical limitations and ethical considerations.

Further detailed information on the management of renal failure can be obtained on the website of the International Renal Interest Society (IRIS, www.iris-kidney.com). This body has established very practical guidelines for the diagnosis, staging and treatment of chronic renal disease in veterinary practice. The stage of renal failure is categorised from I to IV based on serum creatinine concentrations, then substaged based on proteinuria and hypertension. Evidence-based guidelines are then given for the appropriate treatment of each stage.

What if it doesn't get better?

Chronic renal disease is progressive. If clinical signs are difficult to control or progress more rapidly than expected, further investigations should be performed as indicated above, to ensure that therapy is optimal for the individual patient. Eventually, the disease may become so advanced that it is incompatible with a good quality of life and euthanasia should be recommended.

The low-cost option

Phosphate restriction is the most important factor in managing the chronic renal failure patient. If owners are unwilling to pay for a prescription diet, they should be encouraged to use phosphate binders in conjunction with an ordinary diet. The frequency of ongoing monitoring (blood and urine tests, blood pressure) will be influenced by the patient's clinical status and also by the owner's finances. ACE-inhibitors are expensive but are of greatest value in patients with significant proteinuria and/or mild hypertension. Mild dehydration can be treated with subcutaneous fluid therapy on an out-patient basis.

When should I refer?

Most cases of chronic renal disease are managed in general practice. Referral is most likely to be considered if the presentation is unusual (e.g. young animal), or further diagnostics are required such as renal biopsy, renal ultrasound or measurement of glomerular filtration rate (e.g. patients with intermittent mild azotaemia). The prescribing of erythropoietin is best reserved for clinicians with expertise in its use.

Peter Holt

Aetiology and pathogenesis

Prostatic disorders in male dogs are common in veterinary practice. Prostate disease in cats is extremely rare although prostatic malignancies may occur and have the same clinical, radiographic and ultrasonographic features as the canine condition. The major causes of prostatic disease (in order of incidence) are benign enlargement (hyperplasia/metaplasia), prostatitis (acute or chronic), abscessation, prostatic cysts, neoplasia, idiopathic haemorrhage and prostatic displacement into ruptures or hernias. Benign enlargement results from an excess of circulating androgens causing hyperplasia. However, an excess of oestrogens can also cause prostatic enlargement due to squamous metaplasia (especially of the prostatic ducts) and stromal hyperplasia. Severe squamous metaplasia of the ducts can lead to obstruction, predisposing to intraprostatic (prostatic retention) cysts. Prostate cancer is one of the few prostate conditions to affect castrated dogs and some authors believe it may have a higher prevalence in castrated animals.

History and clinical signs

Dogs with prostatic disease may present with haematuria, dysuria, urinary incontinence, dyschezia (difficulty defaecating), abdominal pain and weight loss. These signs are not pathognomonic and must be differentiated from similar signs due to other urinary tract problems, rectal disorders or bleeding disorders.

Specific diagnostic techniques

Differentiation of prostatic disorders by clinical examination alone (i.e. palpation of the prostate *per rectum*) is not possible, although the results of some examinations may suggest certain conditions. Useful differential features include:

- Non-painful, symmetrical enlargement – benign hyperplasia/metaplasia
- Painful prostrate – acute prostatitis, prostatic abscess, neoplasia
- Asymmetrical prostatic enlargement – prostatic abscesses, cysts, tumours
- Small, irregular, painful prostate – seen in some dogs with prostatic tumours
- Immovable prostate fixed in the pelvis – malignant, invasive prostate tumour.

Apart from clinical examination, useful investigative techniques include:

- Urinalysis (including culture if infection is suspected)
- Contrast radiography (especially retrograde positive contrast urethrocystography) – this can demonstrate prostate size and symmetry which is useful in animals in which palpation is difficult. There may also be abnormal filling of the gland with contrast medium from the urethra in cases of prostatic malignancy
- Ultrasonography – this can determine the size and shape of the prostate gland and improves the diagnostic value of fine needle aspirates and biopsies, as they are more likely to be representative of the lesion visualised and less likely to result in iatrogenic trauma
- Cytology ± culture of fine needle aspirates and/or prostatic washes – these can demonstrate inflammatory or neoplastic changes and detect the presence of infection
- Histopathology of biopsies – this can differentiate between inflammatory, hyperplastic or neoplastic changes.

100 Top Consultations in Small Animal General Practice, First Edition
By Peter Hill, Sheena Warman and Geoff Shawcross
© 2011 Blackwell Publishing Ltd

Treatment

The treatment of choice for prostatic hyperplasia in non-breeding dogs is castration as it results in a permanent resolution. The condition also responds to anti-androgen therapy such as osaterone acetate tablets (Ypozane, Virbac, 0.25–0.5 mg/kg once daily for 7 days) or delmadinone acetate injections (Tardak, Pfizer, 1–2 mg/kg, repeated after eight days if no response is seen to the first injection). With both drugs, the lower dose rates are used in larger dogs. Oestrogens may also be used but prolonged oestrogen therapy is contra-indicated since squamous metaplastic prostatic enlargement may result. Alternatively, 5-alpha-reductase inhibitors such as finasteride can be used. These drugs inhibit the conversion of circulating testosterone to the more potent dihydrotestosterone, which binds with androgen receptors in the prostate and can lead to hyperplasia. They can maintain the circulating testosterone levels (and thus libido) of breeding dogs, but they may be teratogenic.

Prostatitis may respond to antibiotics and castration, but care must be taken as to the choice of antibiotics. Potentiated sulphonamides and fluoroquinolones are most likely to have good penetration into prostatic fluid. Other antibiotics such as penicillins may cross the acutely inflamed blood–prostate barrier but may not be effective in chronic cases.

Abscesses and cysts require drainage, either with an ultrasound-guided approach or surgically. The prognosis associated with prostatic cysts and abscesses is guarded and no one form of treatment (marsupialisation, drainage procedures, partial or complete prostatectomy) is 100% successful. Mild cases may respond to castration and repeated needle drainage. Omentalisation of prostatic abscesses has been used with good results. This may be combined with partial resection of the prostate. Total prostatectomy is no longer recommended because of high post-operative morbidity and poor results. A biopsy should always be taken during surgery since a proportion of prostatic cysts and abscesses have a carcinoma of the lining.

Most prostatic tumours are malignant and the prognosis is poor. Total prostatectomy is not recommended although some palliation may be obtained in some animals using tube cystostomies, transurethral debulking and urethral stenting and/or NSAIDs such as meloxicam.

What if it doesn't get better?

If the patient has not responded to treatment for the initial diagnosis, further investigation is required to ensure that nothing has been missed. Other than benign hyperplasia, most prostatic disorders carry a guarded prognosis and owners should be given realistic expectations from the outset.

The low cost option

Benign hyperplasia is very common so it is reasonable to treat presumptively for this in patients with an enlarged, non-painful prostate. If prostatitis is suspected, potentiated sulphonamides are likely to represent the cheapest antibiotic with effective prostatic penetration, although they can be associated with side-effects. Surgical management of cysts and abscesses will incur significant cost, and ultrasound-guided drainage is likely to be a cheaper option. Evaluation and treatment of painful prostatic conditions is likely to incur significant costs.

When should I refer?

With the exception of benign hyperplasia or mild prostatitis, most cases of prostatic disease are best managed by specialist surgeons. In general practice, diagnostic techniques such as ultrasound guided aspiration or biopsy, and surgical techniques such as drainage procedures, omentalisation, and partial prostatectomy may be limited by the facilities and expertise available.

Section 8

Section 9
Reproductive tract problems

Section 9
Reproductive tract problems

Geoff Shawcross

Aetiology and pathogenesis

Pyometra is a purulent inflammation of the uterus associated with bacterial infection of excessive uterine secretions. It is a potentially life-threatening condition. Successive progesterone cycles lead to cystic endometrial hyperplasia and the accumulation of fluid within the uterus which becomes infected by uropathogens. The pus may be retained within the uterus (closed pyometra) or escape from the uterus through the cervix and be visible as a vulval discharge (open pyometra). Bacterial endotoxins migrate into the circulation causing clinical signs of endotoxaemia. Immune complexes also develop which can result in glomerular damage and renal failure. The uterus may rupture spontaneously, leading to peritonitis. The condition is most common in middle-to-old-aged bitches that have never bred but it may occur at any age from puberty onwards. There is a higher incidence in bitches that have received progestogens or oestrogen hormones to control their 'seasons' or treat misalliance.

History and clinical signs

Pyometra is a common condition. Cases usually present during the few weeks following oestrus, although many owners may not have recognised the 'season'. Cases of open pyometra present with a blood-stained, purulent vulval discharge which has a characteristic odour. There is often general malaise and lethargy, with anorexia and polydipsia. Bitches with closed pyometra usually have more severe signs associated with endotoxaemia. In these cases, vomiting is common and they rapidly suffer from dehydration and hypovolaemic shock. Abdominal distension may be present if the uterus is grossly enlarged. Pyrexia is not a common finding and severely depressed dogs may have a subnormal temperature.

Although the classical textbook description of pyometra is one of a severe illness with rapid progression, some cases have a more insidious onset and can present a real diagnostic challenge. For this reason, pyometra should be a differential in all cases of malaise, lethargy, polydipsia or reduced appetite in the unspayed bitch.

Important differentials include other causes of polydipsia, especially diabetes mellitus and renal failure; other causes of abdominal swelling, such as pregnancy, ascites and hepatomegaly; other causes of vomiting, especially poisoning, and gastrointestinal, hepatic or renal disease.

Specific diagnostic techniques

- Abdominal palpation is a necessary part of the clinical examination but should be carried out carefully as excessive pressure on the abdomen may rupture the uterus.
- Haematology: There is often a moderate anaemia but the red cell count can appear normal because of dehydration. In the majority of cases there is a neutrophilia and a left shift. A low white cell count, or the presence of toxic neutrophils, is a sign of severe endotoxaemia and the case carries a more guarded prognosis.
- Biochemistry: A baseline profile is recommended both for diagnostic evaluation and therapeutic guidance. Relevant tests include blood glucose, renal function tests, liver enzyme and function tests, serum proteins, and electrolytes. Blood glucose is often slightly elevated because of stress, but diabetes mellitus can occur concurrently with pyometra.
- Diagnostic imaging: Although it is possible to make a diagnosis based on history and clinical signs in many cases (especially when the pyometra is open), diagnostic imaging may be necessary when the diagnosis is uncertain. Depending on the degree of enlargement, it may be possible to see an enlarged uterus on a radiograph, but it is only possible to differentiate pregnancy from pyometra after 40 days of gestation, when foetal skeletons have started to calcify. Ultrasonography may be used

100 Top Consultations in Small Animal General Practice, First Edition
By Peter Hill, Sheena Warman and Geoff Shawcross
© 2011 Blackwell Publishing Ltd

to demonstrate enlarged uterine horns, which appear as fluid-filled tubular structures within the abdomen, and to differentiate abdominal enlargement caused by fluid accumulation within the abdomen (e.g. ascites) from that caused by pyometra or pregnancy. More expertise is required to detect a less enlarged uterus.

Treatment

Currently, the treatment of choice is ovariohysterectomy as soon as the bitch's condition allows. Aggressive fluid therapy, especially before surgery, will improve the anaesthetic risks by reducing the effects of azotaemia, hypovolaemia and endotoxaemia. Fluids may need to be continued for several days post-operatively. Broad-spectrum antibiotic cover should be given both before and after surgery. Opiates, rather than NSAIDs, should be used perioperatively because of the risk of renal damage associated with NSAIDs in the azotaemic patient. Recovery following surgery is usually rapid and the long-term prognosis is very good.

Several medical protocols have been evaluated but none are currently licensed for the treatment of pyometra in the UK. The basis of medical treatment is the expulsion of the purulent uterine contents through a relaxed cervix, coupled with antibiotic therapy and additional supportive therapy. In most trials, prostaglandins have been used in combination with antiprogestins but generally the drugs have unpleasant and sometimes deleterious side effects. The antiprogestin, aglepristone (Alizin, Virbac) in combination with low-dose cloprostenol has recently shown the most promise for the successful medical treatment of pyometra with fewer undesirable side-effects. Successful pregnancies have occurred following this treatment protocol. However, in the majority of cases treated medically, the condition recurs at a subsequent oestrous cycle, even if there was a satisfactory response initially. There is also a danger that the bitch's condition will deteriorate despite medication, increasing the anaesthetic risk and making the decision for surgery more problematic.

What if it doesn't get better?

Surgical ovariohysterectomy should be curative in cases of pyometra. If the dog remains ill after the operation, further differential diagnoses should be considered for the signs.

The low-cost option

Some of the diagnostic tests are expensive and may be unnecessary if the history and physical signs give a high level of suspicion. Medical therapy may be cheaper than surgery, especially if hospitalisation is not required, but the owner should be cautioned that the response rate and long-term prognosis may not be satisfactory and surgery may become necessary. Euthanasia on welfare grounds should be considered if there are major financial constraints.

When should I refer?

Managing cases of pyometra is usually well within the scope of general practice. Referral may be necessary if there are complications associated with concurrent disease, especially diabetes mellitus or severe endotoxaemia. In such cases, referral would be a matter of urgency.

Geoff Shawcross

General advice about pregnancy

The usual gestation period in bitches is 63–65 days, counted from the first mating, although it is possible for gestation to be between 60–70 days. In most cases, pregnancy passes uneventfully in dogs. However, breeders should be encouraged to have their bitch checked early in pregnancy to ensure that the pregnancy is progressing normally. Relevant advice that can be given at this time includes:

- Diet – bitches require increased nutrition but only towards the last third of pregnancy (approximately 1.5 times normal). Owners should be careful that the animal does not become overweight. As long as the dog is on a balanced diet, there is no need for nutritional supplements. Supplementation with calcium is contraindicated during pregnancy
- Worming – the life-cycle of *Toxacara* spp. is such that previously quiescent visceral larvae within the bitch migrate to the placenta from around day 42 of pregnancy and infect the puppies before they are born. Fenbendazole (Panacur, Intervet/Schering Plough Animal Health) has been shown to be safe and effective in killing these migrating larvae when administered daily from day 40 of pregnancy continuously to 2 days post-whelping at a dose of 25 mg/kg bodyweight
- Vaccination – passive maternal antibodies cross the placenta in the dog. In order that the puppies have a degree of protection against the most serious diseases (parvovirus, distemper, canine infectious hepatitis), the vaccination status of the bitch should be current. If there is a substantial risk that the puppies will be exposed to one of these diseases, or the bitch's vaccination status is out of date, then a booster vaccination should be given in the last third of pregnancy. As a general principle, as far as possible, drugs/vaccines should be avoided during the first third of pregnancy to limit the risk of

teratogenic defects occurring during the differentiation phase of the embryo
- Exercise – should be encouraged throughout pregnancy but jumping and chasing balls, etc. should be discouraged. Some heavily pregnant bitches will find exercise tiring, especially towards the end of pregnancy and should be limited to short but frequent walks.

Diagnosis of pregnancy

This can be achieved in bitches using the following modalities:

- Abdominal palpation – detection of foetal units by abdominal palpation requires experience. It is most reliable in slim bitches that have a relaxed abdomen. Prior to 26 days the foetal units are small and difficult to find; after 32 days they become ill-defined
- Ultrasonography – this is the most reliable technique for the diagnosis of pregnancy and provides information about foetal viability from day 25. It is unreliable for determination of litter size
- Measurement of plasma relaxin – this is best performed from day 28 onwards. Note that small litters of three or less can give false-negative results
- Radiography – this is useful after skeletal ossification has occurred (42 days), and is the most reliable technique for determining litter size. However, the clinician should always warn the breeder that determining litter size (especially in breeds that routinely have large litters) is difficult and that it is not always possible to be accurate.

100 Top Consultations in Small Animal General Practice, First Edition
By Peter Hill, Sheena Warman and Geoff Shawcross
© 2011 Blackwell Publishing Ltd

Complications during pregnancy

Complications during pregnancy are uncommon and most problems occur around the time of parturition. A problem that can occur rarely is abortion. This can be caused by bacterial infections (*E. coli*, staphylococci or *Brucella canis*), herpes virus infection, severe illnesses such as immune-mediated haemolytic anaemia, hypothyroidism, or drugs such as phenylephrine and glucocorticoids (although the latter are not reliable abortifacients in dogs).

Preparations for whelping

Whelping is the term used to describe the process of parturition in dogs. It is a subject on which veterinarians are often asked for advice. Preparations should be made well in advance of the expected parturition date to allow the bitch to familiarise herself with the different environment and routine. The breeder should prepare a whelping box in a quiet place that can be observed easily without having to disturb the bitch. A source of artificial heating should be available but only used when necessary. The heat source should be placed at one corner of the whelping box so that the bitch/puppies can move away from it. The breeder should also be warned that heat lamps, when used incorrectly, can cause serious skin burns. It is also wise to have a canine milk substitute available, together with a feeding bottle or syringe, in case supplementation of the puppies is required.

Inexperienced breeders should be given information on how the normal parturition process should proceed, together with the signs that would indicate that veterinary intervention is necessary (outlined below). It would be helpful if this advice were available as a fact-sheet, as it is likely that the breeder will not remember all of the detailed advice given during a routine consultation.

The normal parturition process

For descriptive purposes, parturition is divided into three stages. First-stage labour is the preparation stage and can be evident for a day or two. Restlessness, nesting behaviour and loss of appetite are common (but inconsistent) signs of first-stage labour and impending parturition. Second-stage labour is the phase during which puppies are delivered. It is generally accepted that the bitch's temperature will drop temporarily a few hours before the onset of second-stage labour. The owner can be encouraged to take the bitch's temperature at frequent intervals through the day: 38.3–38.8°C (101–102°F) is normal, but a sudden drop to 36–37°C (97–99°F) is a sign that parturition is imminent. Third-stage labour is characterised by expulsion of the placentae. The placentae are usually expelled following the delivery of each pup but it is not unusual for puppies to be delivered and their placenta delivered later. Breeders should be encouraged to match the number of pups with the placentae, whenever possible. Following a normal birth, the uterus will contract rapidly and expel blood, fluid and placental debris (lochial fluid). This usually resolves within a few days but occasionally persists for several weeks. These cases rarely need treatment but they should be monitored frequently for pyrexia and signs of sepsis.

Dealing with the umbilical cord

Left to themselves, bitches will chew through the cords and eat the placentae. Often, advice is given to tie the cord and then cut through with scissors. However, the best technique is to apply two pairs of haemostats and then tear them apart. This is less likely to result in haemorrhage and infection. It is unnecessary to apply disinfectants to the cord. Eating the placenta may enhance neurohumoral mechanisms that improve uterine contraction and lactation; certainly, the placenta is a source of nutrients for the bitch. However, eating too many usually results in vomiting and the best advice is to allow the bitch to eat one or two and then dispose of the rest. Breeders may erroneously blame perceived mismanagement of the umbilical cord as the cause of umbilical hernias.

Checking the puppies

Owners should check for umbilical hernias, cleft palates, head/facial distortions, open eyes and other obvious abnormalities. If the veterinary surgeon is asked to make these checks, the owner should be made aware of the limitations of the veterinary examination. Many congenital and hereditary diseases are not obvious within the first few days after birth and developmental problems may only become apparent when there is a failure to grow properly compared to their siblings. Puppies should be weighed at birth and regularly thereafter. Generally, a puppy will double its birth weight within 10 days.

Complications of parturition requiring veterinary intervention

A major problem the clinician faces is deciding when veterinary intervention is necessary. However, it is prudent to examine the bitch promptly and frequently when contacted by a breeder to avoid the risk of being blamed for the fact that puppies have died due to a lack of professional attention.

Some of the complications of parturition which may require veterinary intervention are:

- Prolonged gestation – there are many documented cases where gestation has extended beyond 70 days and resulted in a live litter. However, such gestation periods are exceptional and the clinician should always examine bitches frequently if gestation extends beyond 67 days

- Failure to proceed from stage 1 – again, there are several documented cases where a successful parturition has followed a first-stage labour that has persisted for several days. However, a clinical examination is warranted after 36 hours if purposeful straining has not started. Bitches carrying a single pup or a small number compared with the breed norm may fail to proceed to stage 2
- Hypocalcaemia – eclampsia occurs most commonly 2–3 weeks post-partum when lactation is at its peak, but it can occur towards the end of pregnancy. In the early stages, affected dogs appear anxious, unsettled and pant excessively but the signs can progress rapidly leading to incoordination, convulsions and a life-threatening hyperthermia. Bitches suffering from marginal hypocalcaemia will not show classical signs of eclampsia but the lack of calcium limits the ability of the uterus to contract and is often associated with a failure to complete stage 2 labour
- Dystocia – failure to produce a pup after purposeful straining for more than 20 minutes should be investigated thoroughly as it may indicate dystocia. Relative foetal oversize is common in certain breeds (e.g. English Bulldog, Staffordshire Bull Terrier). Posterior presentations are common and should be considered normal but can result in a protracted delivery, especially when it is the first pup. Because the birth canal of the bitch is comparatively long, if the head or feet are visible at the vulva then the pup has passed completely into the cervix and can be delivered by traction. Delivery needs to be prompt as the placenta has separated and the foetus will die of anoxia. Inexperienced breeders rarely have the confidence to apply the degree of traction required to effect the delivery. Obstetric lubrication should be employed, as the lubricating property of the foetal fluids has usually been lost by the time the clinician is involved. Using instruments to aid delivery (e.g. whelping forceps, loops) should be avoided if the pup is alive because of the high risk of causing substantial trauma to the head or limbs
- Failure to complete stage 2 – this is a common reason for veterinary attention. Often, one or more puppies have been delivered but purposeful straining has stopped. When delivering large litters, it is normal for the bitch to 'rest' during the process. These normal rest periods can last an hour or more; however, they are characterised by normal mothering behaviour with the bitch cleaning and suckling the puppies. If uterine exhaustion has occurred towards the end of the whelping process, (i.e. only one or two puppies remain in utero) and there is no evidence of dystocia, it is worth administering oxytocin to encourage uterine contraction. It is probably better to proceed to caesarean section if this problem occurs early in the parturition process because placental separation is occurring and prolonged delivery jeopardises the puppies

- Metritis and mastitis are not common but are serious and life-threatening when they do occur. A vaginal discharge can occur for several weeks post-partum without significant clinical signs but the bitch needs to be monitored frequently for signs of malaise that could indicate septic metritis has developed. Mastitis is usually characterised by abscessation in one or more glands. Both conditions will result in lactation failure and loss of mothering behaviour. Often, the first signs that there is a problem are restless puppies that are cold, hungry, and failing to gain weight.

Caesarean section

Elective caesarean section should be considered if the bitch has birth canal deformities that would suggest dystocia is likely to occur. Surgery will also be necessary if stage 2 fails, despite oxytocin/calcium treatment. When there is evidence that the uterus is infected following foetal death, hysterectomy is usually a safer procedure than hysterotomy. It should be noted that hysterectomy may have a negative impact on subsequent milk production. The puppies delivered via caesarean section are usually depressed because of a combination of anoxia through placental separation and sedative effects of the anaesthetic. Resuscitation of the pups, comprising removal of fluid from the airway, supplemental oxygen, and vigorous rubbing of the chest, face and perineum, is usually required following delivery. The use of drugs that stimulate the respiratory centre (e.g. doxapram) are contraindicated. Mothering behaviour is often reduced following surgery for the first two days, probably because of the bitch's lack of involvement in the birth process. During surgery, both uterine horns and the birth canal should be checked thoroughly, to ensure that no pup is left behind.

Oestrus control

Oestrus control is an important method for preventing unwanted canine and feline pregnancies. The most common (and permanent) method of oestrus control is surgical ovariohysterectomy (spaying, neutering, de-sexing, see Chapter 3). Non-surgical oestrus control is reversible and allows the animal to return to breeding if that should be desired. Medical control of oestrus can be considered for the following reasons:

- As an alternative to neutering, but this requires long-term medication
- To defer oestrus cycles ('seasons') indefinitely, while retaining the option to breed
- To defer a season that is pending, to a time more convenient to the owner
- To stop a season that has just started
- To prevent signs of false pregnancy.

Adverse effects may be seen with both progestagens and testosterone based drugs, which include:

- Cystic endometrial hyperplasia and development of pyometritis
- Insulin resistance
- Adrenal suppression
- Increased appetite, weight gain and lethargy.

Misalliance (Mésalliance)

Misalliance is an unwanted canine mating. In some circumstances, a bitch may have been seen to have been mated but in many cases a bitch in oestrus has escaped from the premises and been missing for several hours. In these cases there has to be a presumption that the bitch has been mated. Unwanted matings also occur commonly in cats, but these typically go un-noticed until the cat is showing signs of pregnancy, or actually gives birth.

Treatment

A number of drugs are available to control oestrus in the dog and cat (see Table 72.1). The treatment protocols for some of these drugs can be complex and clinicians must consult the relevant data sheet for guidance. When advising clients, the clinician should bear in mind that, because the treatment protocols are complex, owners may not always comply with the regime and this may result in an apparent failure of the treatment. Consideration should also be given to the potential side-effects of treatment with these drugs (especially in the long term) and the cost-effectiveness of long-term therapy. In most cases, the return to normal cycles once medication is stopped is unpredictable.

Treatment

There are two licensed products in the UK for the treatment of misalliance. Low-dose oestradiol benzoate (Mesalin, Intervet) can be given on days 3 and 5, and possibly day 7 after mating. Owners should be warned that it is considered only 95% effective at preventing pregnancy and that the signs of oestrus will be prolonged. The use of Mesalin is contraindicated in the cat.

Aglepristone (a progesterone receptor antagonist: Alizin, Virbac) can be used for the termination of pregnancy in bitches up to 45 days after mating. It is given as two subcutaneous injections 24 hours apart. It is reported to be 99% effective up to day 22, and 94% effective from day 22–45. Care must be taken to avoid self-injection as local reactions can occur, and particular care should be taken by pregnant women.

100 Top Consultations in Small Animal General Practice, First Edition
By Peter Hill, Sheena Warman and Geoff Shawcross
© 2011 Blackwell Publishing Ltd

Table 72.1 Drugs for medical control of the oestrus cycle. Not all drugs are available in all countries. Clinicians should consult the data sheets for precise dosing protocols as they may vary depending on the intended purpose.

Active agent	Trade name	Species	Protocol
Megestrol acetate	Ovarid (Virbac)	Dog and cat	Daily tablets (complex dosing protocols – see data sheet for precise instructions)
Medroxy progesterone acetate	Promone E (Pfizer)	Dog	50 mg by SC injection during anoestrus, followed by injections every 6 months
Proligestone	Delvosterone (Intervet/ Schering Plough)	Dog and cat	10–33 mg/kg by SC injection (complex dosing protocols – see data sheet for precise instructions)
Testosterone esters	Durateston (Intervet/Schering Plough)	Dog and cat	0.5–1.0 ml/10 kg by SC or IM injection every 28 days for up to 6 months
Mibolerone	Cheque drops (Upjohn)	Dog	30 µg/11 kg, PO daily

False pregnancy

False pregnancy (phantom pregnancy, pseudopregnancy, pseudocyesis) is characterised by changes in behaviour and mammary gland development that would suggest that an animal is near a full-term pregnancy or actually nursing, when in fact they are not. False pregnancy is very common in entire bitches and can be considered a normal variation of the reproductive cycle, but it is uncommon in the cat. Affected bitches often have signs that recur after each oestrous cycle. In many individuals, these signs become progressively more intense with each successive cycle.

False pregnancy is caused by a high plasma concentration of prolactin at the end of the luteal phase, when progesterone levels are decreasing. Unlike many domestic species, (e.g. horse, cattle) spontaneous lysis of the corpus luteum does not occur in the dog and cat and there is a physiological 'presumption' that once ovulation has taken place a pregnancy will ensue. Cats are non-spontaneous ovulators so false pregnancies are rare in this species and when they do occur, they usually follow unsuccessful mating.

Clinical signs of false pregnancy include:

- Mammary gland enlargement
- Lactation
- Licking the glands or self-nursing
- Nesting
- Adoption of toys or objects
- Anorexia (this can be very worrying to owners, but dogs can often be enticed to eat in the consulting room).

False pregnancies need to be differentiated from a real pregnancy, impending parturition, pyometra and mastitis.

Treatment

Before suggesting any treatment protocol, the clinician must be confident that the animal is not pregnant. It is unwise to rely on the owner's certainty that the animal could not have been mated. Treatment is not usually necessary, as spontaneous resolution will occur, usually within 14 days.

Nesting behaviour should be discouraged and the nursing of toys etc. actively disrupted. Exercise should be increased but bitches should be kept on a lead as they may bolt for home in an anxious attempt to return to their 'litter'. A reduction in the quality of the diet to one which is high in fibre but low in carbohydrate and protein may have a limiting effect on lactation. Giving advice to limit fluid intake is unwise as there is a risk of causing dehydration that may precipitate subclinical disease, especially in older

Table 72.2 **Drugs for medical control of false pregnancy. Clinicians should consult the data sheets for precise dosing protocols.**

Active agent	Trade name	Mode of action	Protocol
Cabergoline	Galastop (CEVA)	Prolactin inhibitor	0.1 ml/kg PO daily for 4–6 days
Testosterone esters	Durateston (Intervet/Schering Plough)	Pituitary suppression	0.5–1.0 ml/10 kg by SC or IM injection
Proligestone	Delvosterone (Intervet/Schering Plough)	Progestagen	10–33 mg/kg by SC injection

animals. Lactation can be perpetuated by self-nursing and so this should be prevented by using an Elizabethan-type collar, or body-jacket that covers the mammary glands. Self-nursing also increases the risk of mastitis developing. Occasionally, a bitch may become aggressive towards the owner/family if her maternal protective instincts are intense.

Drug therapy should be considered when lactation is severe (leading to discomfort), or physiological changes are so severe that the animal is distressed/aggressive. Drugs that can be used to treat false pregnancy are shown in Table 72.2. Of these, cabergoline is the most effective, but also the most expensive.

Bitches that are prevented from having seasons by using medication (see under Oestrus control, above) rarely exhibit signs of false pregnancy. However, spaying remains the most effective long-term solution for false pregnancy but this should not be carried out during the false pregnancy phase as lactation may be prolonged.

Section 10
Endocrine problems

Sheena Warman

Aetiology and pathogenesis

Hypothyroidism is one of the more common canine endocrine disorders, but there is a tendency for it to be over-diagnosed and an understanding of the clinical signs and diagnostic tests is essential. The most common cause is immune-mediated destruction of the thyroid glands (lymphocytic thyroiditis) but it also occurs due to idiopathic atrophy of the glands. Neoplastic destruction, anti-thyroid drugs and congenital defects can occasionally cause hypothyroidism.

History and clinical signs

Hypothyroidism occurs most commonly in middle-aged dogs, with breed predispositions in Boxers, Golden Retrievers and Dobermann Pinschers. Clinical signs are very variable, and many are non-specific. The most common clinical signs include those associated with a reduced metabolic rate (lethargy, mental dullness, weight gain, cold intolerance) and dermatologic changes (endocrine alopecia, dry hair coat, hyperpigmentation, seborrhoea, pyoderma, otitis externa; Figures 73.1 and 73.2). Less commonly, other signs such as changes in oestrus cycle, neuropathies, bradycardia or ocular changes, may be seen.

Important differential diagnoses

Many of the signs of hypothyroidism are non-specific, e.g. lethargy and mental dullness. Weight gain is more commonly a consequence of excessive caloric intake and lack of exercise. These signs can be mistaken by owners for signs of ageing. Many normal dogs will 'heat-seek' at times. Other causes of endocrine alopecia include hyperadrenocorticism (usually associated with additional clinical signs) and imbalances in sex steroids. Many of the other dermatological changes are not specific to hypothyroidism, but hypothyroidism should be considered in recurrent or poorly-responsive cases.

100 Top Consultations in Small Animal General Practice, First Edition
By Peter Hill, Sheena Warman and Geoff Shawcross
© 2011 Blackwell Publishing Ltd

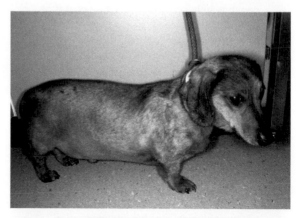

Figure 73.1 **Bilaterally symmetrical alopecia in a Dachshund with hypothyroidism (picture courtesy of Peter Hill)**

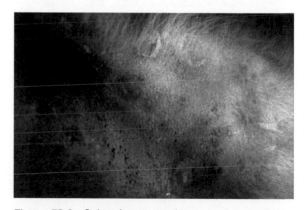

Figure 73.2 **Seborrhoea, pyoderma and comedones in a Shetland Sheepdog with hypothyroidism (picture courtesy of Peter Hill)**

Specific diagnostic techniques

A thorough history and physical examination, paying particular attention to the areas outlined above, is essential. Appropriate historical and clinical features must be present before a diagnosis of hypothyroidism is pursued further. There is no routinely available single diagnostic test which confirms hypothyroidism. Many drugs and non-thyroidal illnesses (euthyroid-sick syndrome) can result in misleading test results.

The following tests are valuable in the investigation of suspected hypothyroidism:

- Haematology – A mild normocytic, normochromic, non-regenerative anaemia may be apparent
- Biochemistry – Hypercholesterolaemia is common in hypothyroidism. Other causes of hypercholesterolaemia include post-prandial sampling, endocrinopathies (diabetes mellitus, hyperadrenocorticism), cholestasis, protein-losing nephropathies, glucocorticoid therapy, inherited conditions and idiopathic
- Tests of thyroid gland function – In order to minimise false-positive results, these should only be performed when consistent clinical signs and supportive haematological/biochemical changes are present, and when non-thyroidal illness is considered unlikely.
  - Total thyroxine (T4): useful as an initial screening test, but often low in dogs with non-thyroidal illness or on medication (phenobarbitone, corticosteroids, NSAIDS, sulphonamides, furosemide).
  - Free T4: useful as an initial screening test if non-thyroidal illness is suspected or if medications listed above cannot be withdrawn prior to testing, as it is less affected than total T4.
  - Canine thyroid-stimulating hormone (TSH) – elevated in most hypothyroid dogs due to loss of negative feedback. However, about 20% of hypothyroid dogs have normal TSH, and it can be elevated in some euthyroid dogs. It should always be interpreted in conjunction with a total or free T4.

In the presence of supportive clinical findings, low total or free T4 in conjunction with high TSH is highly suggestive of hypothyroidism. However, discordant test results are common, and in these situations retesting in 3–6 months is recommended. Alternatively, dynamic testing can be considered (see below) or, if clinical signs are very highly suggestive, trial therapy can be considered. However, many dogs with non-thyroidal disease will show some improvement on thyroid therapy. Thus, in order to confirm a diagnosis, if a positive response is seen, treatment should be gradually discontinued and, if signs recur, hypothyroidism is likely. If a dog has received thyroid supplementation, tests of thyroid function should not be performed until 6–8 weeks after cessation of therapy as the exogenous drug will have suppressed the pituitary/thyroid axis.

Many laboratories offer additional testing. The TSH-stimulation test is the 'gold standard' for differentiating hypothyroid from healthy dogs or those with euthyroid-sick syndrome. Human recombinant TSH (Thyrogen, Genzyme) is available but is expensive; some commercial diagnostic laboratories will supply individual vials on prescription to practices, which can be cost-effective. Non-pharmaceutical grade bovine TSH has been used but there are difficulties regarding supply and safety. The thyrotropin-releasing hormone (TRH) stimulation test is less reliable. Other tests are available to measure antibodies to thyroglobulin, triiodothyronine (T3) or T4, which suggest the presence of lymphocytic thyroiditis. A positive antithyroglobulin result implies thyroid gland inflammation, but does not give any information regarding clinical significance. Dogs with confirmed hypothyroidism can be negative, and euthyroid dogs can be positive. A cautionary note is that anti-T4 antibodies can cross-react with the reagents used in thyroid hormone assays causing falsely elevated total T4 measurements. Therefore, in patients in which the clinical suspicion of hypothyroidism is very high, but total T4 concentrations are normal, T4 auto-antibodies should be measured.

Treatment

Treatment of hypothyroidism is straightforward but lifelong. Sodium-levothyroxine is supplemented at an initial dose of 0.02 mg/kg once or twice daily. Absorption and metabolism vary between individuals, so once daily dosing is adequate in many dogs, and some dogs can be managed on a lower dose. The response to treatment is assessed by monitoring both clinical signs and thyroxine concentrations in the blood. Treatment should be continued for 6–8 weeks before evaluating clinical response. Peak T4 serum concentration is routinely measured 4–6 hours post medication, two weeks after starting therapy or after a change in dose. The aim is to achieve T4 in the upper half of the reference range. There can be marked day to day variation in absorption of oral T4 so it can also be useful to assay TSH concentrations; if T4 supplementation is adequate then TSH should be normal. Signs of over-dosing (thyrotoxicosis) are rare but can include panting, aggression, PUPD, polyphagia and weight loss. If these are noted, supplementation should be reduced or discontinued for a few days.

What if it doesn't get better?

In most cases, a failure to respond to medication indicates that the original diagnosis was incorrect. Dogs that are started on thyroxine usually show an obvious increase in energy and activity levels within the first week. However, owners should be warned that improvement in cutaneous signs such as alopecia can take 3 months before becoming apparent. Genuinely hypothyroid dogs may fail to respond if the dose of thyroxine is inadequate for that individual. This can be verified with pre- and post-pill testing. If the post-pill concentration is too low, an increase in dose is indicated. If the post-pill concentration is acceptable, but the pre-pill concentration is too low, twice daily dosing should be recommended.

When should I refer?

Most cases of hypothyroidism are effectively diagnosed and managed within general practice. However, further advice or referral (e.g. for dynamic function testing) should be sought if there are repeatedly discordant test results, or a lack of response to treatment. A rare complication of hypothyroidism is 'myxoedema coma', which can occur in dogs with undiagnosed hypothyroidism with overwhelming concurrent disease such as heart failure or sepsis. Signs include stupor, coma, hypothermia, respiratory and cardiovascular depression; referral of these rare cases should be considered.

The low-cost option

Although thyroid supplementation is relatively inexpensive, treatment of hypothyroidism is required for the rest of the patient's life. Thus, although it can be tempting to start treatment despite an uncertain diagnosis, it is usually more cost-effective in the long-term to ensure an accurate a diagnosis from the outset by appropriate testing as outlined above. Once a diagnosis is established and treatment initiated, clinical response alone is adequate in many cases to monitor the effectiveness of medication. Some dogs can be managed on a lower dose than that usually recommended.

Sheena Warman

Aetiology and pathogenesis

Canine hyperadrenocorticism (HAC), or Cushing's syndrome, is the result of an excess of circulating glucocorticoids. It occurs spontaneously in two forms:

- Pituitary-dependent hyperadrenocorticism (PDH) – This accounts for 85% of cases and is due to over-production of ACTH from the pituitary gland (usually from a microadenoma) resulting in excessive production of glucocorticoids from the adrenal glands
- Adrenal-dependent hyperadrenocorticism (ADH) – This accounts for 15% of cases and is caused by an adenoma or carcinoma of an adrenal gland.

Hyperadrenocorticism can also be caused by excessive administration of exogenous glucocorticoids (iatrogenic hyperadrenocorticism), although in this syndrome the adrenal glands are underactive rather than overactive.

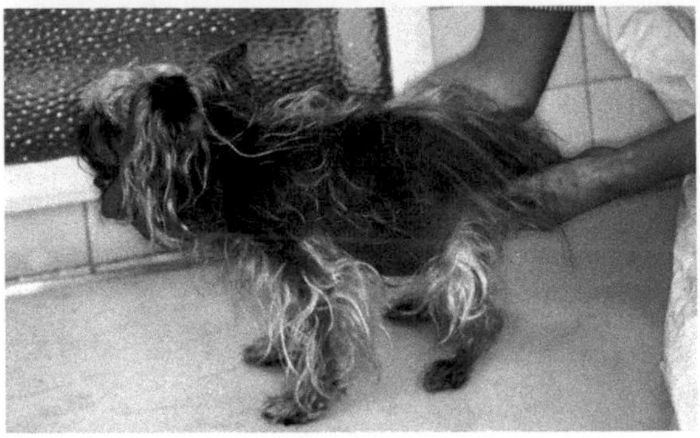

History and clinical signs

Hyperadrenocorticism (PDH or ADH) is a disease of middle-aged to older dogs, although it has occasionally been described in young dogs. In smaller breeds, PDH is most frequently seen, whereas in larger breeds there is a higher incidence of ADH. The clinical signs are a direct consequence of excessive circulating levels of cortisol and include PUPD, polyphagia, pot-bellied appearance (due to muscle weakness, redistribution of fat and hepatomegaly), dermatological changes (endocrine alopecia, calcinosis cutis, hyperpigmentation), excessive panting and exercise intolerance (Figures 74.1, 74.2 and 74.3). Less commonly, neurological signs such as blindness or seizures may occur due to a pituitary macroadenoma. Occasionally, the patient will be presented because of complications of hyperadrenocorticism such as diabetes mellitus, pulmonary thromboembolism, hypertension, urinary tract infections or delayed wound-healing. It is also important to take a full medication history as even topical corticosteroid treatment can occasionally result in signs of HAC.

Figure 74.1 **Bilaterally symmetrical alopecia and 'pot belly' in a Yorkshire Terrier with hyperadrenocorticism (picture courtesy of Peter Hill)**

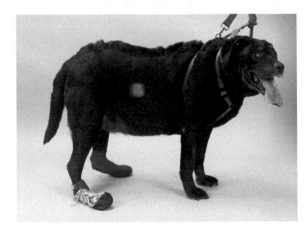

Figure 74.2 **Excessive panting, rotund abdomen and ventral bowing of the spine in a Labrador with iatrogenic hyperadrenocorticism (picture courtesy of Peter Hill)**

100 Top Consultations in Small Animal General Practice, First Edition
By Peter Hill, Sheena Warman and Geoff Shawcross
© 2011 Blackwell Publishing Ltd

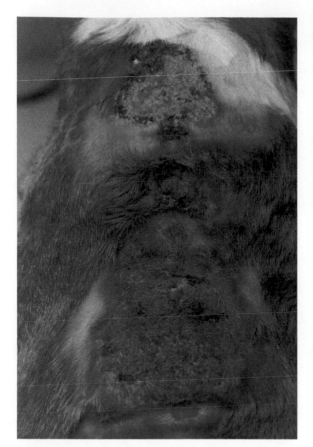

Figure 74.3 **Calcinosis cutis on the back of a dog with hyperadrenocorticism**

Important differential diagnoses

- PUPD – diabetes mellitus, chronic renal disease, pyelonephritis, pyometra, hypoadrenocorticism, hypercalcaemia, hypokalaemia, drugs (e.g. furosemide, glucocorticoids, phenobarbitone). Less commonly hepatic disease, polycythaemia, primary diabetes insipidus, psychogenic polydipsia (see Chapter 6 for approach to PUPD)
- Dermatological changes – hypothyroidism, sex hormone imbalance, follicular dysplasia.

Specific diagnostic techniques

It is essential that some compatible historical and clinical features are present before considering a diagnosis of HAC as no test is 100% accurate. The likelihood of a false-positive diagnosis will increase dramatically in a poorly selected patient population. It is also important to remember that HAC is a progressive disease and the abnormalities detected both clinically and on laboratory tests become more obvious and dramatic with the passage of time. Hence, in an early case, the symptoms can be mild and the laboratory abnormalities can be borderline between normal and abnormal.

Routine laboratory testing

- Haematology – Will usually show a stress leukogram (neutrophilia, monocytosis, eosinopenia, lymphopenia) and occasionally a mild erythrocytosis and/or thrombocytosis
- Biochemistry – Usually ALKP will be increased (steroid-induced isoenzyme). Additionally, there may be elevations in ALT, bile acids, cholesterol, triglycerides and glucose
- Urinalysis – Specific gravity can be highly variable but is usually less than 1.030. Proteinuria may be noted if there is concurrent glomerulonephritis, and glycosuria will be apparent if there is concurrent diabetes mellitus. If HAC is confirmed, urine culture should be performed, even if the sediment examination is normal, as high circulating cortisol concentrations may mask signs of a urinary tract infection.

Tests of the pituitary–adrenocortical axis

These should only be performed in the presence of suggestive history, clinical signs and haematological/biochemical findings. There is no ideal test to confirm HAC. Dogs with non-adrenal illness can have false-positive results, and dogs with HAC can have false-negative results. A combination of tests may be required for the disease to be diagnosed with confidence.

- Screening tests
  - ACTH stimulation test – Serum cortisol is measured before and 1 hour after the administration of exogenous ACTH. In patients with HAC it is expected that post-ACTH cortisol concentrations will be elevated more dramatically than in a normal

dog, usually to greater than 600 nmol/L. It is not a particularly sensitive test (detects 60–80% of cases) but is reasonably specific (i.e. false-positives are unusual if case selection is appropriate, although they can occur, e.g. in the presence of unstable diabetes mellitus). It is useful to **confirm** a diagnosis, and is the only test that can be used to confirm a diagnosis of iatrogenic HAC (flat-line response). It is also useful for monitoring response to treatment.

- Low-dose dexamethasone suppression test (LDDS) – Serum cortisol is measured before and 3 and 8 hours after IV administration of a low-dose (0.01 mg/kg) of dexamethasone. In normal dogs, this results in prolonged suppression of cortisol production, defined as cortisol <40 nmol/l at 3 and 8 hours, and <50% basal levels at both 3 and 8 hours. It is a highly sensitive test (few false-negatives), but not very specific (false-positives are common). It is useful to **exclude** HAC as a diagnosis, and can also distinguish between PDH and ADH in some cases (see below).

- Urinary cortisol:creatinine ratio – high sensitivity but poor specificity. If results are positive, further confirmatory tests would still be required. Should be performed on a free-catch urine sample collected at home.

- Tests to differentiate PDH from ADH – It is only necessary to perform these tests if surgery would be an option for an adrenal tumour, or if the owners would like more information regarding likely disease progression and prognosis.

  - LDDS –All dogs with ADH and some dogs with PDH will fail to show any evidence of suppression as defined above, so a failure to suppress does not allow differentiation of the causes. However some dogs with PDH will meet at least one of the criteria for suppression (typically showing suppression at 3 hours but 'escaping' at 8 hours). If this pattern is seen in a patient with confirmed HAC, a specific diagnosis of PDH can be made.

  - Endogenous ACTH assay – this is probably the most useful test in general practice. However, there are special sampling requirements so the laboratory should be contacted in advance. Most dogs with PDH will have elevated ACTH concentrations, and most dogs with ADH will have undetectable concentrations. However, concentrations in the range of 10–45 pg/ml are unhelpful.

  - High-dose dexamethasone suppression test – Procedure as for LDDS but with 0.1 mg/kg dexamethasone. With this test, suppression of cortisol concentrations at either 3 or 8 hours confirms a diagnosis of PDH. However, 15% of dogs with PDH will still fail to suppress, so they cannot be differentiated from dogs with ADH without further investigation.

  - Imaging – ultrasonography of the adrenal glands, by an experienced operator, can help differentiate PDH from ADH. CT or MRI may be considered to evaluate a pituitary mass.

Treatment

HAC is inevitably a progressive disease, although in many cases progression is very gradual. If the diagnosis is uncertain, the animal should be monitored and re-evaluated one to three months later, repeating tests if necessary.

The only treatment licensed for HAC in many countries is trilostane, an inhibitor of an enzyme required for the production of corticosteroids in the adrenal glands. Treatment is given once daily with food and effectiveness monitored by a combination of clinical improvement and ACTH stimulation tests (performed approximately 4 hours following dosing). Usually PUPD is reduced within 4 weeks, with improved hair growth within 4 months. Some patients require twice daily dosing. It is effective in most cases of PDH, and can help in some cases of ADH. Side-effects of mild diarrhoea or appetite reduction usually respond to lowering of the dose. More severe signs (lethargy, diarrhoea or vomiting) may be a consequence of hypoadrenocorticism. In these cases trilostane should be stopped, an ACTH stimulation test performed, and prednisolone and supportive treatment administered for a few days.

Mitotane is an unlicensed adrenocorticolytic drug which can be useful in cases of PDH or ADH that do not respond to trilostane. Treatment involves an induction phase (25–50 mg/kg daily in divided doses) until PUPD or polyphagia start to improve (usually within 5–10 days; an ACTH stimulation test is performed at this point), followed by a maintenance phase (50 mg/kg weekly in two or three divided doses). Side-effects are common and include vomiting and signs associated with hypoadrenocorticism (lethargy, anorexia, vomiting, diarrhoea, collapse, hyperkalaemia, hyponatraemia, hypotension).

Adrenalectomy is the treatment of choice for ADH unless metastatic lesions are present, the tumour is locally invasive, or the dog is a particularly poor anaesthetic risk. Medical stabilisation is usually attempted prior to surgery. However, there are many potential complications associated with surgery such as haemorrhage, wound breakdown and hypoadrenocorticism, and cases are best dealt with by specialist surgeons and critical care teams.

Successful treatment and reduction of cortisol concentrations can unmask other underlying diseases such as osteoarthritis or atopic dermatitis, or can result in rapid expansion of pituitary tumours and neurological signs. The prognosis for well-managed PDH is fair, with mean survival of about 30 months. Mean survival following successful surgery for ADH is 36 months.

What if it doesn't get better?

The response to treatment in dogs with HAC is monitored both clinically and with ACTH stimulation tests. If the dog is not improving, it usually reflects failure to suppress cortisol production adequately. If the post-stimulation cortisol concentration is too high, the treatment protocol and/or drug dosages should be modified so that better control can be achieved.

If the dog's clinical signs are not improving despite appropriate treatment, other differential diagnoses or complications should be considered to explain the symptoms.

The low-cost option

HAC is an expensive disease to diagnose and treat, particularly since diagnosis is not always straightforward. Haematology, biochemistry and urinalysis should be performed in all cases to investigate other possible causes of PUPD. Following this, if HAC seems likely but the owner will not be able to afford treatment, there is little point in aggressively pursuing a diagnosis. Empirical treatment of suspected HAC without confirmatory testing and subsequent monitoring is dangerous and should never be recommended.

If an owner is not interested in pursuing surgical management of a potential adrenal tumour, then there is little point performing testing to differentiate between PDH and ADH, unless the owner wants this information as a guide to how well the dog is likely to respond to medical management. While HAC is a progressive disease that does impact on quality of life, it is not a painful condition and many dogs will cope with the disease for many months if left untreated. The owner's funds may be better targeted towards managing any complications of the disease (e.g. urinary tract infections), although owners should be made aware of the risk of pulmonary thromboembolism which can result in rapid deterioration and death.

When should I refer?

Most cases of HAC can be diagnosed and treated in general practice, although specialist advice may be valuable, particularly in the interpretation of laboratory results. Referral may be considered for adrenal ultrasound, surgical treatment of an adrenal tumour, or in cases which do not respond as expected to treatment. Specialist advice may be necessary if HAC is associated with complications such as diabetes mellitus, hypertension or protein-losing nephropathy.

Sheena Warman

Aetiology and pathogenesis

Diabetes mellitus (DM) occurs as a result of an absolute or relative deficiency of insulin production by the β-cells of the pancreas. In dogs, the disease is usually the result of destruction of β-cells due to immune-mediated damage or chronic pancreatitis, with some breeds genetically predisposed (e.g. Samoyed, Tibetan Terrier and Cairn Terrier in the UK). In cats, the disease is associated with deposition of amylin in the pancreas. Additional factors that can contribute to insulin resistance and the onset of DM in dogs and cats include obesity, concurrent endocrine disease (HAC, metoestrus-induced growth hormone excess in entire bitches, thyroid disease), pancreatitis, and drugs (progestagens, corticosteroids).

Deficiency of insulin results in hyperglycaemia that exceeds the renal threshold for glucose reabsorption (9–11 mmol/L in dogs; 10–14 mmol/L in cats). This results in glycosuria, leading to an osmotic diuresis, polyuria and polydipsia. Reduced peripheral uptake of glucose by cells results in weight loss despite polyphagia, which occurs due to the inability of glucose to enter the cells of the satiety centre. If the problem is not recognised and treated early enough, mobilisation of fatty acids to ketones can result in diabetic ketoacidosis, a true medical emergency.

History and clinical signs

DM is generally a disease of middle-aged to older animals. Animals with DM are usually presented when the owner notices polyuria and/or polydipsia. Polyphagia and weight loss may also be reported. In entire bitches, it is important to establish the timing of the last season in case the DM is associated with metoestrus, and also because pyometra is an important differential diagnosis for PUPD in an entire bitch. Any drug administration should be noted, along with any clinical signs relating to possible concurrent diseases. Patients with diabetic ketoacidosis are systemically ill and likely to have additional signs such as vomiting, dehydration and possibly collapse. Cats may occasionally have hindlimb weakness and a plantigrade stance due to diabetic neuropathy.

100 Top Consultations in Small Animal General Practice, First Edition
By Peter Hill, Sheena Warman and Geoff Shawcross
© 2011 Blackwell Publishing Ltd

Physical examination does not usually reveal any specific abnormalities unless concurrent diseases are present. Body weight and condition score should be noted. Poor hair coat and hepatomegaly may be evident, and ocular examination may demonstrate the presence of diabetic cataracts, which can occur very rapidly after the onset of the disease.

DM is an important differential diagnosis for PUPD and weight loss, and further information about investigating these signs can be found in Chapters 5 and 6. Other causes of polyphagia include HAC (not usually associated with weight loss), hyperthyroidism in cats, and drug administration (glucocorticoids, phenobarbitone).

Specific diagnostic techniques

The first step in the investigation of PUPD is urinalysis, which in diabetic animals will demonstrate glycosuria. Rarely, glycosuria can be caused due to a renal tubular defect, so confirmation of diabetes mellitus requires demonstration of hyperglycaemia which exceeds the renal threshold for glucose reabsorption (see above). In cats, stress hyperglycaemia is common so persistent hyperglycaemia or glycosuria must be demonstrated. Alternatively, measurement of serum fructosamine concentration can be used to confirm the diagnosis. This is a glycated protein that gives an indication of glucose levels over the previous 2–3 weeks.

Since DM is a disease of older animals, which often have concurrent disorders, further evaluation of the patient's haematology, biochemistry and urinalysis is always indicated. Findings which can be associated with diabetes mellitus include elevated liver enzyme concentrations (due to hepatic lipidosis), hypercholesterolaemia and ketonuria (which may alter the approach to the case – see below). Bacterial culture of the urine is indicated because asymptomatic urinary tract infection is common in diabetic patients. Thyroxine concentration should be measured in cats. Blood pressure should be measured if facilities are available. Measurement of canine or feline pancreatic lipase immunoreactivity should be considered if there is a suspicion of pancreatitis, and measurement of progesterone should be considered in entire bitches in case of metoestrus-associated DM (which may be reversible if the bitch is spayed prior to her next season).

Treatment

The implications of living with a diabetic pet must be fully discussed with the owner. Diet and daily exercise routines should be kept constant, and most pets will require insulin injections once or twice daily for the rest of their life. This requires both financial and time commitments for the owner, which not all clients will be able to achieve. The manufacturers of pet insulin products provide useful support material for clients. Some owners are nervous of injecting their pets so it is useful to have a nurse in the practice who can spend time with them, teaching correct injection technique. Owners must also be aware of the potential complications of diabetes mellitus, particularly hypoglycaemia and, in dogs, the possibility of cataract development. Insulin must be stored in the fridge and should be gently rolled (not shaken) to resuspend the insulin prior to administration. Specific insulin syringes should be used for injection; in particular, it is important to note that different products contain different concentrations of insulin, and use of the appropriate brand of syringe is essential to avoid serious over- or under-dosing.

Dogs

All dogs with DM require insulin injections for effective treatment. Most dogs will require life-long treatment. The only significant exception is entire bitches with metoestrus-associated DM in which the diabetic state may resolve if the bitch is spayed prior to her next season. Despite this, insulin treatment is still required initially. Owners should be warned that it can take several weeks to establish the appropriate insulin dose for their dog. For initial stabilisation of the non-ketotic diabetic dog, a medium-duration acting insulin ('lente' bovine or porcine insulin) is administered once or twice daily at a starting dose of 0.25–0.5 IU/kg. Twice daily injections, with insulin administered every 12 hours at the same time as feeding, leads to quicker and more effective control. With once daily regimes the animal is fed a third of its daily requirement at the time of injection, and the

rest eight hours later. For many owners, the twice daily regime fits better with their daily routine. The diet must be consistent and it is important to calculate the dog's energy requirement at the beginning of treatment (see Appendix 4 for guidance on weight loss). Most dogs will benefit from a high-fibre diet as this helps minimise fluctuations in glucose levels; thin dogs should be fed a normal maintenance diet, and picky dogs should be fed whatever they are used to.

It is helpful to keep the patient in the practice on the first day that insulin is administered. Following this first injection, blood glucose should be checked every 2–3 hours to ensure that the glucose does not drop dangerously low. If it remains >10 mmol/l, the patient can be discharged to continue treatment at home. The owner should monitor appetite, demeanour and water intake, and be aware of the signs and treatment for hypoglycaemia (ataxia, lethargy, seizures, treated by smearing syrup or honey on the dog's gums). The aim is to establish good control of clinical signs with blood glucose concentrations below the renal threshold for most of the day. The dog should be rechecked weekly initially. If PUPD has resolved and weight is stable, then control is likely to be acceptable (and can be confirmed by admitting the dog and checking several blood glucose concentrations during the day). If clinical signs persist, there are two recommended approaches to deciding on initial alterations in insulin dose. A 12-hour glucose curve can be performed, noting the duration of effect of the insulin and the nadir (trough) glucose concentration (Figure 75.1). Alternatively, the blood glucose can be checked every few days at the time of the expected nadir (usually 6–8 h post injection); however, not every patient will respond to insulin in a typical manner. As a guide:

- If the nadir is <3 mmol/L, the insulin dose should be reduced by 50%
- If it is 3–5 mmol/L, the dose should be reduced by 20%
- If it is 5–8 mmol/L, there is no need to change the dose
- If it is >8 mmol/L, the dose can be increased by 20%.

It can take dogs several days to adjust to changes in dosage, so weekly re-evaluation is appropriate in most cases. Most dogs will eventually be controlled with a dose of approximately 1 IU/kg twice daily. It is not appropriate to attempt to stabilise diabetics based on results of morning urine or blood glucose concentrations; duration of action of insulin is less than 12 hours in many dogs, and this approach is very likely to lead to complications associated with overdosage.

In patients with DM and mild ketonuria which are otherwise well, a similar approach to that above can be followed, with the owner monitoring the dog's demeanour and checking urine with ketone dipsticks for worsening of ketosis. Alternatively, the patient can be hospitalised and given short-acting regular (neutral) insulin injections every 8 hours (with food), at a dose of 0.1–0.2 IU/kg, until ketonuria has resolved, followed by stabilisation as outlined above. Patients that show signs of diabetic keto-acidosis (ketonuria, vomiting, dehydration, collapse) are emergencies and require urgent treatment with IV fluids and hourly injections with neutral insulin. They often have significant concurrent disease and require close monitoring; even in referral hospitals, 25% of these patients die or are euthanised. For a full discussion of the management of diabetic keto-acidosis, the reader is referred to emergency medicine texts.

Cats

The principles of insulin administration are similar in cats. However, glucose curves can be unreliable due to stress hyperglycaemia. Monitoring of water intake and weight are essential, and periodic fructosamine assays can be useful to monitor control. Insulin absorption and duration of response is less predictable than in dogs. Some cats, usually those with mild disease or which are overweight, can be managed conservatively with high protein diets (such as Hill's m/d), weight loss, and oral hypoglycaemic drugs such as glipizide, which stimulates release of insulin from any remaining functional β-cells, as well as increasing peripheral sensitivity to insulin. However, this is not successful in the majority of cats. Use of glipizide can cause vomiting, and may increase the risk of β-cell exhaustion due to the toxic effects of ongoing hyperglycaemia. This conservative approach should be reserved for cases in which the owner is unwilling to inject insulin. Some cats, particularly obese patients or those which have been treated with progestagens, have a transient diabetic state which can be reversed following successful initial stabilisation and weight loss; long-term treatment will not be necessary in these cats.

Whilst some dogs can be successfully managed with once daily lente insulin injections, lente insulin must always be administered twice daily in cats. In

some cats, the duration of action of lente insulins is much shorter than in dogs. Alternatively, the longer-acting protamine zinc insulin preparations can be administered, although absorption and duration of action are less predictable.

Long-term monitoring should include water intake, weight, appetite and demeanour by the owner, and 3-monthly veterinary check-ups. In entire bitches, even if the onset of diabetes mellitus was not associated with metoestrus, spaying should be recommended to reduce the risk of the patient becoming unstable around the time of a season.

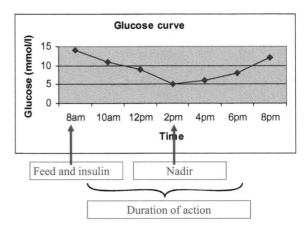

Figure 75.1   **An example of a glucose curve from a diabetic dog**

What if it doesn't get better?

Some diabetics can be challenging to stabilise. Insulin resistance is considered if the dose required is >1.5 IU/kg per injection on twice daily regimes, or >2 IU/kg once daily. If the patient does not appear to be improving despite what would be expected to be an adequate dose of insulin, the first step is to ensure that the insulin is in-date, properly stored, and being correctly administered. If these factors are addressed and the patient still requires excessive doses of insulin, causes of insulin resistance should be considered and investigated as appropriate. Causes of insulin resistance include the Somogyi effect (excessive dose of insulin causing transient hypoglycaemia with rebound, often prolonged, hyperglycaemia), obesity, excessive endogenous or exogenous glucocorticoids or progestagens, bacterial infections (e.g.

dental or urinary tract infections), chronic renal insufficiency, chronic pancreatitis, exocrine pancreatic insufficiency, neoplasia, hypothyroidism (dogs), hyperthyroidism (cats), acromegaly (cats), or anti-insulin antibody development.

The low-cost option

Stabilisation and treatment of diabetes mellitus is expensive. It can be an unpredictable disease, particularly if concurrent diseases are present. Bottles of insulin should be discarded 28 days after opening, but costs can be minimised in small patients by using the 40 IU/ml porcine insulin available in 2.5-ml bottles. Some owners will not be able to treat their pet for financial or lifestyle reasons and euthanasia may need to be discussed as an option following diagnosis.

When should I refer?

Most cases of diabetes mellitus can be managed within general practice. Specialist advice should be sought if patients are proving difficult to stabilise, or in cases complicated by concurrent diseases. Referral may need to be considered for the management of ketoacidotic patients if facilities and expertise are not available within the practice. Dogs with cataracts should be referred to specialist veterinary ophthalmologists for assessment as soon as possible.

Section 10

Andrea Harvey

Aetiology and pathogenesis

Hyperthyroidism is a common endocrinopathy occurring in older cats. In about 98% of cases it is caused by benign adenomatous hyperplasia of the thyroid glands. In the remaining cases, it results from a thyroid carcinoma. The underlying aetiology remains unknown. In approximately 75% of cases, there is bilateral gland involvement. In 10–20% of cases, there may be additional ectopic hyperactive thyroid tissue within the thoracic cavity.

History and clinical signs

The classical history for a hyperthyroid cat is that of weight loss despite a voracious appetite. However, it is becoming common for hyperthyroidism to be detected much earlier, before significant weight loss has occurred. Other clinical signs that may be noticed earlier in the course of the disease include vomiting, restlessness, excessive vocalisation, diarrhoea, polyuria/polydipsia, a poor coat, tremors, weakness, or dyspnoea/panting. Some cats also exhibit what is known as 'apathetic hyperthyroidism' where, rather than being polyphagic and hyperactive, they are inappetent and lethargic. Concurrent illness, which is common in this age group of cats, may also complicate the clinical picture.

On physical examination, a palpable goitre is often the only clinical finding, found in around 90% of hyperthyroid cats. Lack of a palpable goitre does not exclude the diagnosis since the position of the thyroid gland can be very variable, and in some cases intrathoracic ectopic hyperfunctional thyroid tissue may be present. Palpation of a cervical mass is also not pathognomonic for hyperthyroidism, since non-active thyroid nodules can occur, in addition to cervical masses of other origins. Other abnormalities that may be found include a poor body condition score, poor coat condition (Figure 76.1), tachycardia and tachypnoea. Additional cardiac abnormalities such as a murmur or gallop rhythm may be present on auscultation since secondary ventricular hypertrophy is common. Hypertension is common in hyperthyroid patients and evidence of hypertensive retinopathy may be present on ocular examination.

100 Top Consultations in Small Animal General Practice, First Edition
By Peter Hill, Sheena Warman and Geoff Shawcross
© 2011 Blackwell Publishing Ltd

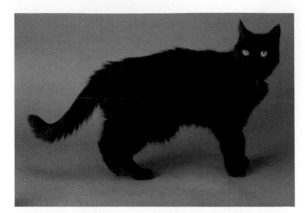

Figure 76.1 A hyperthyroid cat showing an unkempt coat

Common differential diagnoses

- Other conditions causing weight loss, especially chronic renal disease, DM and neoplasia (see Chapter 5)
- Other causes of polyphagia, especially DM and malabsorption (e.g. inflammatory bowel disease, exocrine pancreatic insufficiency, lymphocytic cholangitis)
- Diseases causing PUPD, especially chronic renal failure and DM (see Chapter 6)
- Other causes of vomiting and diarrhoea (see Chapters 38 and 39)
- Other conditions causing inappetence and anorexia (see Chapter 4)

Specific diagnostic techniques

Definitive diagnosis of hyperthyroidism is usually based on the demonstration of an elevated serum total T4 concentration. Although in-house T4 analysers are available, they are sometimes unreliable and samples for T4 measurement are best sent to a reliable external laboratory. Elevated total T4 is very specific for hyperthyroidism, and in more than 90%

of hyperthyroid cats, this alone will be enough to confirm the diagnosis.

Occasionally in hyperthyroid cats, total T4 may be at the top of the normal range. This can be due to normal T4 fluctuations in an early/mild hyperthyroid cat, or because of suppression of T4 concentrations due to a concurrent non-thyroidal illness. If total T4 is within the normal range in a suspected hyperthyroid cat, the following further investigations may be useful:

1. A repeat measurement of total T4 and exclusion of non-thyroidal illness.
2. If the T4 is still in the normal range, measurement of free T4 by equilibrium dialysis.
3. If total and free T4 are still normal, the following can be considered:
   - Waiting, monitoring the cat, and repeating the above steps 2–3 months later.
   - Thyroid scintigraphy. Although usually a referral procedure, it is useful because it provides information on the location of hyperfunctional thyroid tissue, thereby assisting with treatment planning.

Since hyperthyroidism is a disease of older animals that often have concurrent disorders that may influence treatment, additional diagnostic tests should be performed including full haematology, biochemistry, urinalysis and blood pressure measurement. Moderately elevated liver enzymes are commonly present. It is important to assess renal parameters prior to treatment, since treatment of hyperthyroidism can result in elevation of renal parameters due to 'un-masking' of concurrent renal insufficiency. Additional investigations will be dependent on clinical and laboratory findings.

Treatment

Whenever possible, hyperthyroid patients should be stabilised with medical management initially. This allows re-assessment of renal function once the cat has become euthyroid (before pursuing irreversible treatment), and to allow stabilisation of the cat's condition prior to anaesthesia (if thyroidectomy is planned). Licensed treatments in the UK are methimazole (Felimazole, Dechra) and slow-release carbimazole (Vidalta, Intervet Schering Plough). Carbimazole is rapidly metabolised to methimazole after administration. To minimise side effects, it is advised to start on a low dose initially (methimazole 2.5 mg once or twice daily, or carbimazole 10–15 mg once daily), and to increase the dose every 3 weeks as required to achieve euthyroidism, provided that no unacceptable side-effects develop. Side-effects most commonly occur within the first 3 months of therapy. They are generally mild and include inappetence, vomiting and lethargy. More serious side-effects include hepatopathies, facial pruritus and haematological disorders. If any of the latter occur, treatment should be stopped immediately.

Once stabilised, there are three options for long-term management: continuation of medical therapy, surgical thyroidectomy or administration of radioactive iodine. Surgical thyroidectomy is commonly performed in general practice and will often be curative. Disadvantages of thyroidectomy include:

- The requirement for general anaesthesia (which can be a risk in these patients)
- The risk of disease recurrence, especially following unilateral thyroidectomy
- The risk of hypoparathyroidism and subsequent hypocalcaemia if the parathyroid glands are inadvertently damaged/removed during a bilateral thyroidectomy
- Failure to achieve a cure if any ectopic thyroid tissue is present.

Administration of radioactive iodine is an excellent treatment option as it is curative without being dependent on the location of the hyperfunctional thyroid tissue. It is associated with minimal side-effects and there is no requirement for anaesthesia. The disadvantages are the relatively limited availability, and the requirement for 3–4 weeks of hospitalisation post-treatment in a specialist unit because of the excretion of radioactive substances.

Any concurrent disease or secondary complication, such as congestive heart failure or hypertension, may require specific treatment depending on the severity.

What if it doesn't get better?

The majority of cats will be relatively straightforward to stabilise on medical management. The most common cause of treatment failure is lack of owner compliance or difficulty in medicating the cat. If euthyroidism is not easily achieved and poor compliance has been excluded, then other causes for poor response to treatment should be considered. These include the presence of a thyroid carcinoma, or a large volume of hyperfunctional adenomatous thyroid tissue. Thyroid scintigraphy can be useful to evaluate cases responding poorly to medical management.

The low-cost option

Medical management is the cheapest option in the short term, but regular assessments, monitoring of serum T4 and monitoring haematology/biochemistry for side-effects of methimazole or carbimazole treatment are required for optimal stabilisation. Since life-long treatment is required, medical management may end up costing more than surgery or radioactive iodine treatment, depending on the predicted life expectancy of the cat. However, with medical management, the cost is spread over a longer period.

When should I refer?

Most cases of hyperthyroidism can be successfully managed in general practice. Situations in which referral might be offered include:

- If the owner is interested in pursuing radioactive iodine treatment
- If the owner wishes to evaluate the cat more fully (including thyroid scintigraphy) to aid in treatment planning
- If hyperthyroidism is diagnosed but there is lack of a palpable goitre
- If the practice does not have the facilities or expertise to perform thyroidectomy
- If there are concurrent diseases present which the practice does not have facilities or expertise to investigate/manage
- If hyperthyroidism has not resolved or has recurred following a previous thyroidectomy (ectopic thyroid tissue may be present)
- If there are difficulties stabilising the patient with medical management
- If a thyroid carcinoma has been diagnosed on histopathology
- If there is a large/irregular goitre which could be indicative of thyroid carcinoma.

Section 11
Emergencies and trauma

Geoff Shawcross

The road traffic accident (RTA) or hit-by-car (HBC) is a frequent presentation in small animal practice. Dogs, cats and wild animals are frequently involved. When wild animals are involved, it is necessary to be realistic about costs and rehabilitation; if they are to survive when returned to the wild, they will need to have made a full recovery.

Diagnostic approach

The injuries sustained in RTAs can extend from minor bruising and abrasions, to life-threatening internal injuries that need prompt diagnosis and treatment. It is important to establish how much time has elapsed between the RTA and the animal being presented. This, coupled with the animal's demeanour, will give an indication of the severity of the animal's injuries. Patients that are presented several hours following an accident, with a bright demeanour and stable cardiovascular and respiratory signs, are unlikely to have sustained serious injury, but such animals should still be monitored for delayed onset of signs.

The clinical examination should focus on life-threatening injuries first, leaving tests that require palpation, manipulation and assessment of movement (that are often painful) until the end of the examination. The most obvious injuries are often the least important in the short term. Injured animals may be in a lot of pain and very frightened; such cases should be handled cautiously and sympathetically, to avoid being bitten or scratched.

When presented with a confirmed or suspected RTA, the clinician should rapidly assess the patient for haemorrhage, breathing and circulation.

* Haemorrhage – If there is any external arterial bleeding, this should be stopped immediately by application of pressure. This can be achieved temporarily by hand pressure whilst the rest of the examination is undertaken. Minor bleeding from skin wounds can be ignored at this stage
* Breathing – The patient should be checked to ensure that it is breathing and has an adequate airway, and then evaluated for respiratory rate, effort and pattern. Respiratory distress should be presumed to be associated with thoracic injuries, although panting can be the result of fear, stress or pain. Cyanosis is a serious sign, indicative of severe respiratory compromise. Thoracic auscultation and percussion can suggest injuries such as pneumothorax (hyper-resonance dorsally on percussion with reduced lung sounds), haemothorax (muffled heart sounds and absence of lung sounds ventrally; hypo-resonance ventrally on percussion), or pulmonary contusions (crackles)
* Circulation – The circulation should be checked by assessing the heart rate, pulse rate, pulse quality, mucous membrane colour and CRT. Tachycardia, pale mucous membranes, slow CRT and poor pulse quality are highly suggestive of hypovolaemic shock due to haemorrhage (internal or external), which may be ongoing.

Once breathing and circulation have been confirmed (or re-established), the clinician should perform a brief assessment of other body functions:

* Demeanour should be classified as bright/active, depressed or moribund. Severely injured animals may be in a collapsed state because of hypovolaemia, hypoxia, brain injury or multiple orthopaedic injuries (although in the latter case, the patient should still be relatively alert)
* Signs of brain injury include a reduced level of consciousness, seizures or variation in pupil size. Other signs of head trauma which may suggest brain injury include external wounds, jaw fractures, aural or ocular haemorrhage, head tilt or abnormal eye position
* Musculoskeletal injuries are usually recognised by the owner and are often their major concern. However, they are not life-threatening in the short term and should be fully assessed later, when vital signs are stable

100 Top Consultations in Small Animal General Practice, First Edition
By Peter Hill, Sheena Warman and Geoff Shawcross
© 2011 Blackwell Publishing Ltd

- Superficial wounds, like musculoskeletal injuries, may be alarming but can be fully evaluated later.

After the initial clinical examination, it should be possible to categorise the case into:

- Life-threatening injuries needing immediate medical attention (e.g. shock, pneumothorax)
- Serious injuries that will need surgical correction once the animal is stable (e.g. fractured limb)
- Minor injuries that require surgical correction (e.g. skin laceration)
- No surgical treatment necessary, just outpatient care (e.g. minor bruising).

Further investigations that may be indicated in RTA cases (after emergency stabilisation if necessary) include:

- Abdominocentesis – This is a simple, rapid method of discovering if there is free fluid (especially blood) within the abdomen. A 21-gauge needle is inserted in the most dependent part of the abdomen. Any fluid which appears in the hub is collected into EDTA and plain tubes for analysis
- Radiography – Most useful for investigating thoracic and orthopaedic problems
- Ultrasound – This is most useful for detecting free fluid (blood, urine) in the abdomen or blood in the pleural space. Determining the extent of organ damage by ultrasound requires considerable experience with the technique
- Haematology and biochemical profile – For reference and as indicators of liver, kidney, bladder and muscle damage. A minimum database of PCV, total solids, urea, creatinine, glucose and electrolytes can provide valuable information. Blood tests are not always helpful for determining internal haemorrhage, as PCV is usually normal until blood volume has returned to normal.

Treatment

Respiratory stabilisation

If there is evidence of respiratory compromise or hypovolaemic shock, then oxygen should be administered. During assessment and initial stabilisation this can be provided as flow-by, mask or nasal prongs (if tolerated); nasal catheters are ideal for ongoing oxygen therapy. Oxygen cages restrict the ability of the clinician to assess and treat the patient, and are rarely effective. Pulse oximetry can often be helpful to guide therapy.

Pneumothorax cases require close monitoring. Some will improve and resolve spontaneously but if breathing deteriorates, thoracocentesis will be necessary. This is performed with a small gauge butterfly needle attached to a three-way tap and syringe. The skin is surgically prepared. The needle is inserted at the 6–8th intercostal space just above the costo-chondral junction, avoiding the large vessels on the caudal aspect of the rib, with continuous aspiration on the syringe. Once in the pleural space, the needle is directed caudally against the rib cage with the bevel facing inward to minimise the risk of trauma to the lungs.

Cardiovascular stabilisation

If there are clinical signs of hypovolaemic shock, then 'shock' doses of crystalloids are appropriate. These should be given in incremental boluses (20–30 ml/kg in dogs, 10–15 ml/kg in cats, to a total 'shock dose', if necessary, of 60–90 ml/kg in dogs, 40–60 ml/kg in cats), with the patient's cardiovascular and respiratory parameters assessed after each bolus. In patients with internal haemorrhage (abdominal, pleural, pulmonary or intracranial) a compromise is often necessary between providing adequate cardiovascular support whilst minimising ongoing haemorrhage. In particular, if there is evidence of pulmonary contusions (tachypnoea with audible respiratory crackles) much lower doses than this may be necessary to avoid exacerbation of pulmonary haemorrhage.

General care

- Analgesics – All RTAs will be in discomfort and will benefit from analgesics. In critical patients IM pethidine or methadone are useful as initial analgesics whilst the patient is fully assessed. Analgesics that also have a sedative effect should only be used once the demeanour has been fully evaluated. NSAIDs should be

avoided in patients with cardiovascular compromise
- Kennel rest – Confinement will limit further injury and allow the patient to settle. A quiet environment and darkened cage may help
- Antibiotics should be given to all cases with wounds, or likely to undergo surgery. Early antibiosis reduces the opportunity for infection to become established.

Specific injuries that frequently occur include:

- Internal abdominal haemorrhage caused by rupture of the spleen, liver or kidney. These usually require aggressive fluid therapy and prompt surgical intervention to stop ongoing haemorrhage. Ongoing intra-abdominal haemorrhage may be reduced in some cases by placement of a tight abdominal wrap
- Chest injuries such as lung lobe contusions are common and frequently recognised on radiographs. Fractured ribs are most common in large dogs. The condition is very painful and restricts respiratory effort. Effective analgesia is required, but surgical stabilisation is rarely necessary. Diaphragmatic rupture is more common in the cat than the dog. Immediate surgery is rarely advisable and should be deferred until the patient is stable. Oxygen therapy and quiet confinement are important
- Head injuries may be associated with brain injury and the animal's level of consciousness should be closely monitored (for at least 48 hours if head trauma is severe). If raised intra-cranial pressure is suspected (e.g. miosis and/or reduced consciousness), then the head should be elevated by about 20° (e.g. by putting a dog on a tilted stretcher, or a cat on an upturned clipboard), pressure on the jugular veins should be avoided, and procedures which cause coughing or sneezing (e.g. placement of a nasal catheter) should be avoided. Oxygen should be provided and cardiovascular support given to maintain normal arterial blood pressure. Hypertonic saline (7.2% NaCl, 3–5 ml/kg) may be preferable to large volumes of crystalloids. Mannitol is indicated in cases with very severe initial injury or those which

deteriorate despite initial therapy. Treatment with corticosteroids is no longer recommended as studies in people have shown that they may be detrimental when used to treat severe traumatic brain injury
- Facial bone fractures (especially separation of the lower mandible at the symphysis), fractured teeth and lacerated tongues are common. These require appropriate attention once the patient is stable. Nasal haemorrhage is common and usually resolves spontaneously, without complications. Intra-ocular haemorrhage or proptosis usually results in loss of vision and enucleation should be considered
- Limb and pelvic fractures are common and easily recognised on radiographs. The clinician should discuss with the owner the likely expense and prognosis associated with repair as soon as practicable. Inexperienced surgeons would be advised to refer fractures that require internal stabilisation, rather than embarking on a procedure and then getting into difficulties
- Vertebral fractures are less common than vertebral dislocations. Spinal radiographs can be misleading as many dislocations become re-aligned due to muscle contraction, belying the extent of the neurological damage. Evaluation of conscious pain perception is the single, most important assessment to be made in all cases of spinal injury
- Ventral hernia/rupture caused by avulsion of the abdominal muscles from the pubis is a frequent finding in the cat. There may be concurrent pelvic fractures and bladder injury, but it usually occurs without these associations. The extent of this injury is often underestimated and repair is often difficult
- Degloving injuries can lead to extensive skin loss from the distal limbs. Lengthy treatment is required that may involve skin grafts. Although a functional result can be achieved in most cases, amputation may have to be considered if financial resources are limited.
- Frayed claws are common in cats that have been dragged along the road. Although this is not a serious injury in itself, it can be a useful indicator of a road accident in cases where the history is not known.

What if it doesn't get better?

Due to the wide variety and complex nature of non-fatal injuries that may occur in RTAs, the animal must be continuously re-assessed if it is not recovering as well as expected. Some injuries sustained in an RTA can be life-threatening and result in the death of the animal.

The low-cost option

Cost-effective management of RTA patients depends on accurate assessment of the case as soon as possible. Initial treatment involving analgesia, antibiosis and fluid therapy as appropriate will only incur moderate costs but orthopaedic, intra-abdominal and intra-thoracic surgery is likely to be expensive. In cases where the patient is presented without the owner present, treatment should be limited to stabilisation and analgesia. The owner's consent should be sought before embarking on costly procedures as they may need to consider both the long-term prognosis and financial implications. Limb amputation can be a cost-effective treatment for complex fractures, especially if a good, functional outcome is doubtful following conventional repair. Not all cases will make a complete recovery and the owner's expectations/requirements should be taken into account before embarking on expensive procedures that may not yield good, functional results. Euthanasia may have to be considered if the cost of treatment is beyond the resources of the owner and financial help is unavailable.

When should I refer?

Stabilisation of the patient is required at the primary practice, and clinicians must become competent with the initial management and assessment of RTAs. Once stable, surgical cases such as complex orthopaedic and neurological conditions may benefit from specialist management. Early contact with the specialist centre should be sought; their advice could improve the quality of the initial management of the case. Inexperienced surgeons should always consider referral to a more experienced colleague, rather than embarking on an unfamiliar procedure and then getting into difficulties.

Geoff Shawcross

Aetiology and pathogenesis

Pharyngeal foreign bodies are frequently seen in dogs and cats, most commonly in young animals because of their inquisitive behaviour. Pharyngeal foreign bodies usually result from playing with objects, or trying to swallow food items that are too large or irregular in shape. Large objects can occlude the airway, leading to asphyxiation. If a foreign body becomes embedded in the soft tissue structures of the pharynx, there is a likelihood of abscessation that will lead to swelling and, possibly, occlusion of the pharynx.

Differential diagnoses

- Pharyngeal tumour, e.g. tonsillar carcinoma, eustachian tube polyp
- Pharyngeal wound
- Tonsillitis
- Pharyngeal malformations in predisposed breeds
- Upper respiratory tract disease
- Fracture of the hyoid apparatus.

History and clinical signs

Despite the possible differentials, the sudden onset and distressing presentation will always give a high index of suspicion that a pharyngeal foreign body is the cause of the symptoms. The owner may know exactly what the problem is and/or the foreign body may be visible on a simple clinical examination.

The usual signs of a pharyngeal foreign body are acute onset gagging, pawing at the mouth and salivation, which may be blood-stained. If the naso-pharynx is involved, sneezing and respiratory stertor may be present, especially in the cat. Usually, the animal will be reluctant to eat and attempts to do so will trigger a bout of gagging. However, as time passes, the distress caused by small foreign bodies usually settles down and the symptoms become more subtle. These include reluctance to eat, swelling, and pain in the parotid region or throat. If the retropharyngeal lymph nodes become involved, the enlargement can lead to signs that may be confused with

a cervical disc protrusion. Unresolved migrating foreign bodies (e.g. grass seeds) may lead to fibrosis involving the masticatory muscles, making it difficult for the mouth to be opened fully, even under general anaesthesia. If the foreign body is large, e.g. a ball, the pharyngeal occlusion may lead to severe dyspnoea or asphyxiation. Chronic nasopharyngeal foreign bodies may give rise to a muco-purulent nasal discharge.

Specific diagnostic techniques

A foreign body may be visible on a simple clinical examination of the oral cavity in the conscious patient. Where the index of suspicion is high but the foreign body is not visible, or oral examination is resented, a thorough examination should be carried out under general anaesthesia. This allows evaluation of the oro- and naso-pharynx and the investigation of any pharyngeal wounds or sinus tracts. Good illumination is essential and can be provided by a head-lamp, laryngoscope or flexible endoscope. Particular attention should be paid to the tonsillar crypts and the nasopharynx, by reflecting the soft palate.

Radiography will reveal the size and position of metallic or bony foreign bodies, and any displacement of cervical soft tissue structures that has occurred secondary to abscessation. Ultrasonography of the cervical region may help localise a radiolucent foreign body and determine the nature of any swelling around the upper neck. Imaging should always be undertaken if a foreign body is suspected but cannot be seen, or there is a visible penetrating wound.

Treatment

Following identification of the foreign body, treatment is aimed at removal and then controlling potential pharyngeal oedema, pain and infection. It may be possible to remove certain oral foreign bodies in the conscious patient, especially if it is accessible and has

100 Top Consultations in Small Animal General Practice, First Edition
By Peter Hill, Sheena Warman and Geoff Shawcross
© 2011 Blackwell Publishing Ltd

not perforated the oral structures. However, patients with a pharyngeal foreign body usually require a general anaesthetic. Wounds in the pharynx should be thoroughly searched for the remains of any foreign material and then flushed with warm saline. Prior to flushing, a snugly fitting endotracheal tube should be in place and the animal should be tilted head-down, to prevent aspiration into the airway. Broad-spectrum antibiotics should be given if there is damage to the pharyngeal tissues. NSAIDs should be used to reduce tissue swelling and pain. Pharyngeal wounds tend to heal very quickly; very few need to be sutured but if required, only a minimal number of sutures need be placed. If swallowing food appears difficult or painful, most animals will take soft ice cream and once they have started eating, will take other soft foods quite readily.

Specific treatment of common pharyngeal foreign bodies

- **Fish bones, irregular bones (vertebrae).** Fine (cartilaginous) bones are frequently seen in the cat, typically wedged horizontally across the pharynx and embedded in the soft tissues. They are easily removed with artery forceps, although general anaesthesia is usually required. Irregular bones are more commonly seen in the dog and are easy to diagnose and remove. Damage to the tissues is usually minimal.
- **Fishhooks.** Cats are affected when they try to play with 'flies' or eat the bait. Dogs will also try to eat the bait, or catch a moving fishing line. Whenever possible, any line that remains attached to the hook should be preserved and prevented from being swallowed. The barb on the hook makes it very difficult to pull the hook backwards and so it is best removed by pushing it forward through the tissues. If the eye is large or there is not much space to manipulate the hook, it may be necessary to cut the hook in two before it can be removed. However, most fishhooks are made of high tensile steel and can only be cut with proper hardened steel cutters (not nail clippers). Fishhooks that have moved on from the pharynx may become lodged in the oesophagus or stomach. Such cases should be radiographed and examined endoscopically to determine the exact position of the hook and quantify the tissue damage. Some can be removed endoscopically but surgery may be

required. Referral should be considered for such cases if adequate facilities are not available.
- **Needle and thread.** The needle may lodge across the pharynx, or become deeply embedded in the root of the tongue. Unlike fishhooks, they are usually easy to remove with artery forceps. Keeping any thread attached to the needle helps in localising the needle and in manipulating it during removal.
- **Grass seeds, blades of grass, burrs.** Result from self-grooming or eating grass. Grass seeds will often become embedded in the tonsillar crypt and blades of grass frequently lodge in the nasopharynx, behind the soft palate. Grass seeds will start to migrate through the mucous membrane if not diagnosed and removed quickly, making them difficult to find and triggering considerable soft tissue reaction.
- **Balls.** Usually occurs when a dog catches a ball which is too small relative to the size of the dog. The ball becomes trapped behind the fauces of the throat and over the root of the tongue. Breathing is severely compromised and there is a very high risk of death through asphyxiation. By the time they are presented, these cases are usually severely dyspnoeic and every effort should be made to ensure the animal is not frightened or anxious. The ball is best removed under a short-acting general anaesthetic but all the necessary equipment to perform an emergency tracheotomy must be to hand before induction. Once the dog is anaesthetised, the ball can be fixed by external manipulation of the larynx and then grasped with large tissue forceps. A surprising amount of effort is often required to dislodge the ball. During this time, the dog is unlikely to be able to breathe and, unless a tracheotomy has been performed, every effort must be made to remove the obstruction as quickly as possible. The removal of air-filled balls (e.g. tennis balls) may be facilitated by stabbing them first so that they will collapse when grasped.
- **Wood splinters.** These are seen in dogs that play with sticks or are destructive. Although dogs may present with the typical acute signs of gagging and distress, very often these signs have become chronic. Wood splinters are often associated with abscessation in the root of the tongue or upper cervical region but can be difficult to identify and localise. As they are not

radio-opaque, ultrasonography may be a better diagnostic tool than radiography.
- **Stick penetration injuries.** These are quite common and occur when a dog runs onto a stick when playing. These injuries must always be fully evaluated under a general anaesthetic. Tissue damage can be extensive and the wounds are often heavily contaminated.

The low-cost option

Costs are low if the diagnosis is straightforward and the foreign body can be removed in the conscious patient; usually these patients only require minimal medication. Costs will increase if a general anaesthetic is necessary but early diagnosis and treatment will avoid the cost of dealing with the complications associated with an embedded or migrating foreign body.

What if it doesn't get better?

Persistence of signs after a foreign body has been removed should prompt a search for other possible causes. If a foreign body has not been found, but is still suspected, further attempts at finding it should be made.

When should I refer?

Most cases are well within the capacity of general practice. Referral to an experienced surgeon should be considered if surgery in the cervical region is required or there is extensive damage at the back of the throat (usually following a stick injury). Foreign bodies that are oesophageal may require instrumentation or surgical expertise that is not available in the practice.

Section 11

Geoff Shawcross

Aetiology and pathogenesis

Grass-seed foreign bodies are a very common occurrence in both dogs and cats that have access to areas of uncut grass or farmland. Typically, they are most common in the late summer months but undiagnosed grass-seed foreign bodies can cause chronic otitis and chronic draining abscesses throughout the year. Long-coated breeds are more commonly affected as the seeds are easily entangled in the hair. The barbed nature of the seeds facilitates their migration through the tissues and prevents their easy removal.

History and clinical signs

Grass-seed foreign bodies usually affect the ears, eyes, nasal passages, pharynx and interdigital skin, although they can be found in other sites. Symptoms are usually sudden in onset, and often very severe.

Typical clinical signs in the various sites include:

- Ears – Sudden onset headshaking after exercising in fields or long grass. The condition is rare in the cat and most common in dogs with pendulous pinnae. Major differentials would be insect stings and urticarial reactions
- Eyes – Sudden onset blepharospasm and epiphora which rapidly becomes mucopurulent. There may be aggressive rubbing of the affected eye resulting in excoriation of the peri-orbital skin. Usually, only one eye is affected. It is very rare for the problem to be bilateral. Major differentials include corneal injury caused by trauma (e.g. cat scratches) or caustic substances, or idiopathic corneal ulceration. Severe conjunctivitis, uveitis and glaucoma can give similar signs
- Nose – Sudden onset violent sneezing and rubbing of the nose. There may be slight bleeding from one nostril. Although the symptoms persist, the severity reduces after a short time. Other causes of acute-onset sneezing include viral infection (cats), inhalation of irritant chemicals or dusts, and other types of foreign body. Epistaxis may also occur with

trauma, tooth root abscesses, nasal tumours and *Aspergillus* infection, although the latter three conditions usually occur as more chronic problems
- Pharynx – Sudden onset gagging and retching, which may be severe enough to result in regurgitation. The condition is more common in the cat owing to their tendency to eat grass, either directly or when grooming. The grass seed usually becomes lodged in the tonsillar crypt where it becomes reasonably well tolerated in the short term but it may penetrate the mucous membrane and result in a retropharyngeal or parotid abscess. When abscessation occurs, there may be signs of general malaise, swelling and discomfort around the throat and cranial neck, pyrexia and dysphagia. Because the initial clinical signs are severe, the history should give a high level of suspicion that an oro-pharyngeal foreign body exists. However, major differentials should include tonsillitis and pharyngitis caused by infection, tonsillar tumours and nasopharyngeal polyps. When there is swelling in the parotid region, inflammation or tumours involving the regional lymph nodes or salivary glands should also be considered. Dysphagia, pain and swelling around the throat are also associated with damage to the larynx, or fracture of the hyoid apparatus. The pain associated with retropharyngeal abscessation may be confused with cranial cervical disc disease. Occasionally a grass seed can migrate from the pharynx via the trachea into the lungs resulting in a cough, often associated with foul-smelling halitosis
- Interdigital skin – Rapidly developing interdigital swellings that rupture and form a discharging sinus. They are a source of irritation and result in compulsive licking. They frequently affect more than one interdigital web and more than one foot. Left untreated, they can migrate up the leg forming multiple sinuses along their track. They are rare in the cat. The major differentials are interdigital pyogranulomas and interdigital furunculosis which may be caused by bacterial infection or implanted hair shafts
- Other areas – Grass seeds can be the cause of chronic draining sinuses over all areas of the head, neck and trunk. They have also been the cause of preputial and vulval discharges, and abscesses in the

100 Top Consultations in Small Animal General Practice, First Edition
By Peter Hill, Sheena Warman and Geoff Shawcross
© 2011 Blackwell Publishing Ltd

anal sacs, lungs and abdomen. In most of these cases, grass seeds would not be considered as a primary differential as the condition usually presents out of the grass-seed season but their involvement becomes apparent when the condition is surgically explored.

Specific diagnostic techniques

An ability to perform a detailed otoscopic, ophthalmoscopic, nasal or dermatological examination is important when searching for grass seeds. Radiography may be necessary to differentiate nasal and pharyngeal problems.

Treatment

Successful treatment of problems associated with grass seeds requires their removal. Left in situ, grass seeds can lead to chronic problems. Specific treatment recommendations are as follows:

- Ears – Otoscopy should allow the foreign body to be seen, but may be resented if the ear canal is painful. It is not uncommon for both ears to be affected and both should be thoroughly checked. The grass seed can be removed with long crocodile forceps through an open-ended cone on an otoscope that has good magnification and illumination. If at all possible, this should be carried out under sedation or a light, short-acting general anaesthetic such as propofol. Anaesthesia may not be necessary with a co-operative patient and good restraint, but the procedure can be painful and there is a risk of iatrogenic damage to the tympanic membrane if the animal moves at a critical moment. Once the seed is removed, 2–3 days treatment with ear drops containing an anti-inflammatory and antibiotic combination will reduce the discomfort and prevent infection developing
- Eyes – A few drops of an ophthalmic anaesthetic should be instilled into the eye to relieve discomfort and allow a thorough examination of the eye, followed by application of fluorescein. In most cases there is evidence of extensive but shallow ulceration of the cornea, which is not central. Grass seeds

commonly become lodged behind the third eyelid and the tail of the seed can often be seen just protruding from the leading edge. The conjunctival sac should also be carefully searched, especially the ventral fornix. It is unusual for a grass seed to become lodged under the upper eyelid. Only if the patient is uncooperative, or the diagnosis is in doubt, would general anaesthesia be necessary. If seen, the grass seed can be easily grasped with blunt-pointed dressing forceps. The corneal ulceration should be treated with an antibiotic ophthalmic ointment for 3–5 days and usually heals very quickly. Topical corticosteroids should be avoided as they can inhibit healing. An Elizabethan collar may be necessary for a short time if self-mutilation is occurring
- Nose – Investigation requires a general anaesthetic. A well-fitting endotracheal tube should be used. A few drops of local anaesthetic instilled into the nostril can reduce reflex sneezing associated with the sensitive nasal mucous membranes. A narrow cone attached to an otoscope can be inserted into the nostril and used to provide illumination and magnification. If available, a rigid rhinoscope will provide the best visualisation. The instruments must be handled gently to avoid haemorrhage. Foreign bodies tend to enter the ventral meatus and if a grass seed is seen, it can be removed with crocodile forceps. If nothing can be found, the soft palate should be retracted with tissue forceps to examine the choanae, as the seed may have migrated into the pharynx. If the search is still unsuccessful, or the grass seed has fragmented, the nasal cavity should be flushed from both directions with warmed saline to dislodge the material. After removal or flushing, broad-spectrum antibiotic cover should be provided for about 5 days, along with a short course of NSAIDs. In contrast to other sites, nasal grass seeds become well tolerated within a short period of time and it is not unusual for the natural protective mechanisms in the nose to result in the disintegration and ejection of the foreign material
- Pharyngeal – Although it may be possible to see a grass seed lodged in the pharynx on a simple oral examination, its removal will require a general anaesthetic. It is not uncommon for there to be multiple grass seeds and so it is

necessary to search the area carefully for small, draining sinus tracts. After removal, broad-spectrum antibiotics should be given for 3–5 days along with a NSAID

- Interdigital – Owners should be warned that it is difficult to find grass seeds that are causing sinus tracts and it may take several surgical attempts to resolve the problem. The history should give a high level of suspicion and, because of the tendency for the grass seeds to migrate, it is best to make an early assumption that a grass seed is the cause of the swelling or draining sinus tract. The presence of grass seeds lying between the toes, or caught up in the coat, should add confidence to the diagnosis. When cases are presented early, it may be possible to just see the tails of the grass seed at the opening of the tract. Cooperative dogs, together with adequate restraint, may allow gentle searching of a sinus tract with sterile crocodile forceps. More extensive investigation should be done under general anaesthesia. After removal, the wound should be dressed for 3–4 days to keep it clean and prevent further interference, and the dog treated with a short course of broad-spectrum antibiotics. The signs will resolve very quickly if the grass seed has been removed. If a grass seed cannot be found, the wounds should not be sutured. The foot should be dressed for 4 days and the dog treated with a broad-spectrum antibiotic. When the dressing is removed, the dog can be re-examined, if necessary under general anaesthesia. A new tract may have developed which would be highly suggestive that the grass seed has migrated further. Healed or closing tracts can be ignored. For future prophylaxis, the coat can be clipped short in the summer months, especially around the ears and feet, and fields and uncut grassland should be avoided when exercising dogs.

What if it doesn't get better?

If a grass seed can be found and removed, it is very likely that the signs will resolve completely. If a grass seed cannot be found, or if the signs do not resolve completely, other causes of otitis, ocular pain, sneezing, epistaxis, retching, interdigital lesions or chronic discharging sinuses should be considered. Further investigations should be performed to determine the underlying cause of these signs.

The low-cost option

Removal of grass seeds from the ears and eyes is typically a low-cost procedure. Removal of nasal and pharyngeal grass seeds will additionally involve the cost of a general anaesthetic. Repeated searches for interdigital grass seeds can lead to escalating costs so this should only be performed if there is a high index of suspicion. It is not usually necessary to use expensive broad-spectrum antibiotics after removal of grass seeds – ampicillin or amoxicillin are appropriate choices.

When should I refer?

Most grass-seed problems are within the scope of general practice. Referral is appropriate after failing to find the cause of a chronic otitis, blepharospasm, persistent nasal problem or sinus tract, despite several attempts. Investigation and the surgical management of a retropharyngeal, intra-thoracic or intra-abdominal lesion may be beyond the surgical scope of an inexperienced surgeon, or where diagnostic and surgical facilities are limited.

Peter Hill

Aetiology and pathogenesis

Burns can be caused by excessive temperatures (e.g. flames, extreme heat sources, engine parts, scalding water, hot oil, tar), caustic chemicals (e.g. acids, alkalis) or electric currents. Most burns in pets occur on the skin, resulting in various degrees of necrosis and inflammation, but they can also occur in the mouth.

The factors that determine the severity of a thermal burn include the temperature and contact time. A very high temperature can cause serious damage with very short exposures. However, prolonged contact with lower temperatures can also lead to burns, as is seen in anaesthetised pets placed on heating pads. Pressure and ischaemia also contribute to the skin damage in such cases. Chemical burns are caused by the caustic nature of the offending substance which can directly damage the skin. Electrical burns are caused by electrical energy being transformed into heat and would be seen most commonly in pets that have chewed through an electrical cord.

Prolonged exposure to strong sunlight can also cause thermal burns in dogs, especially on the dorsum. However, sun-induced skin damage is usually more of a chronic problem in animals, resulting in solar dermatitis and increased risk of skin cancer. This is a particular problem in white-haired cats that are prone to developing squamous cell carcinomas on their ear tips in response to sun damage.

Depending on their depth, burns may result in serious medical complications such as shock, electrolyte imbalances, respiratory distress, life-threatening sepsis, DIC and death. A specific complication seen with severe burns is compartment syndrome, in which tissue swelling within fascial compartments creates strictures that restrict blood supply to the limbs and inhibit thoracic wall movement.

History and clinical signs

In many cases, the owner will be aware of the incident that resulted in the injury, so diagnosis is usually straightforward. Even if no specific accident has been observed,

100 Top Consultations in Small Animal General Practice, First Edition
By Peter Hill, Sheena Warman and Geoff Shawcross
© 2011 Blackwell Publishing Ltd

the diagnosis can usually be made relatively easily on clinical examination alone. A characteristic of most burns that aids in establishing a diagnosis is the clear demarcation between normal and affected sites. Unusual patterns, lack of symmetry, straight or angular edges, or drip configurations help to distinguish burns from other skin disorders. Owners should be made aware that the full extent of a burn may not become apparent until five days after the initial injury as further tissue necrosis becomes evident. Conditions that may occasionally appear similar to burns include toxic epidermal necrolysis, autoimmune ulcerative diseases and vasculitis.

Specific diagnostic techniques

The abnormalities seen with a burn will depend on the depth of tissue involved. Burns are typically classified as follows:

- **1st degree / superficial burns** only involve damage to the epidermis but they do not cause severe epidermal necrosis. They present with erythema, and the skin is dry and painful (Figure 80.1)
- **2nd degree / superficial partial thickness burns** cause severe necrosis of the epidermis and also involve the superficial dermis. Blisters might be seen transiently, but ulcers are more typical in dogs and cats. The skin will appear red, moist and is very painful. These burns will usually heal with minimal scarring
- **3rd degree / deep partial thickness burns** involve damage to the epidermis, deep dermis and panniculus, causing deeper ulcers which heal slowly by scarring (Figure 80.2)
- **4th degree / full thickness burns** involve complete necrosis of all layers of the skin, including hair follicles and some subcutaneous fat. These burns are often less painful than more superficial burns due to destruction of nerve endings. A thick, coagulated crust of necrotic skin (eschar) may form at the site of the burn (Figure 80.3). This may feel hard to the

touch (like cardboard). This will eventually slough off, leaving a raw ulcerated area. These lesions heal very slowly and often require skin grafts or surgical closure

- **5th degree / subdermal burns** extend down to the subcutaneous fascia, muscle, tendon or even bones. The affected area is insensitive and will be covered in a thick, hard, leathery eschar.

Another important factor in assessing the severity of a burn is by the percentage of total body surface area affected. The more extensive the involvement, the more likely are serious medical complications. A full physical examination should be performed in all burns patients to identify any systemic complications.

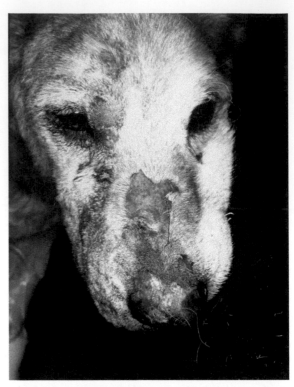

Figure 80.2   Second and third degree burns on the face of a dog that was burnt in a bonfire. Note the well-demarcated edges.

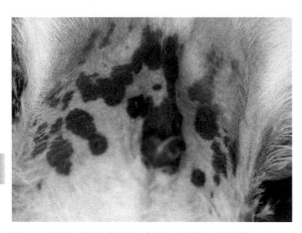

Figure 80.1   First degree burn on the ventral abdomen of a dog that was scalded with hot water

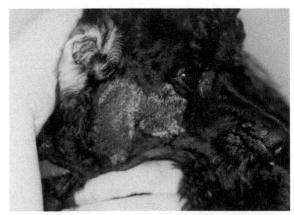

Figure 80.3   Fourth degree burn on the side of a dog's face that came into contact with hot metal. The well-demarcated areas are thickened, hard, and feel like cardboard. These will eventually slough off if not removed

Treatment

Burn patients should be rapidly assessed to determine the extent and depth of tissue damage. First degree burns are usually self-limiting and require minimal treatment. Topical application of a moisturising cream may help to soothe the skin and reduce peeling. If extensive, pain relief can be provided with a short course of NSAIDs. Second and third degree burns should be treated with a topical antimicrobial cream such as silver sulfadiazine, which helps to prevent infection and sepsis. Covering the affected areas with dressings can encourage healing, but Vaseline-impregnated gauzes should be avoided. Silver-impregnated dressings (Acticoat, Smith & Nephew) can be used to combine the antimicrobial effects of the silver within a suitable dressing. If extensive fluid loss is anticipated (for example, if the affected area is large), the dressing can be covered with Intrasite hydrogel and then cling film, to retain moisture within the dressing. Dressings should be changed every 2–7 days, depending on the amount of exudation that is expected. If the lesions are extensive, systemic therapy with broad-spectrum antibiotics is also indicated. Deeper localised burns are likely to require surgical intervention to encourage healing. This may involve removal of eschars, primary closure or skin grafts.

Burns patients suffering from widespread lesions (more than 30% of the body area) require emergency hospitalisation and intensive care. Blood samples should be taken for haematology, biochemistry and a coagulation profile. Intensive IV fluid therapy is indicated to maintain arterial blood pressure and urine output. If extensive protein loss has occurred, judicious use of colloids is indicated to maintain osmotic pressure. Serum electrolytes should be monitored throughout treatment. Broad-spectrum antibiotic treatment should be given if there is any risk of sepsis or pneumonia. If necessary, supplemental oxygen should be provided, especially in cases involving smoke inhalation or pneumonia. Areas amenable to dressing should be covered as described above. Burns involving the limbs should undergo debridement as soon as the patient is sufficiently stable, to prevent strictures or limb ischaemia.

What if it doesn't get better?

Burn injuries will not progress after the first five days. As long as the animal survives, and doesn't develop serious medical complications, a recovery can be expected. However, there may be some loss of function due to scarring. In some cases, the aesthetic consequences of scarring can be dramatic (Figure 80.4).

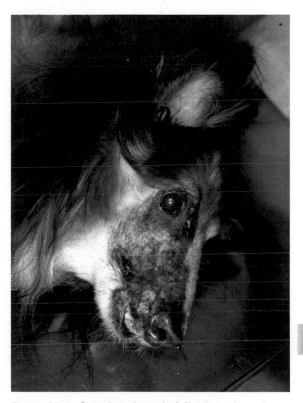

Figure 80.4 **Scarring alopecia following a burn to the side of a dog's face caused by hot kitchen oil**

The low-cost option

Minor burns can be treated as out patients and shouldn't incur high costs. Serious burns will require hospitalisation, intensive care and possibly surgery, which will be expensive. If funds are not available for such care, euthanasia should be considered.

When should I refer?

Minor burns are easily dealt with in the general practice setting. Even more severe burns can be dealt with in most veterinary clinics. Referral should be considered for those cases in which serious medical complications are likely, or have occurred. These cases require intensive care and constant monitoring, along with the expertise needed to make rapid therapeutic decisions. Surgical repair of burn defects by grafting or flaps is best carried out by specialist surgeons.

Section 12
Cancer

Mark Goodfellow

Aetiology and pathogenesis

Neoplasia (cancer/tumour) occurs when cells acquire the ability to divide in an uncontrolled fashion, independently of the requirement for new cells. This is normally the consequence of at least two genetic alterations, one or more of which may be common in a given breed. Unlike benign tumours, malignant cells have the ability to cross basement membranes, invade surrounding tissues and metastasise to distant sites. Benign tumours are denoted by the tissue of origin followed by the suffix -oma (e.g. fibroma). Malignant tumours that arise from epithelial tissue are designated carcinomas; those from glandular epithelial tissue, adenocarcinomas; and those from mesenchymal tissue, sarcomas. The most notable exceptions to this nomenclature are lymphomas (by definition malignant); melanomas and histiocytosis, named malignant when appropriate; and mast cell tumours, which are not typically referred to as mastocytomas and may be benign (in cats) or malignant.

Common tumours of dogs and cats

- Skin tumours – lipoma, sebaceous adenoma, mast cell tumour (see Chapter 26 for full list)
- Haemopoietic tumours – lymphoma (see Chapter 83), leukaemia, multiple myeloma
- Oral cavity tumours – malignant melanoma, squamous cell carcinoma, fibrosarcoma
- Intestinal tract tumours – gastric or intestinal adenoma/carcinoma, lymphoma, leiomyoma/sarcoma
- Liver tumours – hepatic carcinoma, biliary carcinoma, common site of metastasis
- Spleen tumours – haemangiosarcoma, lymphoma
- Kidney tumours – renal carcinoma, lymphoma (especially the cat)
- Bladder tumours – transitional cell carcinoma
- Lung tumours – pulmonary carcinoma, common site of metastasis
- Blood vessel tumours – haemangioma/sarcoma

- Cardiac tumours – heart base tumour
- Skeletal tumours – osteosarcoma, chondrosarcoma
- Testicular tumours – Sertoli cell tumour, interstitial cell tumour
- Tumours of the female reproductive tract – ovarian adenoma/carcinoma, granulosa cell tumour, leiomyoma
- Pituitary tumours – adenoma.

Diagnostic approach

The clinical signs of cancer may be non-specific (e.g. weight loss, inappetence, lethargy), may relate to the organ affected (e.g. lameness, haematuria) or result from factors released by the tumour (e.g. polydipsia associated with humoral hypercalcaemia of malignancy). Owners may have noticed a lump if the affected tissue is superficial (e.g. skin, mammary or oral cavity tumours; lymphoma). Whenever neoplasia is suspected, a complete physical examination is mandatory, including detailed palpation of the lymph nodes and abdominal cavity.

If a mass is detected, early investigation and rapid diagnosis maximises the likelihood of successful treatment. For accessible masses, fine needle aspirates can provide valuable information (see Chapter 26 for skin tumours). However, biopsies obtained surgically or by using a needle core device (e.g. Tru-cut) are required for definitive diagnosis of most tumours.

If a histopathology or cytology report is received that diagnoses neoplasia, it is important to verify that it is both appropriate for the tissue sample submitted and for the patient. An unexpected or unclear diagnosis should be discussed with the pathologist. Biopsy reports should describe any features of malignancy that are present, such as the mitotic index (an indication of the number of cells that are seen to be undergoing division), degree of cellular atypia (abnormal morphological features of the cell or nucleus) or evidence of vascular invasion. They should also report whether the tumour extends to the edge of the submitted sample (i.e. the margins).

100 Top Consultations in Small Animal General Practice, First Edition
By Peter Hill, Sheena Warman and Geoff Shawcross
© 2011 Blackwell Publishing Ltd

If a malignant tumour is present, the extent to which it has disseminated around the rest of the body can be ascertained by staging. This is done using the **TNM** classification:

- **Tumour** – evaluation of the tumour itself, including its extent and consequences
- **Nodes** – determination if the tumour has spread to local or distant lymph nodes
- **Metastasis** – detection of distant metastases.

This process involves investigations such as blood tests, thoracic radiographs, abdominal radiography and ultrasonography, CT or MRI scans, and/or bone marrow aspirates or biopsies. The degree of staging required for a given tumour varies, and may require referral. In some cases, staging merely refers to the process of determining how far a tumour has spread, whereas for certain tumours (e.g. lymphoma) specific classification categories have been defined. Staging is important because it helps to determine the most appropriate treatment for a patient, and the prognosis.

Treatment

Based on their experiences with the human disease, pet owners often associate a diagnosis of cancer with profound morbidity, a reduced life-span, radical surgery and/or toxic treatment protocols. Consequently, a diagnosis of cancer is often met with a more profound emotional response than for other severe chronic diseases, which actually may have a poorer prognosis. With the exception of some surgically excisable tumours, complete cure is rarely achieved. Being prepared to discuss all possible options by gathering accurate information regarding individual tumour behaviour, treatment choices and prognosis prior to a consultation is vital.

Potential treatment options for cancer include:

- Surgical resection
- Chemotherapy
- Radiotherapy.

Selection of appropriate therapy is dependent on tumour type and is vital to optimise outcome. Surgery as a sole therapy is most suitable for control of localised benign disease, such as tumours in the skin or easily accessible organs. In contrast, chemotherapy is a systemic treatment most suitable for dissemi-

nated tumours (e.g. lymphoma). Chemotherapy may also be employed following resection of malignant tumours, for control of distant metastases. Control of radiosensitive tumours (e.g. mast cell tumours, melanoma, meningioma) may involve local radiotherapy alone or follow surgical debulking of disease.

Regardless of the treatment chosen, the ultimate aim is to maximise quality of life. Treatments should be tailored to avoid the severe adverse effects of therapy experienced by humans, which are unacceptable in veterinary patients. Adverse effects are not compatible with a good quality of life and aggressive remedial action should be taken if they occur. Symptomatic and supportive care (anti-emetics, encouragement to eat, etc.) is necessary for all patients, irrespective of the treatment employed, and forms the basis of palliative care.

Decisions regarding definitive or palliative treatment are made on the basis of information obtained from staging and considering the patient's co-morbidities. It is important that the treatment instituted should improve the patient's overall wellbeing. For example, use of a nephrotoxic chemotherapy drug in the face of severe pre-existing renal disease is likely to worsen the patient's condition overall, even if the neoplasia is controlled. Palliative care should be prescribed in all cases, and in some situations may be the only form of treatment employed. This may include such modalities as analgesics, anti-emetics or special diets.

What if it doesn't get better?

The prognosis for patients with cancer will vary from case to case and is influenced by the factors discussed above. Table 81.1 shows the median survival times for some common tumours. Such figures are averages and there will be patients who live substantially shorter periods and those who survive considerably longer. Such information is best presented to owners as no more than a guide, whilst stressing that the quality of life, rather than longevity, is the primary aim of treatment.

Relapse of the disease is likely in many cases, and animals should be carefully monitored during treatment to detect this as soon as possible. Assessment of the patient's quality of life is equally as important as clinical assessment of treatment success. For example, a reduction in tumour size is irrelevant if the patient is anorexic, cachectic and leading a miserable life. Owners should therefore be questioned regarding non-specific indicators of wellbeing such as appetite, activity levels, behaviour and play patterns.

Recurrence of a tumour at a surgical site is indicative of an incomplete excision and residual disease. Repeat surgery or other adjunctive therapy is necessary, which may require referral to a specialist. The appearance of new lesions at a distant site should prompt repeat staging. Lack of response to an appropriate chemotherapy drug at an appropriate dose is indicative of tumour resistance and will occur in all cases during therapy at some point.

Euthanasia is an option at any time following a diagnosis of cancer and owners often request guidance in its timing. Asking owners to gauge if the patient's quality of life is deteriorating or, if on balance, the good periods are no longer out-weighing the bad, will aid this decision.

Table 81.1   Accepted treatment options for some common canine and feline tumours with a guide to median survival time.

Tumour	Surgery	Chemotherapy	Radiation Therapy	Other	Approximate median survival time (months) with definitive therapy	
					Dog	Cat
Multicentric lymphoma*		X			2–13 (see Chapter 83)	1–9
Cutaneous mast cell tumour*	X	X	X	X[1]	Cure achievable (grades I and II) 1–12 months for grade III (see Chapter 31)	Mastocytic forms – wide surgical excision curative, Histiocytic forms – may spontaneously regress
Splenic haemangiosarcoma	X	X			5–6	Rare
Appendicular osteosarcoma	X	X			12	Rare
Mammary gland tumours*	X				1–>24 (see Chapter 82)	10–12
Oral malignant melanoma	X	X	X	X[2]	3–21	Rare
Transitional cell carcinoma of the bladder		X		X[3]	4	Very rare
Testicular tumours	X				Curative in >85% of cases	Rare
Lipoma	X				Curative	Curative

[1]Tyrosine kinase inhibitors.
[2]Immunotherapy.
[3]Cyclooxygenase (COX) inhibitors.
*Subtypes of these tumours differ markedly in behaviour and prognosis.

Section 12

The low-cost option

In common with all chronic diseases, the cumulative cost of long-term care of a patient with cancer can be substantial. In general, palliative care is less expensive than definitive treatment. The cost of treatment can be minimised by performing only diagnostic staging procedures appropriate to the tumour identified and by performing the most efficacious therapy from the outset. In some cases, financial limitations may preclude full staging and optimal treatment of tumours, in which case the clinician should recommend a palliative care programme to maximise the quality of the pet's remaining life. Euthanasia should be offered if a tumour is significantly affecting a patient's quality of life and funds are not available for specific treatment or palliative care.

When should I refer?

Many types of tumour can be dealt with in general practice, especially if surgical resection is likely to effect a complete cure. Specialist advice should be sought if complex surgical techniques or reconstructions are required (e.g. for maxillofacial tumours, liver tumours, mast cell tumours on the distal limb). The use of chemotherapy requires expertise and familiarity with specific agents, and the availability of suitable drug-handling facilities. Some chemotherapy protocols are prescribed in general practice, but referral to an oncologist is advised for complex protocols. Radiotherapy will require referral to an oncologist who has access to this treatment modality. Referral is also recommended if a combination of therapies is the most efficacious treatment for a particular tumour.

The best outcome is achieved by planning and executing definitive treatment on the first occasion, and referral should be offered if this is not likely to happen within the practice. Clinicians should remember that the first surgical resection has the highest likelihood of success and the first chemotherapy-induced remission is the longest.

Mark Goodfellow

Aetiology and pathogenesis

Mammary tumours are common in older bitches (>10 years), and are likely to develop in a quarter of entire bitches. Spaniels, Poodles, Dachshunds and German Shepherd breeds are predisposed. Ovariectomy or ovario-hysterectomy of young bitches reduces the incidence significantly. Those spayed before the first oestrus have a negligible risk of developing mammary neoplasia, whereas those spayed before the second oestrus have a 10-fold reduced risk. Later spaying may reduce the risk of benign tumours but seems to have no effect on the risk of developing malignant tumours. Mammary tumours are rare in entire or castrated male dogs.

Mammary tumour development is, at least in part, hormone driven and treatment of entire females with progestagens to retard oestrus causes an increased incidence of benign but not malignant tumours. Conversely, unlike in the human, a protective effect of early pregnancy or lactation has not been proven.

History and clinical signs

In many cases, the owner will have noticed a mass on the ventral abdomen. However, it is not uncommon for previously unnoticed mammary tumours to be detected on routine annual health checks. At the time of presentation or detection, most mammary tumours are asymptomatic, but in dogs with advanced disease, symptoms associated with metastatic spread may be present (e.g. coughing or dyspnoea due to pulmonary metastasis). Mammary tumours are more common in the caudal mammary glands (4 and 5) and present as masses or nodules of any size. They may be fixed to the overlying skin or underlying tissue and may or may not be associated with a nipple. Half of all cases will present with, or subsequently develop, multiple masses. Inflammatory carcinoma is a highly metastatic form of mammary neoplasia and presents as a very painful, erythematous and oedematous swelling of the mammary glands and often the proximal limbs. The patient often shows systemic signs such as lethargy, so this presentation can be easily confused with acute mastitis.

Specific diagnostic techniques

A thorough history and physical examination will usually allow other differential diagnoses for mammary swellings to be eliminated. In the non-pregnant bitch, hyperplastic nodules can be seen during metoestrus or shortly following progestagen therapy. In the post-parturient bitch, duct ectasia (dilation after blockage) and mastitis also need to be considered. Clinicians should also consider other tumours that may arise in this area, but are not derived from mammary tissue (e.g. mast cell tumours or lipomas).

When a mass is detected, thorough palpation of all the mammary glands is essential, along with the regional lymph nodes (axillary and superficial inguinal). Enlargement of the sublumbar lymph nodes may be detected per rectum. The size of all identified masses should be recorded. Features of mammary tumours which suggest malignant behaviour and a relatively poor prognosis include size greater than 3 cm, history of rapid growth, fixation to surrounding tissues, ulceration and nodularity. However, it is not possible to distinguish between benign and malignant masses on the basis of palpation alone. Furthermore, due to the heterogeneous nature of most mammary tumours, cytology cannot always provide this information. Fine needle aspiration of mammary masses is indicated primarily to exclude other differential diagnoses rather than to determine tumour behaviour. Tumour type, and predictions about probable behaviour can only be made on histological examination (usually performed after excision). The difficulty of differentiating benign from malignant mammary masses without biopsy should not encourage a 'wait and see' approach because there is a progression from benign to malignant behaviour over time. Early intervention at the time of presentation will prevent a small mass, which can be removed with a simple curative surgery, progressing to one for which surgery is complex, or distant metastasis has already occurred.

100 Top Consultations in Small Animal General Practice, First Edition
By Peter Hill, Sheena Warman and Geoff Shawcross
© 2011 Blackwell Publishing Ltd

Treatment

Surgery is the treatment of choice for all mammary tumours, except in cases of inflammatory carcinoma or if distant metastasis is identified. The latter two conditions carry a grave prognosis. Local excision is the most appropriate surgery for small discrete masses (less than 1 cm in diameter). Such a surgery, essentially an excisional biopsy, is likely to be curative for benign lesions and, if appropriately planned, does not prevent future more aggressive surgery should the lesion be later diagnosed as malignant or incompletely excised. If the mass is larger than 1 cm, or exhibiting features of malignancy, a staging procedure is recommended before surgery. Also, excisional surgery should be planned as if the mass is known to be malignant.

Staging for suspected malignant masses includes haematology, serum biochemistry, fine needle aspiration of enlarged draining lymph nodes, thoracic radiographs (looking both for pulmonary metastasis and sternal lymphadenopathy) and abdominal ultrasound. The most common route of metastasis is via the lymphatics and common sites of distant metastasis are lung, sublumbar and sternal lymph nodes, and liver. Incisional biopsy should be performed if the mass is large, if multiple masses are present, or if features of malignancy are present. The information from the biopsies can then be used to aid planning of the most appropriate definitive surgery.

When a single mass greater than 1 cm is present, either partial or complete removal of a mammary gland is appropriate to achieve 2–3 cm margins. Multiple masses may dictate removal of additional glands. It may be less traumatic to remove glands in anatomical units (i.e. glands 4 and 5 together) than to perform multiple partial mastectomies. The superficial inguinal node should be removed en-bloc with gland 5. When there is cytological evidence of spread, if possible the axillary node should be removed with gland 1.

Complete removal of glands 1–5 is indicated if there are multiple tumours affecting multiple glands. This doesn't confer a survival advantage, but it is a less traumatic surgery than several mastectomies. Only in young dogs with multiple masses, and in whom future masses are likely, should removal of both mammary chains be considered as a staged prophylactic procedure. Ovariohysterectomy at the time of mammary mass removal is of questionable benefit and significantly increases the morbidity of the procedure.

If, during surgery, a mass is found to display infiltration or fixation to deeper muscular structures, it should not be removed by simple excision. An incisional biopsy should be performed and after closure, the patient should be referred for advanced imaging and, potentially, reconstructive surgery.

At present, neither radiotherapy nor chemotherapy are preferred treatment choices for mammary tumours. Execution of thorough, pre-surgical evaluation of the patient, and performance of an appropriate first surgery, is the most likely stratagem to achieve a successful outcome. Irrespective of the surgery performed, excised tissue must undergo histopathological evaluation to determine tumour type and margins of excision. In the vast majority of patients, total excision of either benign or low-grade malignant mammary masses when they are small will effect a complete cure.

What if it doesn't get better?

In the neutered bitch, over half of mammary tumours are benign adenomas and histological descriptions (simple, complex, ductular, papillary, fibroadenoma) have no bearing on prognosis. Conversely, for carcinomas, tumours described as simple are likely to be more aggressive than complex or non-infiltrating carcinomas. Sarcomas are more likely to metastasize but are less common than carcinomas. Inflammatory carcinomas have an exceptionally poor prognosis and there are no viable therapeutic options.

If a benign lesion has been fully excised, regular monitoring for de novo tumours is all that is warranted. Similarly, complete excision of a histologically low-grade, well-encapsulated carcinoma is likely to be curative. The median survival time for dogs following complete excision of histologically higher-grade malignant lesions, without evidence of vascular or lymphatic invasion is over a year. Incomplete excision of a benign or of a well-circumscribed malignant tumour dictates the need for further surgery (for example, removal of the entire gland if local excision was performed). Histological evidence of vascular or lymphatic invasion is suggestive of a poor prognosis, with a median survival of about 3 months. Regular re-evaluation is recommended and seeking the advice of a veterinary oncologist as to whether further surgery or adjuvant chemotherapy might be warranted, is also prudent.

The low-cost option

If surgical removal is not financially possible then close monitoring of the patient is essential. Some benign mammary masses can achieve a large size and may then become traumatised, whereas malignant masses may ulcerate. In both cases, wound management techniques are appropriate but these wounds are very unlikely to heal. Analgesia, palliative care and nutritional support are appropriate when managing any case of neoplasia, and are inexpensive.

When should I refer?

Referral should be considered when large, widespread or muscle-infiltrating masses necessitate radical surgery in which reconstructive techniques may be required. The advice of a referral surgeon will also be of benefit when planning a second surgery following an incomplete excision. If there is histological evidence of vascular or lymphatic invasion, or microscopic metastatic disease, an oncologist should be consulted, although chemotherapy is likely to be of limited benefit. Unlike in humans, hormonal therapies (e.g. tamoxifen) are unsuitable for canine patients.

Section 12

Mark Goodfellow

Aetiology and pathogenesis

Lymphomas are a diverse group of neoplasms arising from the cells of the lymphoreticular system. They are the most commonly diagnosed malignancy in the dog. The aetiology of lymphoma is unclear and although multiple factors (e.g. genetic predisposition, herbicide exposure, immunosuppression) have been implicated in its pathogenesis, no strong associations have been proven.

History and clinical signs

Around 80% of cases involve multiple peripheral lymph nodes (multicentric disease), with other sites (cranial mediastinal, gastrointestinal, cutaneous and primary extranodal sites such as eye, nervous system, bone, testis and nose) being less commonly affected. This chapter focuses on multicentric disease.

The majority of patients with multicentric disease are asymptomatic at presentation apart from a generalised peripheral lymphadenopathy. However, 20–40% of patients will present with one or more of the following clinical signs: anorexia, lethargy, weight loss, polydipsia and polyuria, pyrexia, dyspnoea, vomiting or diarrhoea. The presence of these clinical signs dramatically affects the prognosis. On clinical examination, hepatomegaly and/or splenomegaly, pallor, pleural or abdominal effusions, petechiation, or loss of body condition may be detected or suspected, and may indicate involvement of other body systems. On palpation, lymph nodes are typically painless, rubbery, non-fixed and may be dramatically enlarged. Not all peripheral lymph nodes are necessarily involved.

Other differential diagnoses for lymphadenopathy should be considered including systemic bacterial, viral or parasitic infections, immune-mediated disease (e.g. dermatopathies, polyarthritis, systemic lupus erythematosus), or other neoplasia (e.g. leukaemia, multiple myeloma, malignant or systemic histiocytosis or metastatic neoplastic disease).

Specific diagnostic techniques

The aim of the diagnostic evaluation is to confirm the clinical suspicion of disease and to determine the prognosis for a given patient. In the case of lymphoma, clinical stage, anatomical site and histological immunophenotype all affect treatment and prognosis.

Confirming the diagnosis

Lymphoma can often be diagnosed on cytological examination of a fine-needle aspirate from an affected lymph node. During a consultation, aspirates can be taken from any affected node, except the submandibular nodes (which tend to show confounding inflammatory changes due to dental disease, even in healthy dogs). Smearing the aspirated material as gently as possible will minimise rupturing of the fragile neoplastic lymphocytes. Lymph node biopsies are not usually required to confirm the diagnosis but allow the tumour to be immunophenotyped, which has an impact on prognosis.

Staging the disease

If the owner is considering treatment for lymphoma, full staging is recommended to help establish the prognosis and reduce complications associated with treatment. A thorough approach is required to determine which organs are affected by disease, any consequences for their function, and the presence of paraneoplastic syndromes and other co-morbidities. Minimum components of the staging procedure include complete haematology and evaluation of a blood smear, complete biochemical profile, urinalysis and thoracic radiography. A bone marrow aspirate is indicated in cases with haematological abnormalities.

Detection of any of the following adversely affects the prognosis:

* Manifestation of disease in the blood and involvement of the bone marrow
* A systemically unwell patient, often with a T-cell malignancy and often associated with humoral hypercalcaemia of malignancy (HHM)

100 Top Consultations in Small Animal General Practice, First Edition
By Peter Hill, Sheena Warman and Geoff Shawcross
© 2011 Blackwell Publishing Ltd

- T-cell immunophenotype (performed, on request, by most diagnostic pathology services)
- Cranial mediastinal lymphadenopathy
- Prolonged pre-treatment with steroids.

If HHM is detected, it should be treated aggressively with saline diuresis whilst awaiting cytological confirmation of diagnosis. On instigation of definitive therapy, HHM will usually resolve rapidly.

Treatment

If no treatment is given, most dogs will succumb to the disease within 4–6 weeks. However, treatment of this type of cancer is relatively rewarding as most cases will show a good response and achieve remission. Despite this, owners should be made aware that even with treatment, almost all dogs will die of their disease eventually, due to the development of chemotherapy resistance.

Lymphoma is a systemic disease and as such requires systemic treatment. A number of chemotherapeutic protocols are available and most involve initial treatment at a high intensity (induction) to achieve a response (Table 83.1). The choice of protocol is based on the patient's clinical condition and temperament, cost, time commitment, efficacy, toxicity and the experience of the clinician. Clinicians should consult more detailed texts if they wish to use these protocols to ensure they are sufficiently well informed. Alternatively, these patients can be referred to veterinary oncologists. Prior to starting treatment, clients must be educated about the precautions that must be taken in handling cytotoxic drugs and the patient's urine and faeces. This is par-ticularly important for pregnant women, small children, and immunosuppressed individuals, and in such households chemotherapy may not be an appropriate option.

The chemotherapy agents are given either PO or IV. If they are handled inappropriately there is a risk of toxicity to the patient, clinician and owner. Each drug has a unique toxicity spectrum but in general all cytotoxic drugs cause myelosuppression (manifested by neutropenia and thrombocytopenia), a slowing of hair growth (except in breeds with continually growing coats in which alopecia may occur) and gastrointestinal disturbances (ranging from anorexia to vomiting and/or diarrhoea). Cyclophosphamide can also cause a sterile haemorrhagic cystitis. Owners should be provided with anti-emetics such as maropitant to be given if signs of nausea appear. Any vomiting or diarrhoea should be treated aggressively as dehydration will increase the toxicity spectrum of the drugs. Many of the drugs administered IV are vesicants and use of an IV cannula placed aseptically is mandatory. Neutropenia is expected 5–7 days after administration of a myelosuppressive drug and so blood sampling for haematology and the confirmation of an adequate neutrophil count is essential prior to the administration of further myelosuppressive drugs. Typically, this is performed 24–48 hours prior to drug administration and thus necessitates an additional visit to the practice. A neutrophil count of less than 3×10^9/L should result in the withholding of myelosuppressive drugs and retesting in 72 hours.

Lymphadenopathy is expected to reduce within days of commencing treatment, along with associated clinical signs such as those attributable to HHM. In most cases, complete resolution of lymphadenopathy is expected (complete remission).

Table 83.1 Three commonly used chemotherapy protocols for the treatment of multicentric lymphoma. Clinicians should consult more detailed texts if they wish to administer these protocols so that they are familiar with doses, administration frequencies, and adverse effects and their management.

Protocol	Length of protocol (weeks)	No. visits to vet practice in a typical 3-week period	Potential for causing adverse effects	Dogs achieving remission (%)	Median remission time (months)	Median survival time (months)
'COP'[1]	continuous	3–6	Lowest	70–75	4–5	7
Doxorubicin alone	15	2	Medium	75–80	4–5	7
'CHOP'[2]	12–27	4–6	Highest	70–90	4–9	7–13

[1]COP: Cyclophosphamide (PO), Vincristine (IV), Prednisolone (PO).
[2]CHOP: Cyclophosphamide (PO), Doxorubicin (IV), Vincristine (IV), Prednisolone (PO); multiple variants.

What if it doesn't get better?

Recurrence of clinical signs (relapse) after a period of remission is indicative of developing multi-drug resistance and, if repeating the original induction protocol is unsuccessful, an alternative treatment protocol should be chosen which contains novel drugs (rescue protocols). Similarly, lack of response to chemotherapy initially, in the face of appropriate drug dose and administration, suggests resistance to the chosen protocol and alternatives should be considered.

The low-cost option

Prednisolone is a lymphotoxic drug and will kill neoplastic lymphocytes. Typically, a patient treated with prednisolone alone would be expected to achieve remission for a short period (1–2 months). However, owners should be cautioned that treatment with prednisolone alone will markedly reduce the efficacy of subsequent treatments should they change their mind and opt for chemotherapy.

When should I refer?

Referral is best considered when the clinician is unfamiliar with the drugs employed, the delivery techniques, and/or the prevention and management of adverse effects that may occur. Many referral centres schedule drug administration in partnership with practices, enabling veterinarians to use drugs they are already familiar with, whilst allowing administration and handling of the more toxic drugs in a referral situation where appropriate facilities and expertise exists. Referral is also appropriate when considering rescue therapy in dogs which have a relapse of their disease.

Section 13
Neurological problems

Sheena Warman

Seizures are the clinical manifestation of excessive or abnormal neuronal activity within the cerebral hemispheres. They can occur as a consequence of intracranial or extracranial disease. Idiopathic epilepsy is the most common cause of recurrent seizures in dogs. This is a functional disorder in which the seizure threshold is reduced. Some breeds are predisposed (e.g. German Shepherd dogs, Labrador Retrievers, Golden Retrievers, Collies).

Differential diagnoses

- Intracranial
  - Functional – idiopathic epilepsy
  - Structural – neoplasia (primary or secondary), inflammatory/infectious lesions, congenital abnormalities (e.g. hydrocephalus), trauma, haemorrhage, infarcts, metabolic storage diseases, scar tissue
- Extracranial
  - Toxins (e.g. metaldehyde, lead, organophosphates, ethylene glycol), hypoglycaemia, hypocalcaemia, heat stroke, hepatic encephalopathy, electrolyte abnormalities, hyperviscosity.

Seizures need to be differentiated from syncope, which is caused by reduced delivery of oxygen or glucose to the brain (due to e.g. hypotension, cardiac arrhythmia, hypoxaemia, or hypoglycaemia) or less common causes of paroxysmal signs such as myasthenia gravis, acute vestibular episodes, narcolepsy–cataplexy or movement disorders.

Diagnostic approach

The first stage of history taking is to ascertain if the patient is having a genuine seizure or another paroxysmal disorder. Owners use terms such as 'fit', 'seizure', 'convulsion' or 'funny turn' to describe any paroxysmal event. Asking the owner to carefully describe the dog's behaviour before, during and after the event should help establish the true nature of the

100 Top Consultations in Small Animal General Practice, First Edition
By Peter Hill, Sheena Warman and Geoff Shawcross
© 2011 Blackwell Publishing Ltd

episodes. Animals with syncope usually look 'floppy', whereas animals suffering seizures usually look 'stiff'.

With true seizures, the generalised tonic–clonic form is most common, characterised by bilaterally symmetric movement of the limbs, jaw and face, loss of consciousness, and often autonomic signs such as salivation, urination and/or defecation. Less commonly, dogs exhibit focal partial motor seizures, arising from one side of the cerebral hemisphere, with asymmetric signs such as turning of the head or muscle twitching. Occasionally focal seizures manifest as episodic altered consciousness or bizarre behaviour (e.g. fly-catching). Partial seizures can progress to generalised seizures.

Seizures can occur as isolated events, as clusters (>1 seizure in 24 hours), or develop into status epilepticus (continuous seizure activity lasting >5 minutes). Some dogs exhibit a 'prodromal phase' for hours or days prior to a seizure, with unusual behaviour such as attention seeking. The seizure itself ('ictus') can last for seconds to minutes. The post-ictal period can last for several hours, with dogs sometimes showing altered behaviours, disorientation, or increased thirst or appetite.

Once it is established that the dog is having seizures, further questioning is aimed at identifying the likely underlying cause. Information should be sought regarding age of onset, duration and frequency of seizures, description of the seizure and the post-ictal period, any abnormalities during the inter-ictal period, and any knowledge of seizures in related dogs. In cases with an acute history, any possible access to toxins should be established. The owner should be asked if the dog has suffered any previous head trauma. The general health of the dog should also be discussed, as this may help point towards extra-cranial causes. A full physical examination should be performed to investigate any concurrent or underlying diseases.

Dogs with idiopathic epilepsy usually have their first seizure between 6 months and 5 years of age. The seizure is usually tonic–clonic in nature, lasts 1–2 minutes and most commonly happens when the animal is at rest. Epileptic dogs should be normal between seizures, with the interval between initial seizures at least 4–6 weeks, although cluster seizures may occur early in some breeds such as Border Collies and Dalmatians.

Patients that don't meet these criteria are more likely to be suffering from extracranial disease or structural intracranial disease. Young dogs are most likely to have a congenital abnormality while older dogs are more likely to have a tumour, vascular abnormality or extra-cranial disease. Dogs with extracranial disease are likely to have additional clinical signs. Dogs with structural intracranial disease may have persistent neurologic abnormalities between seizures, associated with forebrain disease, e.g. circling, hemiparesis, or altered behaviour, although they are not always present. Primary tumours which have metastasised to the brain (e.g. mammary or prostatic tumours) may be apparent. Inflammatory diseases are often rapidly progressive.

It is essential that a full neurological examination is performed in patients with seizures. In the immediate post-ictal period there may be some temporary neurologic abnormalities such as blindness or proprioceptive deficits; if this is the case then neurologic examination should be repeated several days later. If these abnormalities persist a structural intracranial lesion should be suspected, but a normal neurologic examination does not exclude extra-cranial or structural intra-cranial disease. Fundic examination may allow detection of papilloedema associated with raised intracranial pressure, or retinal lesions associated with inflammatory conditions.

All patients with a history of seizures should have full haematology and biochemistry performed to rule out many of the extra-cranial causes of seizures. It is important to include dynamic bile acids as occasionally seizures are the only presenting sign in patients with hepatic dysfunction such as porto-systemic shunts.

Further investigations depend on the patient. Once extra-cranial causes have been excluded, further investigation of intra-cranial disease requires advanced imaging (MRI or CT), and possibly CSF fluid analysis (Figure 84.1). This is not usually necessary in dogs with classic signs of idiopathic epilepsy, although some owners will be keen to rule out structural diseases. Owners should be encouraged to pursue advanced imaging in dogs whose first seizure occurs at less than 6 months or more than 5 years of age, or those with persistent neurological abnormalities between seizures, in which extra-cranial causes have been excluded.

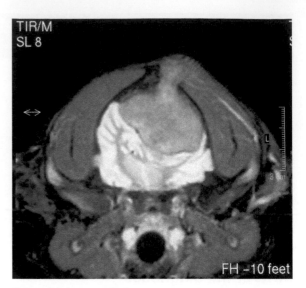

Figure 84.1   An MRI from a young dog that presented with seizures. A large tumour, originating from the skull, is compressing the brain

Treatment

Idiopathic epilepsy

Treatment of idiopathic epilepsy is life-long and requires significant financial and personal commitment from the owner. There are various websites and groups which offer support to owners of epileptic dogs. Owners should be encouraged to keep a 'seizure diary' to help monitor any changes in the dog's condition. When a seizure occurs in the home, the owners should be encouraged to remain calm and quiet, move any furniture that is likely to result in the dog injuring itself, and try to note the duration of the seizure. They should not try to restrain the dog in any way, and children should not be allowed near the dog until its demeanour has returned to normal. Most seizures will stop spontaneously within a minute or two, although the post-ictal phase may last a few hours. Owners are often reassured if it is explained to them that epileptic seizures usually happen at rest, and that they are unlikely to have to deal with a seizuring dog whilst out on a walk.

The aim of treatment of idiopathic epilepsy is to reduce seizure frequency to an acceptable level; it is unrealistic to expect to prevent seizures completely.

Good seizure control can be achieved in 70–80% of dogs. Anticonvulsant therapy should be started if seizures are occurring more than every 3–4 months, have increased in frequency or severity, or if there have been any episodes of cluster seizures or status epilepticus.

The first-choice anticonvulsant therapy in most cases is phenobarbitone. Treatment is started at 2–3 mg/kg twice daily. The owner should be warned that side-effects of PUPD, polyphagia, ataxia and sedation are common, particularly in the first week or so. PUPD and polyphagia may persist, and owners should be warned not to overfeed their pet. Pre-pill (trough) serum phenobarbitone concentrations should be measured after 2–3 weeks, and the dose increased until the drug level is within the therapeutic range (25–35 μg/ml or 107–150 μmol/L in dogs). Once seizure control is acceptable, the dog should be reassessed every 6 months. Phenobarbitone levels, haematology and biochemistry should be monitored. Hepatic enzyme induction (with moderate elevations in ALT and ALKP) is an expected consequence of phenobarbitone therapy, and is not clinically significant. Since hepatotoxicity is an occasional complication of phenobarbitone therapy (particularly at higher therapeutic levels), it is important to monitor liver function specifically with albumin and dynamic bile acids. Phenobarbitone has also been associated with immune-mediated blood dyscrasias. If therapy needs to be discontinued this must be done very gradually to reduce the risk of 'rebound' seizures.

If seizure control remains unacceptable even with levels at the high end of the therapeutic range, then additional drug therapy is likely to be necessary. In most cases potassium bromide is added to treatment. Bromide can also be used as a single agent in dogs with hepatic dysfunction. It should not be given to cats. Bromide has a long half-life and steady state serum concentrations may not be reached for 3–4 months. The initial dose is 20–40 mg/kg daily, given in divided doses with food, although loading doses of 200 mg/kg once daily for 5 days can be used if blood levels need to be raised rapidly. Dietary salt increases renal excretion of bromide so it is important that the diet is kept constant. Target therapeutic concentrations are 1–2 mg/ml (10–20 mmol/L) when used as add-on therapy, and should be measured 4 weeks after starting therapy, 2–3 months later when steady state levels are reached, and then annually. Side-effects include PUPD, polyphagia and pancreatitis. Ataxia and sedation are expected if loading doses are used.

In patients which are prone to cluster seizures, owners can be taught to administer rectal diazepam (0.5–1.0 mg/kg per rectum; up to three doses in 24 hours) when they notice pro-dromal signs, or after the first seizure. This should reduce the risk of further seizures or status epilepticus.

Other causes of seizures

Dogs with extra-cranial or structural intra-cranial disease require specific treatment. Dogs with intra-cranial disease should also receive anti-convulsant therapy as outlined above.

Status epilepticus

Patients presenting in status epilepticus represent a genuine emergency. Attempts should be made to determine the cause of the seizure, and to treat conditions such as hypoglycaemia, hypocalcaemia, or hepatic encephalopathy, if appropriate. Anticonvulsant therapy should be administered to stop seizure activity. Initially, diazepam should be administered (0.5–1.0 mg/kg IV or rectally), and this can be repeated up to four times if necessary until the seizure is controlled. If there is no response, IV propofol is usually effective. In patients not already on treatment with phenobarbitone, a loading dose of phenobarbitone can then be given 12 mg/kg IV then, if required, two further doses of 3 mg/kg IV at 20 minute intervals, to a maximum total dose of 18 mg/kg. If the dog is already receiving oral phenobarbitone therapy, a single 2–4 mg/kg IV or IM dose may result in an effective increase in serum levels. If seizure activity persists, constant-rate infusions of diazepam and/or propofol may be required. Supportive therapy should be provided, with oxygen and fluid therapy. A patent airway must be maintained. Attention should be paid to body temperature; hyperthermia of >41.5°C requires specific cooling measures (e.g. cool water enemas, application of wet towels, fans).

What if it doesn't get better?

About 20% of dogs with idiopathic epilepsy do not achieve adequate seizure control with standard therapy. Alternative add-on drugs are available but specialist advice should be sought prior to their use. It is also important to ensure that underlying causes have been fully investigated.

The low-cost option

The drugs used for management of idiopathic epilepsy are relatively inexpensive. However, lifelong treatment will be required and, with the need for frequent veterinary examinations and blood tests, significant costs will be incurred. Some owners are unable to cope with the financial and personal demands of living with an epileptic dog, and may elect for euthanasia early in the course of the disease.

Advanced imaging is necessary for confirmation or exclusion of structural intra-cranial disease. However, if the dog is considered likely to have idiopathic epilepsy then it is reasonable to proceed with treatment without definitively ruling out structural lesions. Equally, if a patient is considered likely to have structural disease but financial limitations preclude further investigation or specific treatment, then it is reasonable to provide anticonvulsant therapy for as long as quality of life remains acceptable.

When should I refer?

Referral may be necessary for advanced imaging to be performed in patients which are considered likely to have structural intra-cranial disease, or if owners of a dog likely to have idiopathic epilepsy are keen to exclude other possibilities. Referral is likely to be necessary if owners are keen to treat identified intracranial disease. For example treatment of brain tumours with surgery and/or radiation therapy can be very rewarding. Some extra-cranial causes of seizures may require referral for diagnosis and/or treatment, e.g. portosystemic shunts. It may also be necessary to refer epileptic dogs that do not respond to standard therapy, as the input of a specialist can be invaluable in these cases, both in tailoring treatment protocols and managing owner expectations.

Martin Owen

Hindlimb ataxia is the loss of the ability to coordinate normal muscular movement and occurs when proprioceptive function, motor function and/or neuromuscular function is abnormal. In dogs and cats, hindlimb ataxia is often due to compromise of neuronal structures affecting the sensory and motor pathways. Whilst ataxia is typically a neurological or neuromuscular problem, signs of weakness and apparent ataxia may occur in animals with a loss of muscle strength secondary to disuse atrophy due to chronic hindlimb discomfort. Ataxia (usually without weakness) can also occur with vestibular and cerebellar diseases. Hindlimb or generalised weakness can also occur as a result of severe systemic disease, cardiovascular disease or metabolic disorders such as hypoglycaemia or anaemia.

Common differential diagnoses

Spinal cord compromise

- Compression – intervertebral disc herniation (see Chapter 52), tumour, cyst, cervical spondylopathy
- Contusion
- Degeneration – canine degenerative radiculomyelopathy (CDRM)
- Inflammatory – meningitis, granulomatous meningoencephalitis (GME)
- Vascular – fibrocartilaginous embolus (FCE)/ ischaemic myelopathy

Lower motor neuron compromise

- Lumbosacral disease
- Neuromuscular disease
- Peripheral neuropathy
- Myopathy
- Myasthenia gravis (intermittent clinical signs)

Orthopaedic disease

- Bilateral hip osteoarthritis
- Bilateral cruciate disease
- Pelvic fracture

100 Top Consultations in Small Animal General Practice, First Edition
By Peter Hill, Sheena Warman and Geoff Shawcross
© 2011 Blackwell Publishing Ltd

Diagnostic approach

Consideration should be given to the age and breed of the patient since several of the differential diagnoses are over represented in certain breeds and ages (e.g. intervertebral disc disease in Dachshunds). A detailed history should be obtained from the owner because clinical signs referable to other body systems may be relevant in refining the differential diagnoses. It is important to establish the onset, duration and severity of the problem and the nature of its progression. For example, intervertebral disc extrusion, spinal contusion, ischaemic myelopathy and meningitis can lead to acute signs whereas intervertebral disc protrusions, degenerative myelopathy and lumbosacral disease tend to have a more gradual onset. Neuromuscular disease, peripheral neuropathy, myopathies and myasthenia gravis may present with acute or progressive onset of signs.

A full clinical examination of all the body systems should be performed prior to completing an assessment of the patient's locomotor and neurological function. It is helpful to observe the patient moving in a controlled manner, observing the gait closely for evidence of lameness or uncoordinated movement. A systematic orthopaedic examination should be performed followed by a structured neurological exam, starting with postural and proprioceptive tests to characterise fully the limbs affected and the severity of the ataxia/weakness.

The 'paw position' test should be performed on each hindfoot separately. The paw should be gently lifted and then flexed prior to being placed gently onto the floor, with the dorsum of the paw contacting the floor. A normal response results in the dog/cat almost instantly repositioning the paw into a normal resting position. Failure to reposition the paw properly, multiple imperfect attempts to reposition the paw or delayed repositioning all indicate proprioceptive deficits.

If any doubt remains regarding the presence/ absence of neurological dysfunction, the 'reflex-stepping' test should be performed. A smooth, non-grip floor is required for this test. Each hindlimb is tested separately. The paw is gently lifted and placed onto a piece of paper, with the limb in a normal standing position. The paper is steadily and slowly withdrawn laterally, forcing the tested hindlimb to abduct passively. In a normal response, the dog/cat lifts and replaces the hindlimb into a normal standing position almost instantly. Animals with proprioceptive deficits are slow to replace their limb, or when there are marked deficits, the limb may become markedly displaced, with the animal almost collapsing.

'Hopping' is a third test for proprioceptive deficits. The hindlimb tested remains in a normal standing position whilst the contralateral hind paw is elevated and pushed towards the midline, displacing the centre of gravity of the hindquarters, causing the standing pelvic limb to overbalance. To remain balanced, the dog/cat must 'hop' away from the clinician. A normal response results in several small hops that keep the dog/cat carefully balanced on the standing pelvic limb. Proprioceptive deficits result in delayed hops, each with a large displacement of the standing limb, or no hops, in which case the dog/cat overbalances.

The vertebral column should then be tested for painful lesions. The physical examination findings should give a suspicion of the localisation of disease causing the ataxia/weakness (see Table 85.1). Upper motor neuron (UMN) lesions cause weakness/paralysis, with normal to increased muscle tone, intact (although sometimes enhanced) local reflexes and minimal muscle atrophy. Lower motor neuron (LMN) lesions cause weakness/paralysis with absent or reduced muscle tone and reduced/absent local reflexes, and with muscle atrophy which can be severe. An appropriate radiological examination is a sensible initial investigation, since some features are useful indicators of disease. For example:

- Narrowed or mineralised intervertebral disc space, indicative of intervertebral disc herniation
- Irregular disc space, indicative of discospondylitis
- Bone destruction or proliferation, indicative of neoplastic lesion
- Fracture or vertebral displacement, indicative of spinal trauma.

Routine haematological analysis and serum biochemistry testing is helpful to look for disease in other body systems.

Table 85.1 Neurolocalisation of causes of hindlimb ataxia and weakness.

Lesion location	Forelimbs	Hindlimbs
Brain	UMN	UMN
C1–C5	UMN	UMN
C6–T2	LMN	UMN
T3–L3	Normal	UMN
L4–S2	Normal	LMN
S1–S3	Normal	Partial LMN (+ absent perineal reflex and atonic bladder)
Generalised peripheral neuropathy	LMN	LMN

UPN = upper motor neuron signs; LMN = lower motor neuron signs.

Treatment

The findings of the diagnostic investigations detailed above will dictate the most appropriate course of action for initial management. If the patient is painful, control of pain takes priority over other clinical considerations. Effective analgesia should be provided using NSAIDs where appropriate, and using a multimodal approach when indicated. Strict restriction of activity should be enforced if the differential diagnoses include diseases worsened by activity (e.g. intervertebral disc disease). Unfortunately, few of the conditions causing hindlimb ataxia/weakness can be diagnosed with certainty using the investigative facilities of first opinion practice. Hence, if a definitive diagnosis is not reached considering the patient's signalment and the findings of radiological examinations and blood tests, specialist advice should be sought.

What if it doesn't get better?

Ataxia indicates a mild compromise of neurological and/or neuromuscular function and can be the initial presenting sign of serious disease that has the potential for irreversible disruption of neurological/neuromuscular integrity and complete loss of hindlimb function. Consequently, following initial investigation and diagnosis, the patient's neurological function should be closely monitored to ensure that the clinical response to treatment is satisfactory and in accordance with what is expected based on the diagnosis made. Patients that do not respond to treatment as expected should be re-examined, the findings of diagnostic investigations should be checked and specialist advice should be sought so that further investigation and, if necessary, specialist intervention can be offered before there is significant irreversible medical deterioration. An accurate diagnosis is critical in all cases that do not respond to initial treatment since serious, non-recoverable disease is relatively common in cases of hindlimb weakness. Where there is a certain diagnosis of a condition that is expected to deteriorate (e.g. CDRM), only supportive treatment and counselling may be offered.

and routine blood tests) should be performed to check for signs that support the presumptive diagnosis and for signs giving confounding evidence of unexpected disease. Some diseases causing hindlimb ataxia do not require, or do not benefit from, costly surgical intervention (e.g. CDRM, ischaemic myelopathy, mild spinal trauma) and often the progression of these diseases is reliably predictable. For example:

- Cases of CDRM always steadily and progressively deteriorate
- Dogs with mild ischaemic myelopathic lesions usually regain ambulatory function
- Dogs with mild signs of spinal trauma generally recover normal function
- Limbs without deep pain sensation often do not recover.

Consequently, if the clinical findings support such a presumptive diagnosis, the patient can be managed conservatively (with restricted activity and analgesia, as appropriate) carefully monitoring the disease recovery/progression. Any departure from the expected recovery/progression is an indication for re-evaluation and further investigation.

The low-cost option

For a small proportion of cases of hindlimb ataxia, a presumptive diagnosis can be made with a reasonable level of accuracy based on signalment, and a pathognomonic history with classical clinical signs. For example, pelvic limb weakness in association with signs of back pain in a chondrodystrophic breed is most often due to intervertebral disc herniation; sudden onset pelvic limb ataxia that occurs at exercise, without trauma, in a non-chondrodystrophoid dog is highly suggestive of an ischaemic myelopathic event. In such cases, a limited investigation (radiology

When should I refer?

Specialist advice or referral should be sought if a diagnosis is not clear following initial investigations. Frequent checks on clinical progress should be made to establish that the clinical progression meets expectations, especially when only a presumptive diagnosis has been made, or the case is being treated conservatively. If at any stage, there is departure from the anticipated clinical recovery/progression, referral should be sought promptly in order to maximise the opportunity to successfully treat the problem. For information regarding referral of cases with suspected disc disease, see Chapter 52.

Section 13

Sheena Warman

Aetiology and pathogenesis

The vestibular system is responsible for control of balance and the position of the head and eyes. Abnormalities causing clinical signs can occur in either the peripheral nervous system (vestibular labyrinth and vestibular portion of cranial nerve VIII) or central nervous system (vestibular nuclei in the medulla oblongata and the flocculonodular lobe of the cerebellum). Clinical signs of vestibular disease are a relatively common presentation in dogs, and are also seen in cats.

The most common cause of peripheral vestibular disease (PVD) is idiopathic, but it can also be caused by otitis interna, head trauma, neoplasia, polyps, aggressive ear cleaning or aminoglycoside toxicity. Hypothyroidism has been reported as a possible cause, but a true cause and effect relationship has yet to be established. It has been reported as a congenital disease in some breeds (e.g. German Shepherds, Doberman Pinschers, English Cocker Spaniels, Siamese and Burmese cats). Central vestibular disease (CVD) is much less common but can be caused by meningoencephalitis, neoplasia, head trauma, thiamine deficiency, cerebrovascular disorders or metronidazole toxicity.

History and clinical signs

It is important to question the owner regarding the speed of onset, duration and progression of signs, any history of ear disease or medication, any recent drug administration, and any possible history of trauma.

The clinical signs of vestibular disease are usually quite dramatic and typified by head tilt (Figure 86.1), nystagmus and ataxia (circling, rolling or falling). Vomiting may be a feature in acute disease. Differentiating between peripheral and central disease helps guide investigation and treatment and can usually be done following a thorough neurological examination (see Table 86.1). Certain clinical signs (particularly positional vertical nystagmus and hemiparesis) are indicative of CVD; however if these are not present a central lesion cannot be excluded.

Idiopathic vestibular syndrome is common in geriatric dogs and young cats, although it can be seen in any age of pet. The clinical signs can be dramatic and distressing to both pet and owners. There will be no evidence of facial nerve paralysis or Horner's syndrome.

Otitis interna is a less common cause of peripheral vestibular disease, as a consequence of infection from the external ear canals or via the Eustachian tube. Associated otitis media may lead to Horner's syndrome and facial nerve paralysis.

Rarely, vestibular disease is bilateral (e.g. bilateral otitis media/interna, occasionally with idiopathic disease). In these cases head tilt may be absent but the animal has a wide, swinging head movement from side to side, and may fall, roll or circle to either side. There may be loss of normal physiologic nystagmus.

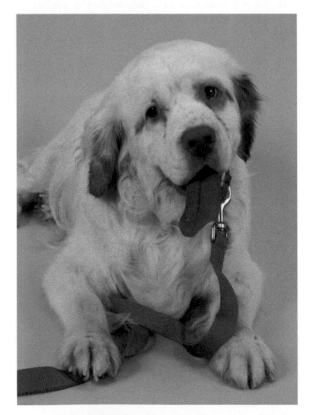

Figure 86.1 **A Clumber Spaniel with a severe head tilt**

100 Top Consultations in Small Animal General Practice, First Edition
By Peter Hill, Sheena Warman and Geoff Shawcross
© 2011 Blackwell Publishing Ltd

Table 86.1 Differentiating between peripheral and central vestibular disease.

Sign	Peripheral disease	Central disease
Head tilt	Towards side of lesion ('tilt to the trouble')	Usually towards side of lesion
Ataxia (circling, rolling or falling)	Towards side of lesion	Present
Nystagmus (not always present)	Horizontal or rotatory, fast phase away from side of lesion	Horizontal, rotatory, vertical or positional
Other signs that may be seen	Facial nerve paralysis (cranial nerve VII) Horner's syndrome (miosis, ptosis and enophthalmos)	Depression/stupor Deficits in conscious proprioception (on side of lesion) Hemiparesis (on side of lesion) Deficits in cranial nerves (other than VII)

In some cases of CVD there is involvement of the flocculonodular node of the cerebellum. In these cases the circling and head tilt can be away from the side of the lesion ('paradoxical' vestibular signs), but any weakness and proprioceptive deficits are ipsilateral to the lesion. Ipsilateral limb hypermetria may also be noted.

Specific diagnostic techniques

In addition to a full physical examination, animals with vestibular signs should receive a detailed otoscopic examination and a full neurological examination, to differentiate between central and peripheral disease and to assess for any evidence of multifocal disease (e.g. some cases of granulomatous meningoencephalitis).

Normal physiologic nystagmus is induced in patients by moving the head from side to side, with the fast phase of eye movement being towards the direction of head movement. Spontaneous nystagmus is abnormal. Subtle nystagmus is sometimes more easy to detect using an ophthalmoscope to look at the retina. A vertical or positional nystagmus indicates CVD. Positional nystagmus is most reliably detected by placing the pet in dorsal recumbency. Conscious proprioception is tested by carefully 'knuckling' each paw whilst supporting the weight of the pet with the other hand. Normal animals will place the paw back in the normal position almost immediately.

The ears should be examined otoscopically for evidence of otitis externa or otitis media (bulging or ruptured tympanic membrane) which could have spread to the inner ear. Evidence of facial nerve paralysis (facial asymmetry, loss of blink, inability to move facial muscles) or Horner's syndrome (ptosis, miosis, enophthalmos and protrusion of the third eyelid) should be assessed. In geriatric patients with signs of PVD and no obvious evidence of otitis it is reasonable to treat supportively for idiopathic vestibular disease for 72 hours. Further investigations should be performed if there is no improvement, or in cats or younger dogs presenting with PVD. A more complete examination of the ear canals and tympanic bullae is required in such cases. Under general anaesthesia, a thorough otoscopic examination should be performed, and the pharynx carefully examined for tumours or polyps. It is important to note that a normal external ear canal does not rule out the possibility of otitis interna, and equally, the presence of otitis externa does not necessarily mean that the vestibular signs are caused by otitis interna. Radiography of the tympanic bullae may demonstrate increased fluid density or osteomyelitis consistent with otitis media. If there is evidence of otitis media, myringotomy can be performed to obtain a fluid sample for cytology and bacterial culture and sensitivity. MRI is the most sensitive technique for detecting otitis media/interna. It will also demonstrate the presence of tumours or polyps, and identify any central lesions.

Haematology and serum biochemistry can be useful to provide evidence of systemic disease. In dogs with additional evidence of hypothyroidism, specific endocrine testing is indicated (see Chapter 73), although it is not clear whether there is a true cause-and-effect relationship between vestibular signs and hypothyroidism.

Further investigation of central vestibular disease usually requires advanced imaging (CT or MRI) and, in cases of suspected meningoencephalitis, CSF analysis. Survey radiographs of the thorax and abdomen, and abdominal ultrasound, can be useful to detect systemic diseases such as neoplasia, which may have resulted in metastases to the central nervous system.

Treatment

Treatment of idiopathic vestibular disease is supportive, with most cases showing a dramatic improvement within 72 hours. Nystagmus usually resolves within the first few days, with other clinical signs improving within seven days, although a mild head tilt may persist. The clinical signs can be very dramatic and upsetting to the owner, so it is important to emphasise that the prognosis in most cases is good. Many owners are worried that their pet has had a 'stroke', resulting in an unnecessarily pessimistic view of the likely prognosis. Some owners may request that their pet be hospitalised until some improvement is seen. Chlorpromazine or maropitant can be useful to treat any associated vomiting, and some animals benefit from mild sedation with a benzodiazepine such as diazepam or an antihistamine such as diphenhydramine. Owners should be warned that the dog may be prone to recurrent episodes, often a year or so later.

Effective treatment of otitis interna requires a prolonged course (4–6 weeks) of an appropriate antibiotic. If otitis media is also present the choice of antibiotic should be determined following culture and sensitivity testing of fluid obtained by myringotomy. If this is not possible, cefalexin would usually be an appropriate empirical choice. It is essential that the treatment course is completed even if clinical signs resolve rapidly, as chronic or recurring infections become progressively more difficult to treat. For this reason, it is advised not to routinely give short courses of antibiotics to patients with vestibular disease 'in case' otitis interna is present. For further information regarding the treatment of concurrent otitis media/externa see Chapter 24.

Treatment of other causes of vestibular disease is tailored according to the diagnosis.

What if it doesn't get better?

If there is no improvement within 72 hours or if signs recur or relapse, then further investigations should be outlined as indicated above. In patients with signs of PVD, it may be that there is an underlying cause such as otitis interna or polyp, or possibly CVD without specific clinical signs. Patients with otitis media/interna may have residual facial nerve paralysis/Horner's syndrome but usually learn to compensate well.

The low-cost option

Patients with idiopathic vestibular syndrome can often be managed as outpatients, incurring minimal expense. Some patients with otitis interna may respond to less expensive antibiotics such as potentiated sulphonamides. Further investigation of CVD requires advanced imaging which incurs significant expense, and most of the causes of CVD represent serious disease. If MRI or CT is not an option for a patient with CVD, it is sensible to allow a few days on symptomatic treatment in case the pet improves (e.g. cerebrovascular accident), but euthanasia may be necessary.

When should I refer?

The main indication for referral of patients with vestibular disease is for advanced imaging to be performed. Although a diagnosis of otitis media/interna can often be made following otoscopy and radiography, MRI and CT are more sensitive techniques and some owners may prefer early referral for this to be performed. MRI or CT is also indicated for further investigation of CVD. Referral is also advised for the treatment of middle-ear infections in which video-otoscopy is indicated to facilitate flushing of the tympanic bullae.

Section 14
Behavioural problems

Jon Bowen

Aggressive behaviour is a normal element of canine communication. Aggression may be normal or abnormal. Normal aggression is highly ritualised, so that each posture and vocalisation has a specific meaning. Signals increase in intensity to convey increasing threat and a greater probability of physical injury, beginning with growling and moving through snarling, snapping and on to biting. These aggressive signals are accompanied by body postures that show the confidence of the animal. A low, hunched posture indicates fear and uncertainty, and an erect posture generally indicates confidence and confrontation.

Prior to becoming aggressive, dogs will usually show signs that they are stressed, anxious, fearful or in emotional conflict. These include lip-licking, yawning, paw lifting, curling the tail under the body, indirect eye contact and a low or hunched body posture. In general, bites only occur after all of these signals have been ignored and the dog remains under pressure. Even then, aggression is usually well controlled, involving a single bite and then withdrawal. Signalling will be curtailed if the dog has learned, through previous encounters, that its signals are generally ignored and therefore purposeless.

In dogs with physical or emotional abnormalities this ritualised pattern may not be followed. Aggression may occur with little or no warning or provocation, and involve a sustained attack with multiple bites. These dogs present a greater danger.

Risk assessment

Before treating a dog that has shown aggression, a risk assessment should be carried out.

Important factors include:

- Signalling – Dogs that launch into an attack without warning (growling, etc.) are much more dangerous than those which bite only after a full sequence of communication. Lack of signalling and rapid escalation to biting can be indications of an impulse control problem

- Bite type – Dogs that inflict multiple bites during an attack, or which hold on after biting, are more dangerous
- Bite severity
- Target – If the dog specifically targets children or elderly people the risk of serious injury is higher
- Predictability – Management relies on the dog's behaviour being predictable, i.e. it must be possible to anticipate and control situations when the dog might pose a risk
- Group behaviour – Risk is greatly increased in multi-dog households where the dogs have a history of attacking as a group
- Redirection – When frustrated or threatened, some dogs will redirect their aggression from the main target of the behaviour (such as another dog) to another nearby dog or person. This can result from the use of punishment to suppress behaviour in a fearful dog, and can make management and treatment hazardous
- Owner responsibility – The dog should not be treated if the owner cannot be relied upon to follow basic management advice such as muzzling.

If the animal poses an unacceptable risk, euthanasia should be advised.

Common differential diagnoses

The main behavioural differentials for aggression are predatory behaviour and play behaviour:

- Predatory behaviour is uncommon, usually targeted at other pets, rarely targeted at people, and involves no signalling to the target (no growling, barking, etc)
- Play behaviour is very common and frequently confused with aggression, especially in young dogs playing with children. It involves specific play communication.

Play can appear highly aggressive, cause injuries, and be superficially difficult to differentiate from real aggression. However, during play, dogs will intersperse their playful aggression with 'metacommunication' signals that reassure the other individual that no threat is intended. These include play-bows, a generally loose body posture and a 'play face' in which the teeth are mostly shielded by the lips and the mouth is open.

100 Top Consultations in Small Animal General Practice, First Edition
By Peter Hill, Sheena Warman and Geoff Shawcross
© 2011 Blackwell Publishing Ltd

Diagnostic approach

Pain, illness and debilitation tend to increase defensiveness and irritability in all species. It should be assumed that any mature adult dog that shows an abrupt or uncharacteristic change in personality or behaviour may be unwell.

Behavioural history-taking can be very lengthy for aggression cases, but for the purposes of a short consultation can be cut down to information about:

- The target of the aggression: species, age, sex, appearance, relationship to the dog (known, unfamiliar), and what they did before, during and after the incident(s)
- Posture and communication: vocalisation, behaviour and body posture before, during and after the incident(s)
- The situation in which the incident(s) occurred: in the home, outside, presence of stressors (such as noise)
- Whether the dog has other known fears or phobias that may be relevant to the incident(s).

This information is used to place the problem within one of the main classes of aggression:

- Fear related: Where the target is an unfamiliar individual, the dog's posture and behaviour are typical of fear
- Territorial: The target is an unfamiliar individual entering, or within, the dog's territory. The posture is erect. The dog may behave normally outside this context
- Possessive: Food or object guarding. The dog may show fearful or confident body posture
- Redirected: Occurs when the dog becomes frustrated or is punished whilst displaying aggression. The aggression is then redirected onto a third party such as the owner. This can greatly increase the risk associated with the treatment of inter-dog or territorial aggression
- Maternal: Can occur in bitches with puppies, or with false pregnancy
- Inter-male canine aggression
- Owner/family directed aggression. The target is a familiar person. Signalling may be fearful, confident or may change during incidents and over time.

Dominance aggression is considered a redundant term, as owner/family directed aggression usually involves ambivalent rather than dominant body posturing and analysis of case histories always reveals fear, anxiety or emotional conflict as an underlying cause. In cases where aggression is owner directed, the dog's posture and behaviour during the incident will indicate its emotional motivation.

Initial management

Circumstances that might lead to aggression should be identified and avoided. The dog should be trained to wear a muzzle, to provide additional safety. Dogs that represent an unacceptable risk should be euthanised.

Underlying medical factors should be treated before treating other causes of the aggression. Specific treatment depends on the reason for aggression. In the majority of cases, referral to a specialist veterinary behaviourist is likely to be required to obtain meaningful results, as the recommendations required cannot be discussed within a routine veterinary consultation. However, some measures that can help in dealing with the various forms of aggression are:

- A dog with territorial aggression should not meet visitors without supervision by an adult able to control it
- Possessive dogs should be fed in an area where they are undisturbed, and objects that the dog may guard should be kept out of its reach
- Dogs with aggression resulting from false pregnancy should be treated with cabergoline (Galastop, CEVA Animal Health)
- Fear-related aggression can be treated using desensitisation and counter-conditioning methods
- Dogs that show owner-directed aggression should not be challenged and may require extensive specialist behavioural modification.

There is currently no evidence that neutering is generally beneficial in cases of aggression, and it should not be recommended as a primary method of treatment. The precise cause or motivation for the behaviour should be assessed first.

Drugs such as selegiline and fluoxetine may be used to reduce fear or anxiety, if these are underlying emotional motivations for aggression. Selective serotonin reuptake inhibitor drugs, such as fluoxetine, can also be used to reduce impulsiveness in dogs that show a lack of signalling, or a rapid escalation of aggressive behaviour. However, the same drugs can produce increased confidence and disinhibition which can make the dog's behaviour more dangerous. Since no drug is licensed for the treatment of aggression, caution is advised.

The low-cost option

Aggressive dogs can often be managed by avoiding the situations that incite aggression and using sensible precautions such as muzzling. However, specific treatment requires additional expertise and may therefore be lengthy and expensive.

What if it doesn't get better?

A dog that has a history of aggressive behaviour can, in law, be considered to have a propensity for this behaviour. If such a dog is allowed to cause, or threaten to cause, injury then the owner may be held to be strictly liable for the dog's actions and there is the prospect of criminal prosecution. A dog that has been aggressive cannot therefore be regarded as 'safe' or 'cured'; the owner will always need to behave responsibly in order to manage the dog safely. However, very significant improvements are seen in many cases of aggression, and properly assessed, successfully managed dogs need not represent a danger.

If a case does not improve or there are concerns over safety, then referral is advised.

Euthanasia should be considered if the dog's pattern of behaviour becomes more risky or unpredictable.

When should I refer?

Altering the behaviour of an aggressive dog requires specific and precise recommendations. As it is often impossible to deal adequately with these issues during routine veterinary consultations, a referral to a veterinary behaviourist is generally recommended. Specific indications for referral would include cases in which:

- The target of the aggression is vulnerable (an elderly person or young child)
- Injuries from bites have been severe
- The pattern of aggression is unpredictable or confusing
- The case may involve legal action
- There is owner-directed aggression and a risk of injury.

Jon Bowen

Fear is the emotional basis for many, if not most, behavioural problems. Typical signs of fear are:

- Fixed attention on the fearful stimulus
- Low body posture
- Barking/growling
- Attempts to escape
- Trembling, panting.

The level of fear relates to the level of threat and tends to decrease with repeated experience; the animal will become less fearful if the stimulus turns out not to be hazardous. Commonly occurring fears are of people, other dogs, noises and traffic. In the clinical setting, dogs will often show signs of fear when they see a stethoscope, thermometer or syringe.

When fearful, immature dogs tend to show avoidant behaviour such as trying to escape from the threat, or seeking reassurance from another individual such as the owner. As the dog approaches adulthood this usually transforms into fear-related aggression, so it is important to treat fear of people and other dogs at the earliest opportunity.

Dogs that were reared in a non-domestic environment (kennel, barn, outbuilding) are at greater risk of developing a range of fear and aggression problems, as are dogs with limited socialisation. Owners may confirm or reinforce fearful behaviour by attempting to soothe the dog when it is afraid.

Common differential diagnoses

The common behavioural differentials for fear are anxiety and phobia. Anxiety is the apprehensive anticipation of threat or danger. It occurs in situations in which no actual threat is present but the dog is in a place that either has fearful associations or is unfamiliar and, therefore, makes the dog feel insecure. Typical signs of anxiety are:

- Loss of appetite
- Trembling, panting
- Lip-licking
- Yawning
- Increased vigilance or scanning behaviour

100 Top Consultations in Small Animal General Practice, First Edition
By Peter Hill, Sheena Warman and Geoff Shawcross
© 2011 Blackwell Publishing Ltd

- Difficulty focussing attention (for example, on commands).

Anxious dogs are difficult to train because they cannot concentrate and they find food rewards unappealing. When anxious, dogs are easily startled, inclined to misinterpret events as threatening and will over-react to what happens to them (perhaps by becoming aggressive or bolting).

Phobic fear is debilitating and progressive. It tends to generalise between stimuli. A dog that is phobic of one noise is likely to become phobic of other similar noises. Typical signs of phobia are:

- The fear does not diminish with repeated normal exposure to the stimulus. In fact, with phobic fear, the problem tends to get worse over time
- The fear is disproportionate to the threat and persists long after the threat has gone. A noise-phobic dog will react with intense fear even to an almost inaudible gunshot sound
- Bolting or panic reactions.

Dogs may experience fear and/or anxiety as part of an overall behavioural problem. However, it is important to differentiate between fearful, phobic and anxious responses to stimuli because they need to be treated differently.

Diagnostic approach

Dogs that are unwell may be both more fearful and more defensive so it is important to rule out underlying medical factors. This is particularly important when there is a sudden change in behaviour, but more insidious changes can still be indicative of the onset of chronic illness or pain.

If the dog is otherwise healthy, the diagnosis is based on the type of behaviours that the dog is showing. The following information is needed to determine the extent of the problem:

- The specific stimuli that evoke fear (person, dog, noise, object)

- The features of those stimuli that alter the severity of the dog's reaction (age or sex of a person or dog, proximity, intensity, movement, size, markings, clothing, etc)
- Whether the dog's response is worse, or better, in certain locations such as in a street or park (i.e. does the dog show increased anxiety in certain locations).

Treatment

It is best to reduce uncontrolled exposure to fearful stimuli, in order to improve the dog's welfare. This also reduces the risk of aggression and makes progress with treatment easier because it reduces the psychological impact of further frightening experiences. Owners should be told not to try to comfort the dog when it is afraid. Clinicians should use information about the dog's fear responses to:

- Determine a means of easily presenting the stimulus at below the threshold that will trigger fear (sound or video recording, at increased distance, or partly disguised)
- Find a location for training in which the dog will be relaxed and not anxious
- Repeatedly expose the dog to these stimuli in a controlled manner using desensitisation or counter-conditioning approaches.

Desensitisation involves repeated exposure to the fear-eliciting stimulus, on its own, at below the level that triggers fear, and in a context in which the dog is relaxed. The advantage of this method is that all training can be done in a single location and the effects will transfer to any other setting. Desensitisation is the first step in treating phobias, because exposure levels must be very low in order to avoid triggering fear. Standardised behavioural programmes are available for the treatment of phobias of fireworks and other noises (Sounds Scary, Sound Therapy 4 Pets Ltd).

Counter-conditioning involves linking the fearful stimulus with something the dog unconditionally likes. Just as the fearful stimulus appears, the dog is presented with an opportunity to play or get food until the stimulus has gone away. This approach works well for dogs that are highly motivated by food or play, but the training must be done in several different places (i.e. different parts of the house, different buildings or parks) in order for what the dog has learned to become generalised to all situations.

It is also important to provide the dog with a means of coping with a fearful stimulus, so that it has control over its own level of exposure (for example, allowing the dog the opportunity to avoid or escape from the perceived threat). This is particularly important in situations where exposure to the fearful stimulus is unavoidable, such as the arrival of an infant into the home of a dog that is known to be afraid of children. If such a dog can retreat to a safe place that is inaccessible to the child, it will become used to the presence of the child much more quickly, and is less likely to become aggressive.

Another application is in the case of dogs with noise phobia. During phobic events, such as thunderstorms and fireworks, these dogs should be given free access to a quiet, dark hiding place with comfortable bedding, water, food and familiar objects such as toys and pieces of the owner's clothing. Ideally this hiding place should be prepared a week before the anticipated event, and it can be made more calming by the use of a pheromone diffuser (DAP, CEVA Animal Health). Short term anxiolytic drugs, such as diazepam or alprazolam, may be used to reduce the dog's emotional response to the phobic event. Acepromazine (ACP) is not recommended, as it produces sedation without anxiolysis, leaving the dog in the same emotional state but reducing its ability to move around and seek refuge. For more detailed information on the use of medication to treat noise phobias, see the BSAVA policy statement (BSAVA.com).

What if it doesn't get better?

For an individual stimulus, improvements should be seen within 4–6 weeks if behavioural therapy is performed daily. Supportive treatment with pheromones (DAP, CEVA Animal Health) or a licensed psychoactive drug, such as selegiline (Selgian, CEVA Animal Health), may be necessary for more severe cases.

The low-cost option

With a methodical approach, most fear problems can be treated successfully at low cost.

When should I refer?

Referral should be considered when:

- Aggression is involved
- The dog is fearful of many different stimuli
- The dog also shows anxiety in a number of different contexts
- The dog fails to respond to therapy.

Jon Bowen

Many dogs are destructive or noisy when they are left alone, but true separation anxiety, resulting from excessive attachment to a person, is uncommon.

Common differential diagnoses

- Opportunism and boredom – Young dogs will often amuse themselves by raiding bins or cupboards, chewing furniture and stripping fabric or wallpaper
- Frustration – Dogs that falsely expect that they will be going out with their owners may show a brief intense period of destructiveness and vocalisation for a few minutes after the owner leaves
- Anxious anticipation of the owner returning – Dogs that have been repeatedly punished for destructiveness will often become anxious as a result of anticipating further punishment when the owner comes home. They are often submissive when the owner returns home
- Fear or phobia – If a dog has experienced a fearful or phobic event when confined in a particular room, it may be anxious and attempt to escape when left in this place while the owner is away
- Cognitive disorder (senility) – Senility affects the dog's ability to cope with its environment so that it becomes more dependent on the owner. These dogs may be very anxious when left alone
- True separation anxiety – Separation anxiety is most often seen in young dogs, but it can also develop after events that disrupt the dog's attachment relationships. These include re-homing or when an owner returns to work after a long period of illness or unemployment.

Diagnostic approach

A diagnosis is established by careful analysis of the dog's behaviours as outlined above. Age of onset, history of other fears and phobias, and signs of excessive attachment are critical to making a diagnosis. To make a diagnosis of separation anxiety the dog must show a consistent pattern of:

- Signs of anxiety as the owner prepares to leave the home
- Becoming distressed when separated from the owner even for short periods, such as when the owner uses the bathroom
- Following and trying to stay close to the owner at all times
- Anxiety *every time* the owner is away, even when the dog is looked after by another person
- Anxiety *throughout* the time when the owner is away (pacing, crying, panting, trembling, loss of continence, drooling)
- Destructiveness that is targeted at trying to escape.

Dogs that are only intermittently anxious when alone and show few other signs of hyperattachment are probably suffering from one of the other problems outlined above.

Where possible, the diagnosis should be supported with video evidence of the dog's behaviour on at least two occasions when left alone for around 40 minutes. The video should include the dog's reactions as the owner prepares to leave.

100 Top Consultations in Small Animal General Practice, First Edition
By Peter Hill, Sheena Warman and Geoff Shawcross
© 2011 Blackwell Publishing Ltd

Initial management

Opportunism and boredom can be remedied by providing the dog with plenty of things to destroy while the owner is out, including cardboard to rip up, chews and activity feeders (Kong®, Activity Ball®). Owners should be advised not to punish dogs that are fearful of the owner returning. Phobias or fearful events that lead to anxiety and attempts to escape from a particular room can be treated with a DAP diffuser (CEVA Animal Health) and benzodiazepine drugs.

Behavioural therapy for separation anxiety is more likely to be effective when accompanied by pheromone treatment with a DAP diffuser or the drug clomipramine (Clomicalm, Novartis). DAP diffusers should be installed close to the location where the dog usually rests. The diffuser must be left switched on at all times, not just when the owner is away, and positioned at a height that permits the dog to get very close to and sniff it. Clomipramine takes 4–6 weeks to produce an effect. The dog may also gain some benefit from having a dog walker or minder.

A number of behavioural approaches are effective:

- Reduce the importance of the person the dog is attached to, by getting other people to feed, play games with, and walk the dog
- Provide activities that encourage independence, such as regular play with dogs during walks
- Give the dog its own bed where it is encouraged to rest and sleep away from physical contact with the owner
- Desensitise the dog to signs that the owner is leaving (picking keys up, putting hat, coat or shoes on, locking windows or switching the television off). This is done by doing these same things many times each day but without going out. Gradually the dog takes less notice of these departure cues
- Practise going out of the house for short periods (i.e. less than a couple of minutes) many times each day.

What if it doesn't get better?

When used with DAP or clomipramine, behavioural therapy should produce improvements within 6–8 weeks. If there is no improvement the case should be reassessed and referral considered.

The low-cost option

Treatment of separation anxiety is rarely cheap or straightforward, as it often requires treatment with DAP or a psychoactive drug such as clomipramine, and the support of dog minders/walkers.

When should I refer?

Referral should be considered:

- If the dog's vocalisation may lead to a prosecution for noise nuisance
- If the dog is very destructive or distressed
- If the dog fails to respond to therapy or the owner is considering re-homing.

If drug therapy is involved, these cases must be referred to a behaviourist who is also a qualified veterinary surgeon.

Jon Bowen

Puppies and kittens learn to choose an appropriate latrine location by observing the behaviour of their mother. They are programmed to acquire substrate and location preferences, which persist for the rest of their lives. Housetraining should seek to mimic these natural processes. From the outset, puppies should be taken outside to go to the toilet, as this produces the strongest and most appropriate preferences. The use of positive reinforcement enhances learning. Cats prefer sandy substrates and secluded latrine locations, so kittens should be provided with several easily accessible litter trays until they have developed a strong substrate preference and have outdoor access.

The use of 'training pads' or newspaper as temporary indoor latrines for dogs and cats should be discouraged, as they can encourage indoor elimination.

Once a proper preference has been established, dogs and cats will usually remain housetrained throughout their life, only soiling indoors when they are distressed, ill or cannot reach a preferred latrine when they need to eliminate. While they are awake, dogs can be expected to remain clean if left alone for 4–5 hours at a time.

Common differential diagnoses

Inappropriate elimination can result from:

- Incomplete housetraining
- Indoor scent marking
- Senility
- Polyuria/polydipsia
- Incontinence: Urine leakage while the animal is asleep or resting, or frequent urination in the bed are indicators of incontinence
- Diarrhoea: Many owners will fail to mention that the animal has soft, high volume stools when they report inappropriate elimination
- Anxiety: This can increase the frequency of urination, as well as produce loose stools
- Fear: animals that are afraid of fireworks or traffic may be reluctant to go to the toilet outside and, therefore, soil more often in the house
- Fear of the owner: animals that have been repeatedly punished for house-soiling may be

reluctant to go to the toilet when the owner is nearby; cats may be wary of using a litter tray when the owner is present, and dogs may be wary of eliminating during a walk.

Diagnostic approach

The patient's age, sex, history and clinical signs should be used to determine the contribution of:

- Medical factors – Senility, incontinence, PUPD, etc
- Emotional factors – Fears, phobias and anxieties
- Learning – Housetraining.

If several animals share the home, video evidence may be needed to confirm the identity of the culprit. Alternatively, the animal can be fed material that can be used to identify its urine or faeces. Sweetcorn makes a good faecal marker, as it is relatively indigestible, and ingested fluorescein dye will make the animal's urine fluoresce under UV light.

In cats, it is particularly important to differentiate between scent marking (e.g. spraying) and elimination, as these are treated differently. When spray-marking, cats will usually choose a highly visible location, and pass small volumes of musty smelling urine while standing up. Whilst spraying, the cat usually has a glazed expression, and the tip of its tail twitches. When urinating, cats choose more discrete locations, and tend to squat and pass large volumes of urine. However, cats with interstitial cystitis may urinate whilst standing up, and pass small volumes of urine.

Spray-marking in cats is a response to social stress, either due to competition with other cats in the household, or outside. Owner should draw a diagram of the location and volume of all the urine spots found in the home. In general, when the majority of spray marks are around windows and external doors this tends to indicate that stress is due to competition with cats outside. When most spray marks are around internal doors and corridors this indicates conflict between cats sharing the household.

100 Top Consultations in Small Animal General Practice, First Edition
By Peter Hill, Sheena Warman and Geoff Shawcross
© 2011 Blackwell Publishing Ltd

Treatment

Potential underlying medical problems should be investigated and treated. The areas where the animal has soiled should be thoroughly cleaned to remove odours that identify locations within the home as latrines or scent-marking spots. Odour-free biological cleaners should be used, and each spot should be washed on at least three separate occasions before considering it clean. The animal should be provided with better access to suitable latrines (more outdoor access, more litter trays etc).

Indoor elimination in dogs

In all cases, it is preferable to train dogs to go to the toilet *on command,* and also give them opportunities to go to the toilet just before the owner goes to bed or goes out. Putting the dog out into the garden unsupervised is no guarantee that it will go to the toilet. Dogs should be taken to go to the toilet in locations where they feel safe and are not going to be frightened or distracted by noises, other dogs, or threats to their territory.

A typical housetraining routine that can be given to dog owners is as follows:

- Take the dog on the leash, to a suitable spot in the garden every 90 minutes, and after every meal and period of sleep
- Circle the spot 2–3 times and then stand still
- As the dog begins to eliminate, quietly give the command phrase of your choice (e.g. *'dog's name*, be clean')
- Immediately after the dog finishes, give praise, a food treat and let it off leash to play and explore the garden for a few minutes
- If the dog does not eliminate within 5–10 minutes, then lead it back into the house without comment
- As is becomes apparent which times the dog prefers to go to the toilet, phase out those times when it does not
- Gradually make the command louder, and say it as you reach the toilet location, rather than as the dog is going to the toilet
- At all other times the dog should be supervised to avoid allowing opportunities for it to soil in the house. When the dog cannot be supervised, an indoor kennel may be used to confine the dog to its bed, where it is less likely to eliminate

- If the dog urinates or defecates in the home while the owner is present, the owner should calmly say 'no' or clap their hands, and lead the dog to the correct toilet place to finish off. Punishment is unnecessary and can cause greater problems
- Dogs should never be punished when owners discover evidence of house-soiling some time after it has happened (such as when they return home).

For most dogs this training takes 2–3 weeks.

Indoor elimination in cats

This is best resolved by providing latrines that conform to the cat's innate preferences:

- Separate litter trays for urine and faeces
- Enough litter trays to provide each cat in the household with its own latrine
- Privacy: litter trays should not be in busy places, close to food bowls etc
- Substrate: sandy, mineral-based litter filled to a depth of 2–3 cm. Wood, wood-pulp and scented litters are deterrent to many cats
- Open litter trays are preferred to covered ones.

Once the cat has stopped eliminating in inappropriate locations, less-used litter trays may be removed, and the remaining ones gradually moved to locations the owner finds less unsightly.

Many cats with outdoor access still find difficulty finding a suitable latrine location, because gardens are paved or provide little privacy. Owners should be encouraged to provide their cats with outdoor latrines around the border of the garden. These are simply constructed by digging 30-cm deep holes and filling them with soft sand.

Indoor marking in cats

Sources of stress should be identified and rectified. If there is conflict between cats sharing a home, tension is significantly reduced by improving available resources:

- Provide outdoor access at all times
- Feed cats ad-libitum from several locations within the home, so that cats can eat whenever they want to
- Increase the number of resting and sleeping places available to the cats

- Provide greater access to high resting places, such as dedicated cat furniture or on shelves
- Increase the number of available litter trays.

The use of pheromone products such as Feliway (CEVA Animal Health) has been shown to significantly reduce inter-cat conflict and indoor marking problems. Feliway diffusers should be used at the manufacturer's recommended rate, and used until indoor marking has stopped for at least 6 weeks.

The same recommendations should be implemented if the source of stress is conflict with non-resident cats. In addition, the owner should install an electronic cat door that prevents non-resident cats from entering the home. Where the resident cat has spray marked close to windows, the external view should be temporarily blocked by applying a coating to the windows (glass etch spray or plastic film). This prevents resident cats from being intimidated by cats outside.

On the first day of treatment, all locations where the cat has previously spray marked should be cleaned thoroughly several times using a scent-free biological cleaner. These sites should then be cleaned weekly, and whenever they are soiled, until the problem has resolved. This prevents the build-up of scent signals that attract re-marking.

What if it doesn't get better?

Dogs that have regularly soiled in the house for months or years and were never properly house-trained may always need to be managed, because they have not learned an appropriate toilet location preference.

With cats, failure to improve may mean that some underlying medical cause, such as cystitis, has been overlooked, or training has not been implemented correctly, or the animal has an emotional disorder (fear or anxiety). Feline indoor marking problems are more difficult to resolve when there is a high population density of cats, and in homes where four or more cats are resident. In some cases, rehoming one or more cats may be the most realistic option.

The low-cost option

Housetraining and increasing the availability of resources are simple and cheap.

When should I refer?

Dogs should be referred when there is a medical cause that cannot be managed by the practice, or when standard treatment has failed. Cats should be referred when indoor marking occurs in households with more than four cats, or where standard treatment has failed.

Section 15
Poisonings

Geoff Shawcross

Poisoning is not an uncommon presentation in companion animal practice. Dogs (especially youngsters) are most commonly affected because of their inquisitive/mischievous behaviour. Cats are less commonly affected because they are more fastidious but symptoms are often very severe in this species. Poisoning usually occurs by ingestion but can also occur by absorption through the skin or by inhalation. Cats are particularly prone to ingesting toxins when cleaning/grooming themselves following contamination of the fur, or eating rodents that have been poisoned.

The large majority of cases are accidental but the clinician should be aware that malicious poisoning does occur and may involve a criminal investigation. In such cases, thorough documentation of clinical (and post-mortem) findings is paramount, together with the correct preservation of suspect material and tissue samples for possible forensic analysis. When presented with the sudden death of their pet, owners often suspect poisoning as the cause. In such circumstances, a thorough post-mortem examination will usually reveal the cause. If post-mortem findings are suggestive of poisoning, tissue samples and gastric contents should be preserved for further analysis. Owners should be warned in advance that the cost of analysing material for suspected toxins can be very expensive.

The clinician should be extremely cautious about giving the client an optimistic prognosis when dealing with any case of poisoning as the full effects of the poisoning may not be apparent immediately. Some poisons have delayed or long-term effects (e.g. non-regenerative anaemia following ingestion of oestrogens, renal failure following ingestion of NSAIDs), which can turn the successful management of the acute symptoms into a disappointing failure.

The practice should be prepared in advance for poisoning cases by having:

- Telephone numbers of a national poison unit (in the UK, this would be the Veterinary Poisons Information Service which needs prior membership), the local

hospital pharmacy, and laboratories prepared to analyse material for toxins
- Antidotes for specific poisons, e.g. vitamin K1
- Reliable emetics. For dogs, an injection of apomorphine is recommended; for cats, intramuscular xylazine is useful
- GI tract demulcents and adsorbents. Activated charcoal in suspension is the most useful and widely available
- Stomach tubes of varying sizes for gastric lavage
- Access to a good toxicology reference textbook, veterinary medicine datasheets and, if possible, human medicine datasheets to determine the active constituents of human drugs.

Poisoning should be considered as a cause of illness when:

- The owner has specific evidence, e.g. chewed containers, accidental administration of the wrong drugs
- There is severe vomiting/diarrhoea, without prior signs of malaise. Vomitus may contain abnormal material or be abnormally coloured
- There are acute CNS signs, e.g. hyperexcitability, seizures, stupor or unconsciousness
- Significant clinical findings that do not fit a common presentation, e.g. haemorrhage into tissues with warfarin. Some poisons give both severe GI tract and neurological signs, which is an uncommon presentation for an infectious disease.

Signs of acute toxicity are usually sudden in onset and progress very rapidly compared with infectious diseases. Prodromal signs are usually absent. Common sources of poisons causing acute signs include (see Table 91.1):

- Human medical drugs such as birth-control tablets, paracetamol, NSAIDS, asthma inhalers, psychoactive drugs
- Veterinary drugs, especially overdosing or the inappropriate use of ectoparasiticidal drugs
- Household products such as disinfectants, paints, solvents, wood preservatives, resulting in coat contamination, or ethylene glycol (antifreeze) which is often ingested
- Garden products such as herbicides, insecticides, and molluscicides. These products often contaminate water sources that the animal drinks

100 Top Consultations in Small Animal General Practice, First Edition
By Peter Hill, Sheena Warman and Geoff Shawcross
© 2011 Blackwell Publishing Ltd

- Vermin-controlling drugs, e.g. coumarin derivatives. Baits are often attractive to non-target species
- Recreational drugs (misuse of controlled substances). In these cases, anamnesis is not always reliable; owners are unlikely to admit to knowing that their

pet has ingested recreational drugs or controlled substances
- Plants or foodstuffs that are poisonous to cats or dogs, e.g. lilies, chocolate, grapes and raisins.

Table 91.1   Summary of clinical signs and treatment of various toxicoses. The prevalence of these poisonings varies widely in different geographical areas. Note that induction of emesis is normally only valuable within the first 3 hours after ingestion. Gastric lavage can be used as an alternative if induction of emesis is unsuccessful.

Toxin	Clinical signs	Specific antidote	General treatment
Acid/Alkali	Corrosive burns on the skin or in the mouth Ptyalism Vomiting Diarrhoea	Water	Wash skin, mouth or eyes with copious amounts of water GI protection with sucralfate and H2 receptor antagonists
Anticoagulant rodenticides	See Chapter 92	Vitamin K1	See Chapter 92
Arsenic	Vomiting Abdominal pain Watery diarrhoea Hypothermia Weak pulses Dehydration	Dimercaptosuccinic acid – use if signs are progressive or with very high exposure	Control shock, acid base and electrolyte disturbances Control hypothermia Induce emesis Activated charcoal Management of vomiting and diarrhoea
Chocolate	Bloating Vomiting Diarrhoea Polydipsia Agitation Tachycardia Tachypnoea Cardiac arrhythmias Hypertension Ataxia Tremors Seizures	None	Control neurological signs Control cardiac arrhythmias Reduce body temperature Induce emesis or gastric lavage Activated charcoal
Ethylene glycol	Stupor Stumbling Ataxia Collapse 'Animals appear drunk' Polydipsia Polyuria Vomiting Acute renal failure	Fomepizole Ethanol	Induce emesis Control acid base disturbances Aggressive fluid therapy

Table 91.1 (*Continued*)

Toxin	Clinical signs	Specific antidote	General treatment
Grapes and raisins	Vomiting Anorexia Diarrhoea Abdominal pain Acute renal failure	None	Induce emesis Activated charcoal Treatment of acute renal failure
Lead	Anorexia Tremors Seizures Vomiting Diarrhoea Abdominal pain	Succimer (meso-2,3 dimercaptosuccinic acid, DMSA) Ca-EDTA	Manage seizures Induce emesis
Lilies	Only seen in cats Vomiting Anorexia Lethargy Polyuria Polydipsia Acute renal failure Seizures	None	Induce emesis Activated charcoal Intravenous fluids Treatment of acute renal failure
Macadamia nuts	Vomiting Diarrhoea Hindlimb weakness	None	Induce emesis Activated charcoal Supportive care
Marijuana	Ataxia CNS depression Tremors Vomiting Urinary incontinence Bradycardia Hypothermia Mydriasis	None	Induce emesis Supportive care Control CNS signs
Metaldehyde 'slug pellets'	Muscle tremors Extensor rigidity Seizures Hyperthermia	None	Induce emesis Activated charcoal Control tremors/seizures Control hyperthermia Supportive care
Non-steroidal anti-inflammatory drugs	Vomiting Haematemesis Diarrhoea (melaena) Polydipsia Polyuria Pale mucous membranes	None	Induce emesis Activated charcoal H2 receptor antagonists Sucralfate Fluid therapy Supportive care

(*Continued*)

Section 15

Table 91.1 (*Continued*)

Toxin	Clinical signs	Specific antidote	General treatment
Onion/garlic	Vomiting Lethargy Pale mucous membranes and brown urine due to haemolytic anaemia	None	Induce emesis Activated charcoal Fluid therapy Blood transfusion if necessary
Paracetamol (acetaminophen)	Lethargy Depression Inappetence Dyspnoea Vomiting Pale, blue or brown mucous membranes Keratoconjunctivitis sicca	N-acetylcysteine	Induce emesis S-adenosyl methionine Cimetidine Vitamin C Supportive care
Petroleum products and turpentine	Salivation Excessive licking Vomiting Inflamed skin or oral cavity Panting Wheezing Coughing	None	Respiratory support Fluid therapy Pain relief Management of aspiration pneumonia Antibiotics Bathing to remove products from skin
Pyrethroids	Mainly cats Tremors Ataxia Hyperexcitability Seizures Hyperthermia Hypersalivation	None	Bathing to remove topically applied products Induce emesis if ingested Control CNS signs Supportive care
Yew	Vomiting Muscle weakness Seizures Bradycardia or Tachycardia Respiratory distress Coma Death	None	Induce emesis Treat cardiac dysrhythmias

Treatment

There is no specific antidote for most poisonous substances and treatment is symptomatic (Table 91.1). The client should be urged to bring the animal to the surgery as soon as possible. There is little merit in advising the use of household products to induce emesis (e.g. washing soda, mustard) as their efficacy is poor and simply leads to a delay in starting proper treatment.

Treatment must be directed towards the following:

- Limiting further contact with the poison. If the coat is contaminated, apply an Elizabethan collar to prevent self-grooming. Clip the coat if the fur is heavily contaminated. Solvents should not be used to remove coat contamination
- Preventing further absorption of the poison. Although this is a logical step, emetics and gastric lavage are only effective if instigated within 3 hours of ingestion. Emesis should not be induced if:
  - the toxin is corrosive in nature
  - if severe CNS depression is apparent, due to the risk of inhalation pneumonia
  - if the animal is seizuring
  - if the animal has a reduced gag reflex
  - if the animal is bradycardic.

Apomorphine (0.04 mg/kg IM or IV) is an extremely effective emetic for dogs but can lead to prolonged and distressing retching. Oral administration of hydrogen peroxide is an alternative (0.25–0.5 ml/kg of a 3% solution). Xylazine is effective for cats but has a sedative effect and should not be used if the toxin itself has a sedative effect. Gastric lavage should be used if emesis is unsuccessful (or contraindicated) and requires general anaesthesia so that the airway can be protected with an endotracheal tube. Only small quantities of lavage fluid (warm water or saline at 5–10 ml/kg) should be used at a time and it should then be drained from the stomach, as this reduces the possibility of increasing gastric pressure and forcing toxic material through the pylorus into the small intestines. The irrigation process should be repeated several times, ideally until the lavage fluid is clear. Activated charcoal may be valuable if administered within a few hours after ingestion of the toxin. It can be given orally, or via the stomach tube in patients undergoing gastric lavage

- Administering a specific antidote whenever possible (Table 91.1). The clinician must refer to a toxicology centre, textbook or the internet for further details of specific antidotes and their use. Obtaining specific antidotes urgently may be problematic and the practice should consider contacting their local hospital pharmacy to establish a channel of communication
- Providing symptomatic treatment. This is one of the most important aspects in the treatment of most cases of suspected poisoning. Where appropriate, anti-emetics should be given to reduce electrolyte loss and dehydration. Sedation and general anaesthesia should be considered if there are signs of hyper-excitability or seizures as prolonged seizure activity leads to hyperthermia, exhaustion, dehydration, electrolyte disturbances and muscle damage. GI tract demulcents such as sucralfate should be given where appropriate. If cardiac arrhythmias are present they should be treated appropriately
- Providing supportive therapy. Vital signs should be monitored frequently. Intravenous fluids should be used to correct fluid and electrolyte deficits, replace ongoing losses and increase renal excretion of toxins and their metabolites. Recumbent patients should be turned frequently to prevent bedsores. Extra warmth or cooling may be necessary to maintain a normal body temperature
- Maintaining a patent airway and providing supplemental oxygenation if the patient is unconscious or in respiratory distress
- Monitoring basic biochemistry, especially hepatic and renal function, electrolytes and haematology on a frequent basis during treatment, to detect and quantify organ damage, and help provide a prognosis.

Section 15

What if it doesn't get better?

Where the diagnosis is certain, a poor response to treatment is usually a sign of progressive organ damage and failure, and represents a poor or grave prognosis. If the diagnosis is uncertain, a review of the clinical signs, biochemistry and haematology is appropriate.

When should I refer?

Referral should be considered if the diagnosis is uncertain and the case is not responding to empirical treatment. A referral centre will have the facilities for a comprehensive investigation. Referral should also be considered if intensive care facilities are necessary but not available at the practice.

The low-cost option

Poisoning cases can be challenging to diagnose and treat. Mild cases may recover uneventfully without major intervention. In severe cases, overall costs are likely to be minimised by treating aggressively from the outset, in an attempt to limit organ damage. Unless there is a significant reason for doing so, specialist analysis for toxins need not be undertaken. If the prognosis is poor, and funds are limited, euthanasia may have to be considered.

Sheena Warman

Aetiology and pathogenesis

Anticoagulant rodenticides are a common cause of poisoning in dogs and cats. The toxins fall into two main groups, the hydroxycoumarin group and the indandione group. Newer forms, classified as 'second-generation' rodenticides, have been developed to overcome resistance to the original chemicals. Examples of hydroxycoumarins include the first-generation drugs warfarin and dicoumarin, and the second-generation drugs brodifacoum, bromadiolone and difenacoum. First-generation indandiones include diphacinone and chlorphacinone.

Clotting factors II, VII, IX and X require the active hydroquinone form of vitamin K for the enzymatic processes that convert them into their functional forms. Vitamin K itself, which is absorbed from the small intestine and stored in hepatocytes, is converted into its active form by a series of enzymatic reactions, one of which is impaired by the anticoagulant rodenticides. Rodenticide toxicity leads to a deficiency in the activated form of vitamin K, and thus a deficiency in the activated forms of clotting factors II, VII, IX and X. This causes a dramatic impairment of secondary haemostasis (i.e. impairment of the conversion of fibrinogen to fibrin via the clotting cascade).

History and clinical signs

In some but not all cases, there will be a known history of exposure to rodenticides and in the case of known toxin ingestion, veterinary attention may be sought before clinical signs have developed. The first-generation compounds are less potent and usually need to be ingested over a period of time in order to cause problems; clinical signs are unlikely to develop until 4–5 days following ingestion (sooner with some indandione products). Clinical problems can persist for 1–5 weeks, depending on the half-life of the compound. On the other hand, second-generation products are highly potent; a single dose can cause clinical signs within 24 hours, and toxic doses can be ingested by the consumption of poisoned rodents. Toxicity is likely to persist for several weeks.

Clinical signs are those associated with defective secondary haemostasis, i.e. acute haemorrhage into body cavities such as the pleural space, mediastinum, pericardium, abdomen and joints. There may also be evidence of subcutaneous bleeding (particularly at any injection sites) and bleeding from mucosal surfaces. Patients will frequently present with signs of hypovolaemic shock associated with acute blood loss, with no external evidence of haemorrhage. Clinical signs such as cough, dyspnoea or lameness may give clues as to the source of haemorrhage. Petechial haemorrhages are uncommon, although some patients will have mild to marked thrombocytopenia of unknown aetiology associated with rodenticide toxicity.

Important differential diagnoses

Other causes of intra-cavitary haemorrhage:

* Trauma
* Neoplasia, e.g. ruptured splenic haemangiosarcoma, diffuse tumours such as mesothelioma
* Pericardial disease.

Other disorders of secondary haemostasis:

* Hepatic disease (the liver is responsible for the synthesis of most clotting factors, as well as being the site of activation of the vitamin-K dependent factors)
* Disseminated intravascular coagulation
* *Angiostrongylus vasorum* infection
* Inherited coagulopathies (e.g. Haemophilia A and B)
* Vitamin K deficiency (due to failure to absorb vitamin K from the small intestine, e.g. EPI, severe inflammatory bowel disease, bile duct obstruction).

Disorders of primary haemostasis:

* Although clinical signs of disorders of secondary haemostasis are usually apparent, there can be some overlap with clinical signs associated with defects in primary haemostasis, i.e. the vascular and platelet response to bleeding, defects which commonly cause bleeding from mucosal surfaces and petechial/ecchymotic haemorrhages. These may be:
  * Thrombocytopenia: destruction of platelets (e.g. immune-mediated thrombocytopenia),

100 Top Consultations in Small Animal General Practice, First Edition
By Peter Hill, Sheena Warman and Geoff Shawcross
© 2011 Blackwell Publishing Ltd

sequestration of platelets (e.g. DIC, vasculitis), or lack of production (bone marrow disease)

- Impaired platelet function: inherited disorders (e.g. von Willebrand's disease) or acquired disorders (e.g. ehrlichiosis, hepatic disease, pancreatitis, DIC).

Specific diagnostic techniques

In cases with a reliable history of toxin exposure and obvious clinical signs, no further diagnostic tests may be necessary. In other situations, further diagnostic procedures may be required. Haematology and evaluation of haemostasis should be performed in any patient with suspected rodenticide toxicity, even if they are clinically normal.

- Haematology – A minimum of measurement of PCV and total solids should be performed in-house, with an EDTA blood sample and fresh smears submitted to an external laboratory for full haematological analysis. Any anaemia should become regenerative within 3–5 days following bleeding (demonstrated by anisocytosis, polychromasia and increased reticulocyte count). Note that some patients with rodenticide poisoning will be thrombocytopenic for unknown reasons
- Evaluation of haemostasis – Prothrombin time (PT) and activated partial thromboplastin time (APTT) should be measured. This usually requires blood to be collected into citrate tubes and submitted to an external laboratory. Activated clotting time (ACT) can be performed rapidly in-house if appropriate equipment is available. In most cases PT, APTT and ACT will all be prolonged, although initially in mild cases, PT alone may be prolonged
- Search for source of haemorrhage – Careful history taking and physical examination will identify a source of haemorrhage in many patients. Further investigations may need to be considered including abdominal ultrasound or thoracic/abdominal radiography
- Confirmation of exposure to anticoagulant rodenticides – This is not always straightforward. In cases with recent exposure, emesis may result in the appearance of toxin in the vomitus. In cases with clinical signs of haemorrhage it may be necessary to exclude other causes of haemorrhage or secondary haemostatic disorders using results of history,

physical examination, full haematology, serum biochemistry (including liver function tests), imaging, and possibly specific clotting factor assays in at-risk breeds. However, it should be remembered that rodenticide toxicity is by far the commonest cause of disorders of secondary haemostasis encountered in general practice. Some laboratories offer a PIVKA assay ('proteins induced by vitamin K antagonism'), but an increase in PIVKA concentration is not 100% specific for anticoagulant toxicity. Toxicology laboratories may be able to detect specific anticoagulants on fluid or tissue samples.

Treatment

Gastric decontamination

Induction of emesis and/or gastric lavage, and administration of adsorbents (e.g. activated charcoal) are indicated only in patients which are known to have ingested toxin within the last 3 hours. Once coagulopathies have developed, these procedures are not beneficial and may precipitate further bleeding.

Vitamin K

Treatment with the correct form of vitamin K (vitamin K_1) is highly effective for the treatment of anticoagulant toxicity. Abnormalities in coagulation parameters return to normal within two days of treatment, but treatment must be continued for the duration of the time that the toxin remains in the body (as little as a week for warfarin; up to several weeks for some of the 2nd generation products). Treatment is usually initiated with subcutaneous injections (using a 23 g needle) at several sites, followed by oral therapy (with a fatty meal) as indicated in Table 92.1. Vitamin K_1 should never be given intravenously due to the risk of anaphylaxis.

Supportive care

The risk of further haemorrhage can be reduced if the patient is cage-rested and procedures such as injections can be avoided. Oxygen should be provided to dyspnoeic patients. Drainage of blood from body cavities is not usually recommended due to the risk of causing further bleeding. The exception to this is thoracocentesis in patients with life-threatening dyspnoea due to haemothorax, and pericardiocente-

Table 92.1 Treatment schedule for vitamin K₁ therapy following rodenticide poisoning.

Toxin	Initial dose of vitamin K_1	Ongoing treatment with vitamin K_1
Known 1st generation hydroxycoumarin ingestion	5 mg/kg SC at several sites	2.5 mg/kg PO divided q8–12 h for 5–7 days
Known indandione or 2nd generation hydroxycoumarin ingestion; unknown anticoagulant toxin	5 mg/kg SC at several sites	5 mg/kg PO divided q8–12 h for 2–3 weeks. Recheck PT 2 days after end of treatment; continue for further 2 weeks if PT still prolonged

sis in patients with life-threatening cardiac tamponade. Patients with clinical signs of hypovolaemic shock will benefit from intravenous crystalloids ± colloids. In some cases the anaemia is severe enough to warrant treatment with blood products or haemoglobin solutions. If available, packed red cells, or fresh or stored whole blood can be given to provide red blood cells, and fresh or stored whole blood or plasma can be used to provide the vitamin-K dependent clotting factors.

The low-cost option

If the toxin is unknown and the owner will not permit ongoing monitoring of coagulation parameters, then treatment with vitamin K_1 should be continued for 3 weeks and the animal strictly rested for a further week. Vitamin K_3 is available but, although it is much cheaper than vitamin K_1, it is far less effective and should not be used. Patients showing clinical signs of hypovolaemic shock are likely to need aggressive fluid therapy ± treatment with blood products, which will inevitably incur expense.

What if it doesn't get better?

Inadequate dose or duration of treatment with vitamin K_1 is likely to be the commonest cause of complications and/or death in these patients. It is also important to ensure that the source of the toxin has been identified and removed. If a patient is receiving adequate treatment but is continuing to bleed, then the diagnosis should be reconsidered and other possible causes of bleeding disorders investigated.

When should I refer?

Most cases of anticoagulant rodenticide toxicity can be dealt with in general practice. Note that injectable preparations of vitamin K_1 are available in different concentrations and it is important to ensure that adequate stocks are maintained to treat large dogs effectively. Referral should be considered if facilities are not available for patients requiring intensive care and/or treatment with blood products, or if the diagnosis is unclear and there is no response to initial treatment.

Section 15

Section 16
Problems in non dog/cat species

Sharon Redrobe

Rabbits are now the third most popular pet in the UK and knowledge of their diseases and management has increased dramatically over recent years. This chapter is only intended to provide a brief overview of the approach to a 'sick' rabbit and readers are urged to consult more detailed texts for specific details on diagnosis and management of the many diseases from which rabbits suffer.

In general, the approach to a sick rabbit is the same as that applied to dogs and cats, but there are two major differences. First, the clinical signs of illness in rabbits are generally not as organ-specific as they are in dogs and cats. Rabbits are therefore often presented with non-specific signs such as lethargy and anorexia. Second, some owners of rabbits may not be prepared to pay as much for tests or treatment as they would for dogs and cats. However, this should always be clarified early in the consultation and not taken for granted. Pet rabbits can become close members of the family and some owners will request the same level of veterinary care as they would for a pet dog or cat.

Common presentations and conditions affecting rabbits

- Dental disease – overgrown teeth, malocclusion, dentoalveolar abscesses, periodontal disease (Figures 93.1 and 93.2)
- Subcutaneous abscesses
- Myiasis (attack by fly larvae/maggots)
- Skin disease (see Chapter 35)
- Head tilt (Figure 93.3) – *Encephalitozoon cuniculi* infection, toxoplasmosis, larval cestode infection, meningitis/encephalitis/brain abscess caused by *Pasteurella* or other bacteria, middle ear infection, ear mites, head trauma
- Lethargy and anorexia – ileus, pneumonia/rhinitis/middle ear infection, blindness/ocular disease, syphilis, early/mild myxomatosis, dental disease
- Weakness or collapse – ileus, hypoglycaemia, hypocalcaemia, lead poisoning, septicaemia, pneumonia, liver disease, renal disease, heart disease, neoplasia, traumatic fractures, *En. cuniculi* infection, toxoplasmosis, heat stroke

100 Top Consultations in Small Animal General Practice, First Edition
By Peter Hill, Sheena Warman and Geoff Shawcross
© 2011 Blackwell Publishing Ltd

- Rhinitis
- Pneumonia (bacterial, aspergillosis)
- Dacryocystitis
- Eye ulcers – bacterial, fungal, mycoplasmal, viral infections
- Syphilis (*Treponema cuniculi* infection)

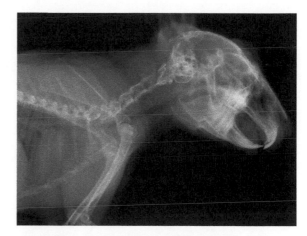

Figure 93.1 Radiograph showing normal rabbit dentition

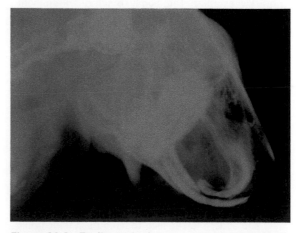

Figure 93.2 Radiograph showing overgrown incisors in a rabbit

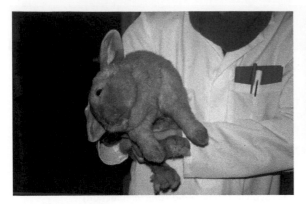

Figure 93.3   Rabbit with a head tilt

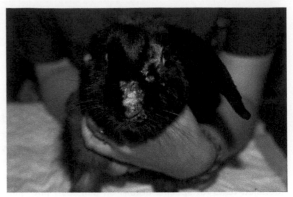

Figure 93.4   Rabbit with syphilis (*Treponema cuniculi*)

- Myxomatosis (Myxoma virus infection transmitted by fleas, mosquitoes)
- Neoplasia
- Bone problems – fractures, arthritis, osteomyelitis
- Ectoparasitic infestations – ear mites, fleas, Cheyletiella
- Diarrhoea – infections with *E. coli*, *Salmonella*, *Yersinia*, rotavirus in young rabbits. True diarrhoea in adult rabbits is rare and is often actually a lack of caecotrophy.

Diagnostic approach

As with dogs and cats, clues to the diagnosis should be obtained from the history and physical examination. Rabbits should be physically restrained with care to avoid iatrogenic injuries. Initial palpation can quickly establish the bodily condition. Prominent bones of the shoulder or hip region would indicate that the rabbit is underweight or emaciated. Nasal discharges can be seen with rhinitis, and the presence of an ocular discharge should prompt a thorough eye examination. A complete examination of a rabbit's mouth can only be performed under sedation or general anaesthesia, but a cursory inspection may detect the presence of overgrown incisors or malocclusion, and allow examination of the tongue and mucosae. The presence of petechiae can indicate septicaemia. The rabbit's skin should be thoroughly examined for the presence of abscesses, maggots, wounds and swellings. Myxomatosis produces erythematous swelling of the eyelids, nares, lips, genitalia and anus, and can lead to tumours in the chronic form. Rabbit syphilis causes lesions at similar sites,

but erosions, oozing and brownish crusts can also be seen (Figure 93.4). The skeleton should be examined for evidence of fractures or pain, and the joints tested for range of movement. Abdominal palpation is relatively easy in rabbits and should allow detection of palpable masses (Figure 93.5). Ileus is characterised by lack of faecal pellet production or, in its earlier stages, the production of smaller and fewer droppings. On palpation, the abdomen may feel gassy or be tense due to pain. The heart and lungs can be easily auscultated in rabbits but complete investigation of these organs requires radiography and ultrasonography. An elevated rectal temperature (normal 39°C) may be seen with infectious disease or pain, but hyperthermia can also occur at environmental temperatures above 22°C.

For most of the conditions listed above, the clinical signs are not specific enough to allow a diagnosis to be made based on history and clinical examination alone. In many cases, a minimum requirement will be a blood test and/or radiography. In a very sick rabbit, a minimal blood database would be a PCV, total protein and glucose. However, full haematology and biochemistry including calcium, phosphorus, CK, AST, albumin and globulin provides a more complete picture. Radiography is useful, as in other mammals, especially in the diagnosis of pneumonia, skeletal diseases, neoplasia and urinary tract diseases (particularly urolithiasis; Figure 93.6). In rabbits, it is most appropriate to obtain lateral and dorsoventral radiographs of the chest and abdomen.

Diagnosing the cause of head tilt can be challenging, and may require serology for *Toxoplasma* and *En. cuniculi*, skull radiographs, ear examination and possibly MRI and CSF analysis.

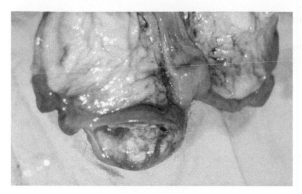

Figure 93.5   Uterine adenocarcinoma in a rabbit

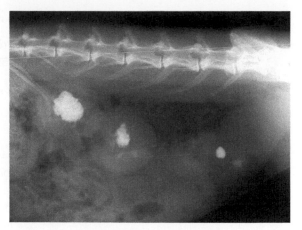

Figure 93.6   Radiograph showing nephro- and urolithiasis in a rabbit

Treatment

Precise treatment of sick rabbits is based on establishing a precise diagnosis, which is likely to require blood tests and radiography. However, initial stabilisation of the patient is important whilst the diagnostic evaluation is underway. Very sick rabbits will benefit from IV administration of glucose and saline via the auricular or cephalic vein, or directly into the femur (see Table 93.1). Isolation in a warm cage or incubator is beneficial, but at no more than 21°C because rabbits are prone to heat stroke at higher temperatures. If facilities are available, a relative humidity of 55% should be maintained as too dry an environment contributes to dehydration and respiratory disease. The rabbit needs to be fed (artificially if required) to prevent further starvation and to prevent or reverse hepatic lipidosis. Placement of a nasogastric tube is the easiest way to achieve this.

Many sick rabbits (for whatever reason) develop a potentially fatal ileus and bloat. Initial supportive treatment includes administration of prokinetics, fluids, pain relief (with buprenorphine or butorphanol) and anti-ulcer treatment (with ranitidine or cimetidine). However, as ileus may also be associated with neoplasia, organ failure or gastric or intestinal obstruction, a rapid diagnosis of the underlying cause is required to effect appropriate treatment. Radiography and/or ultrasonography should be used to investigate the possibility of an intestinal blockage as prokinetics would be contraindicated in those cases.

If a disease is suspected that is caused by (or results in) bacterial infection, it is appropriate to initiate treatment with antibiotics (see Table 93.1), but a definitive diagnosis should be sought to ensure an appropriate drug regime is prescribed, and to allow a prognosis to be established. For rabbits with respiratory infections, nebulisation therapy may be used as well as parenteral therapy. Clinicians should note that pneumonia in rabbits can be caused by *Aspergillus* as well as bacteria, requiring specific antifungal regimes (Table 93.1). *En. cuniculi* infections should be treated with fenbendazole and toxoplasmosis should be treated with potentiated sulphonamides. There is no cure for myxomatosis, but some rabbits recover with supportive care. The judicious use of penicillins is indicated in the treatment of osteomyelitis and small abscesses, but these should be given parenterally rather than orally to avoid dysbiosis. However, subcutaneous abscesses in rabbits contain caseated pus and cannot be effectively lanced as in dogs and cats. Complete surgical excision offers the best prognosis.

Overgrown or maloccluded teeth can be managed by periodic trimming using a dental cutting wheel. Cutting the incisors with nail clippers should be avoided as it can lead to tooth fractures. As rabbits have continuously growing teeth, severe dental problems are usually dealt with by extraction. However, even with extraction, the management of tooth root abscesses can be particularly challenging and the prognosis is guarded. Trauma and skeletal injuries in rabbits require the same approach as orthopaedic repair in domestic mammals, with attention to specific rabbit anatomy.

Table 93.1   Basic treatments for use in rabbits (this is not a comprehensive formulary).

Drug	Dosage	Route	Frequency	Comment
Antimicrobials				
Ceftazidime	50 mg/kg	IM/IV	4 × daily	Effective against aerobic and anaerobic bacteria – frequency of treatment makes impractical unless intensive care case. Risk of dysbiosis
Enilconazole (Imaverol, Janssen)	Dilute 1:10 solution	Nebulise for 30 min	1–2 × daily for 6 weeks	Combine with relevant oral treatment for aspergillosis
Enrofloxacin	20 mg/kg	SC	Once daily for 6 weeks	Treatment for pasteurellosis. Can produce anorexia, not effective against anaerobes, oral treatment less effective
Fenbendazole	20–50 mg/kg daily for 3–5 days. *En. cuniculi* treatment 20 mg/kg for 28 days	PO	As noted	Toxicity has been suspected following small overdose or recommended doses
F10 (antifungal disinfectant that can be inhaled)	Dilute 1:200	Nebulise for 30 min	1–2 × daily for 6 weeks	Combine with relevant oral treatment for Aspergillosis or bacterial respiratory disease
Gentamicin	5–10 mg/kg	IM	Twice daily for 5 days	Especially *Pseudomonas* pneumonia, maintain hydration status – can be nebulised
Itraconazole	10 mg/kg	PO	Once daily for 6 weeks	For aspergillosis; combine with nebulisation for optimum effect
Penicillin G (or other pure penicillin)	20–40 mg/kg	SC	Once a week for 4 doses	For venereal spirochaetosis (syphilis). Risk of dysbiosis – monitor faecal output and demeanour; if affected, stop/delay dosing and use probiotics and high-fibre diet during treatment
Potentiated sulphonamide	30 mg/kg	SC	Twice daily	
Metronidazole	25–50 mg/kg	IM or PO	Daily for 5 doses	Effective against anaerobes and flagellates
Sulphadimidine	1 g/L drinking water	PO	Continuous for 7 days, stop for 7 days then repeat	Coccidiosis

Table 93.1 (*Continued*)

Drug	Dosage	Route	Frequency	Comment
Pain relief				
Buprenorphine	0.05 mg/kg	IV or SC	Every 3–4 h	As required
Butorphanol	3–4 mg/kg	IV or SC	Every 6 h	For pre-emptive surgical pain or management of painful conditions
Meloxicam	0.2–0.4 mg/kg	PO or SC	Once daily	
Sedation/anaesthesia				
Hypnorm (fentanyl/ fluanisone)	0.2–0.5 ml/kg	SC	Once	Sedation or prior to addition of midazolam for general anaesthesia
Isoflurane	2–4%	Mask, then intubate	Maintenance of anaesthesia	Swiftly induces anaesthesia, induction and recovery usually within 1 min
Ketamine and medetomidine	Ketamine: 5 mg/kg, Med: 75 µg/kg	IM	Once	5 min to maximum effect of deep sedation or anaesthesia, duration up to 2 h. Intubate and deliver oxygen/isoflurane
Midazolam	0.5–2 mg/kg	IV to effect	Repeat as required	Duration 15–20 min; useful for sedation for non-painful sampling, imaging
Miscellaneous				
Calcium EDTA	25 mg/kg	SC	Every 6 h for 5 days	To treat lead toxicity
Ivermectin	0.2 mg/kg	SC or IM	Once or repeat weekly × 4 for mites	To treat worms. Toxicity reported with overdosing
Metoclopramide	0.5 mg/kg	SC	Twice daily	To treat ileus
Ranitidine	20 mg/kg	PO	1–2 × daily	To treat ulcers, ileus
Fluid therapy				
Lactated Ringers	3–5% bodyweight per day	IO or IV	Maintenance of fluid balance	Required if rabbit >5% dehydrated or weak. Monitor PCV and urea
Oral fluids	3–5% bodyweight per day	PO	Maintenance	Useful in an anorexic rabbit but only if <5% dehydrated

IO = intra-osseous.
Note: Antibiotics should be used with care in rabbits as they are prone to caecal dysbiosis and clostridial overgrowth if inappropriate drugs, doses and routes are used. In general, the parenteral route is safer and often has better pharmacodynamics than the oral route. Few drug dosages are based on scientific investigation. The drugs listed above are used routinely by the author with clinical success. Note that many of these drugs are not licensed for use in rabbits. Oral therapy, if necessary, should be given directly from a syringe or a piece of favourite food, as it is rarely taken effectively if placed in water or feed bowls.

What if it doesn't get better?

If a specific diagnosis is made, many conditions in rabbits will respond to appropriate treatment, allowing a full recovery. In most cases, failure to respond to treatment indicates that an accurate diagnosis has not been established. Further investigations are required in such cases. However, some conditions in rabbits inherently carry a poor prognosis such as myxomatosis, organ failure, nephroliths, some abscesses, and osteomyelitis (if associated with anorexia and pain that cannot be controlled). Euthanasia should be recommended if an acceptable response is not seen. Euthanasia in rabbits is performed by an intravenous, hepatic or renal injection of barbiturate, or induction of general anaesthesia followed by an intracardiac injection of barbiturate.

to an anorexic rabbit in the absence of a diagnosis may provide temporary benefit whilst a potentially treatable underlying condition is worsening, thus making a cure less likely.

If clients refuse a full diagnostic evaluation, the clinician will need to make a judgement based on the above principles. Fluid therapy with a glucose solution (monitored using a hand-held glucometer) plus multimodal ileus treatment can be life-saving in the short term. A blood smear, PCV and basic biochemistry can be performed relatively cheaply and provide essential information, allowing steps to be made towards a precise diagnosis and thus prognosis. If empirical treatment is prescribed, clinicians should be ready to offer euthanasia if there is not an appropriate response and the rabbit's quality of life is poor.

The low-cost option

As stated earlier, financial limitations may limit the diagnostic and therapeutic options when dealing with rabbits. Clinicians may therefore feel pressurised into providing treatment based on a tentative diagnosis, obtained from the history and physical examination alone. Such a diagnosis may not be accurate, and clients must be made aware that the prognosis is uncertain. Clinicians should always place the welfare of the rabbit first, and bear in mind that empirical supportive care may keep a rabbit alive when it is actually suffering from a fatal disease such as terminal renal failure. Clinicians should also note that providing antibiotics, fluids and assisted feeding

When should I refer?

Many clinicians now have specialist expertise in the management of rabbit diseases. Veterinarians who are not confident at treating rabbits should always consider referral to such a specialist as an option, particularly when owner expectations are high. Referral in such cases should be arranged early, and not after the rabbit has failed to respond to non-specific therapy. As with dogs and cats, referral should also be considered if a diagnosis has not been made following in-house diagnostic investigations and/or the practice does not have the equipment or expertise to perform and interpret more advanced procedures. If treatment has been prescribed, and the rabbit does not appear to be getting better after 24–48 h, referral should definitely be offered.

Sharon Redrobe

This chapter is only intended to provide a brief overview of the approach to a 'sick' hamster, and readers are urged to consult more detailed texts for specific information on the diagnosis and management of the many diseases from which hamsters suffer.

The approach to a sick hamster differs from that applied to dogs and cats in four main ways. First, less information can be gained from the history and physical examination in hamsters than in dogs and cats. This is because owners are less likely to observe specific clinical signs, and their small size precludes certain aspects of physical examination. Second, the clinical signs of illness in hamsters are generally not as organ specific as they are in dogs and cats. Hamsters are therefore often presented with vague signs such as lethargy and anorexia. Third, it is unlikely that owners of hamsters will be prepared to pay as much for tests or treatment as they would for dogs and cats. Fourth, the common golden or Syrian hamster has a lifespan of only 1–3 years. This shorter longevity has to be born in mind, and irreversible 'old age' conditions are common.

Common presentations and conditions affecting hamsters

- Respiratory disease – bacterial, fungal, mycoplasmal, viral
- Diarrhoea – proliferative ileitis (*Campylobacter*, *E.coli*, *Chlamydophila*, *Desulfovibrio*), dietary indiscretion, clostridial overgrowth, coccidiosis
- Lethargy and anorexia – pneumonia, ocular disease, organ failure (old age)
- Weakness or collapse – hypoglycaemia, hypocalcaemia, hypothermia, lead poisoning, septicaemia, liver disease, renal disease, heart disease, neoplasia, ovarian disease, traumatic fractures
- Bone problems – fractures, arthritis, osteomyelitis
- Dental disease – overgrowth, caries, periodontal disease

- Oral cavity disease – impacted cheek pouch, oral tumours
- Alopecia – mites, hypothyroidism, hyperadrenocorticism, cutaneous lymphoma (see Chapter 35).

Diagnostic approach

When dealing with hamsters, a rapid determination should be made as to whether or not treatment is likely to be successful, or if euthanasia is indicated. Hamsters are a short-lived species and if the owner has had the hamster for over 12 months, there is an increasing risk of old-age problems occurring, with an attendant poor prognosis. The exact age of the hamster should be ascertained (if known), its sex and how long it has been ill. The owner may be able to describe some specific symptoms they have noticed (such as diarrhoea), but this is less typical than with dogs and cats. The owner should also be asked about the hamster's diet, (including treats and differentiating what is offered from what is eaten) as inappropriate items can lead to diarrhoea.

Clinical examination should be performed with care and appropriate restraint, bearing in mind that hamsters can bite. The body condition and state of hydration should be quickly assessed. Tenting of the skin indicates 10% dehydration, which should be quickly corrected with subcutaneous or intraperitoneal fluids. Prominent bones in the shoulder or hip region indicate that the hamster is thin or emaciated, which carries a poor prognosis. The nostrils, eyes and prepuce/vagina should be checked for discharges. Note that females in oestrus have a discharge that resembles purulent material. The perineum should be checked for evidence of diarrhoea ('wet tail'). The oral mucosa should be checked for signs of septicaemia, indicated by petechiation. The teeth, tongue and oral cavity should be checked for lesions or discharges. An impacted cheek pouch can readily be emptied under anaesthesia, but oral tumours can present in the same way and need to be differentiated by careful examination. The respiratory rate and effort should be noted, but auscultation of the thorax

100 Top Consultations in Small Animal General Practice, First Edition
By Peter Hill, Sheena Warman and Geoff Shawcross
© 2011 Blackwell Publishing Ltd

is not very rewarding in hamsters. The abdomen should be gently palpated to check for masses. The legs and feet should be examined for injuries, full range of movement or deformities. The skin should be examined for evidence of pruritus or hair loss.

For some of the conditions listed above, a diagnosis and appropriate treatment may require a blood sample (a few drops can be obtained from the lateral saphenous vein) or bacteriological culture (via a rectal swab if diarrhoea is present). A limited range of tests in a very sick hamster would be a PCV, total protein and glucose, but a fuller biochemical profile is required to detect abdominal organ failure.

Initial management

Initial stabilisation of the patient is important whilst a diagnostic evaluation is underway. Very sick hamsters will benefit from glucose and saline given SC or IP (see Table 94.1) and isolation in a warm cage or incubator at 25–30°C. If facilities are available, a relative humidity of 55% should be maintained as too dry an environment contributes to dehydration and respiratory disease. Anorexic hamsters need food to

prevent and reverse hepatic lipidosis. This can be achieved by repeated stomach tubing with vegetable puree mixed in an oral electrolyte solution, given at a volume of 1 ml every 3–4 hours. This procedure is difficult but can be achieved using a straight metal crop tube as is used for birds.

Empirical antibiotic treatment (see Table 94.1) should not be used routinely in hamsters as some conditions do not require antibiotics, and dysbiosis and fatal diarrhoea may result. Respiratory infections can be treated with injectable antibiotics such as enrofloxacin (for *Pasteurella* or *Mycoplasma* pneumonia). Nebulisation therapy with appropriate antibiotics such as fluroquinolones or aminogycosides can be used as well as, or instead of, parenteral therapy (see Table 94.1). Diarrhoea can often be treated with fluid therapy and glucose alone, given orally or parenterally (SC or IP), as most causes are self-limiting. It is the dehydration that is usually life-threatening.

The common dental abnormalities seen in hamsters are incisor fractures or over-growth. Incisors can be removed entirely or trimmed using a high-speed dental burr. Obvious trauma such as leg fractures can either be dealt with by amputation (hamsters do very well with one fore or hind limb removed) or limited orthopaedic repair (using external fixators made from needles and dental acrylic).

Table 94.1 Basic treatments for use in hamsters (this is not a comprehensive formulary).

Drug	Dosage	Route	Frequency	Comment
Antimicrobials				
Enrofloxacin	20 mg/kg	SC	Once daily for up to 6 weeks	Treatment of bacterial infections. Can produce anorexia; not effective against anaerobes; oral treatment less effective
Fenbendazole	20–50 mg/kg	PO	Daily for 3–5 days	Care – toxicity has been suspected even at recommended doses
F10 (an antifungal disinfectant that can be given as an inhalant)	Dilute 1:200	Nebulise for 30 min	1–2 × daily for 6 weeks	Combine with relevant oral treatment for bacterial respiratory disease

Table 94.1 (*Continued*)

Drug	Dosage	Route	Frequency	Comment
Gentamicin	5–10 mg/kg	IM	Twice daily for 5 days	Especially *Pseudomonas* pneumonia; maintain hydration status; can be nebulised
Potentiated sulphonamide	30 mg/kg	SC	Twice daily	
Metronidazole	25–50 mg/kg	IM or PO	Once daily for 5 days	Effective against anaerobes and flagellates
Sulphadimidine	1 g/L drinking water	PO	Continuous for 7 days, stop for 7 days then repeat	Coccidiosis
Pain relief				
Buprenorphine	0.05 mg/kg	SC	Every 3–4 hours	As required
Butorphanol	3–4 mg/kg	SC	Every 4–6 hours	For pre-emptive surgical pain or management of painful conditions
Sedation/anaesthesia				
Isoflurane	2–4%	Mask	Maintenance of anaesthesia	Swiftly induces anaesthesia, induction and recovery usually within 1 min
Miscellaneous				
Calcium EDTA	25 mg/kg	SC	Every 6 hours for 5 days	To treat lead toxicity
Ivermectin	0.2 mg/kg	SC or IM	Once or repeat weekly × 4 for mites	To treat worms. Toxicity reported with overdosing
Ranitidine	20 mg/kg	PO	1–2 times daily	To treat ulcers
Fluid therapy				
Lactated Ringers	3–5% bodyweight per day	IO or SC, IP	Maintenance of fluid balance	Required if hamster > 5% dehydrated or weak. Monitor PCV and urea if possible
Oral fluids	3–5% bodyweight per day	PO	Maintenance of fluid balance	Not if > 5% dehydrated. Otherwise, useful in an anorexic hamster

Note: Antibiotics should be used with care in hamsters as they are prone to caecal dysbiosis and clostridial overgrowth if inappropriate drugs, doses and routes are used. In general, the parenteral route is safer and often has better pharmacodynamics than the oral route. Few drug dosages are based upon scientific investigation. The drugs listed above are used routinely by the author with clinical success. Oral therapy, unless given directly from a syringe or a piece of favourite food, is rarely taken effectively if placed in water or feed bowls and is not recommended.

What if it doesn't get better?

If an accurate diagnosis has not been established, and the hamster fails to respond to appropriate supportive care, further diagnostic evaluation is required. This may entail blood work and diagnostic imaging such as radiography, ultrasonography of the abdomen to look for masses, peritoneal fluid etc. and oral endoscopy to fully evaluate the mouth

If a hamster is not responding to treatment for a known diagnosis, or diagnostic evaluation is not permitted, euthanasia should be performed. This can be carried out by an intra-hepatic injection of barbiturate (quicker than IP), or induction of general anaesthesia using a gaseous anaesthetic followed by an intracardiac injection of barbiturate.

The low-cost option

Financial limitations may limit the diagnostic and therapeutic options when dealing with hamsters. Clinicians may therefore have to prescribe treatment based on a tentative diagnosis, obtained from the history and physical examination alone. Such a diagnosis may not be accurate, and clients must be made aware that the prognosis is uncertain. Clinicians should always place the welfare of the hamster first, and bear in mind that empirical supportive care may keep a hamster alive when it is actually suffering from a fatal disease such as terminal renal failure. If the only option permitted by the client is to try supportive care, the hamster should be monitored for a rapid response. Euthanasia should be recommended if there is no improvement within an hour.

When should I refer?

In many cases, referral of a hamster will not be an option. However, some owners might consider this if there were a specialist within an appropriate distance. Note that some avid hamster breeders have higher value animals. Any illness in a hamster would benefit from being diagnosed and treated by a clinician with specific expertise and facilities for dealing with this species.

Sharon Redrobe

This chapter is only intended to provide a brief overview of the approach to a 'sick' Guinea pig, and readers are urged to consult more detailed texts for specific details on the diagnosis and management of the many diseases from which Guinea pigs suffer.

The approach to a sick Guinea pig differs from that applied to dogs and cats in three main ways. First, less information can be gained from the history and physical examination in Guinea pigs than in dogs and cats. This is because owners are less likely to observe specific clinical signs, and their small size precludes certain aspects of the physical examination. Second, the clinical signs of illness in Guinea pigs are generally not as organ-specific as they are in dogs and cats. Guinea pigs are therefore often presented with vague signs such as lethargy and anorexia. Third, it is unlikely that owners of Guinea pigs will be prepared to pay as much for tests or treatment as they would for dogs and cats.

Common presentations and conditions affecting Guinea pigs

- Respiratory disease – bacterial, fungal, mycoplasmal, viral. Guinea pigs do not cope well with respiratory disease and so may present collapsed and require immediate care. Presentation with chronic respiratory disease is less common than in the rabbit
- Diarrhoea – most common in young animals, especially around weaning time, due to coccidiosis, yersiniosis, salmonellosis. Rare in adults but can be seen with vitamin C deficiency
- Lethargy and anorexia – pneumonia, blindness/ocular disease, ovarian disease, ileus, any severe illness
- Weakness or collapse – hypoglycaemia, hypocalcaemia, lead poisoning, septicaemia, liver disease, renal disease, heart disease, neoplasia, ovarian disease, traumatic fractures, dystocia, urolithiasis
- Bone problems – fractures, arthritis, osteomyelitis

- Dental disease – caries, periodontal disease, overgrowth (Figure 95.1), malocclusion
- Vitamin C deficiency – dental disease, arthritis, bleeding into joints and under skin, poor skin healing, diarrhoea
- Skin disease – *Trixacarus caviae* (Figure 95.2), dermatophytosis (see Chapter 35).

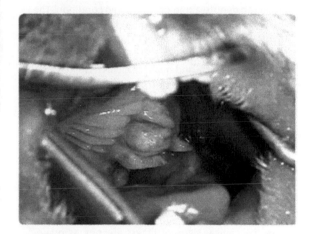

Figure 95.1 Dental spur in a Guinea pig

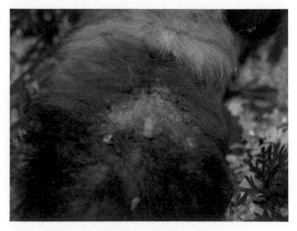

Figure 95.2 *Trixacarus caviae* infestation in a Guinea pig, showing typical scaling

100 Top Consultations in Small Animal General Practice, First Edition
By Peter Hill, Sheena Warman and Geoff Shawcross
© 2011 Blackwell Publishing Ltd

Diagnostic approach

When dealing with Guinea pigs, a rapid determination should be made as to whether or not treatment is likely to be successful, or if euthanasia is indicated. The age of the Guinea pig should be ascertained (if known), its sex and how long it has been ill. The owner may be able to describe some specific symptoms they have noticed (such as respiratory disease), but this is less typical than with dogs and cats. The owner should also be asked about the Guinea pig's diet, (including treats and differentiating what is offered from what is eaten) as inappropriate items can lead to diarrhoea.

Clinical examination should quickly establish the body condition. Prominent bones of the shoulder or hip region denote a thin or emaciated condition. The nostrils, eyes and prepuce/vagina should be checked for discharges and blockages. The tongue and oral cavity should be checked for lesions, discharges, dental overgrowth, and malocclusion. In Guinea pigs, the rear molars can overgrow and trap the tongue, making swallowing difficult and predisposing to aspiration. The oral mucosa should be checked for signs of septicaemia, indicated by petechiation. The skin, head, legs and feet should be examined for injuries, full range of movement or deformities. The heart and lungs can be easily auscultated. The abdomen should be gently palpated to check for masses. The skin should be examined for evidence of pruritus or hair loss.

As the clinical signs of illness are not as organ-specific as they are in dogs and cats, a minimum database of information is required to make a diagnosis and start useful treatment. This should include lateral and dorsoventral radiographs (Figure 95.3), haematology and blood biochemistry. Biochemistry should include glucose, calcium, phosphorus, urea, creatinine, CK, AST, albumin and globulin (total protein). As a minimum in the very sick animal, PCV and total protein are required, but ultrasonography can also be valuable in Guinea pigs.

A specific entity seen in Guinea pigs that isn't seen in rabbits or hamsters is vitamin C deficiency. This is a very common condition as Guinea pigs lack the enzyme L-gulonolactone oxidase and so require pre-formed vitamin C in the diet in order to make collagen and bile acids. Vitamin C deficiency affects joints, skin, healing, teeth, digestion and the urinary tract and can, therefore, result in lameness, skin disease, dental problems, diarrhoea, cystitis and urolithiasis. Vitamin C deficiency can be precipitated by the stress of pregnancy, lactation, advanced age, environmental stressors or concurrent disease.

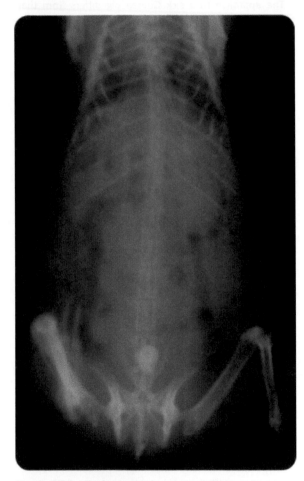

Figure 95.3 **Radograph showing urolithiasis in a Guinea pig**

Treatment

Initial stabilisation of the patient is important whilst a diagnostic evaluation is underway. Very sick Guinea pigs will benefit from glucose and saline Given SC or IP (see Table 95.1) and isolation in a warm cage or incubator at 25–30°C. If facilities are available, a relative humidity of 55% should be maintained as too dry an environment contributes to dehydration and respiratory disease. Anorexic Guinea pigs need food to prevent and reverse hepatic lipidosis. This can be achieved by repeated stomach tubing with vegetable puree mixed in an oral electrolyte solution, given at a volume of 10 ml every 3–4 hours. This should be done with care as Guinea pigs are prone to aspiration. Placement of a pharyngostomy tube can be easier in the long term.

Blanket antibiotic treatment (see Table 95.1) may be initiated if an infectious disease is suspected, but the diagnosis should be substantiated as soon as possible so that the correct drug, dose and treatment course can be prescribed. Respiratory infections can be treated with injectable antibiotics, such as enrofloxacin (for *Pasteurella* or *Mycoplasma* pneumonia). Nebulisation therapy with appropriate antibiotics such as fluoroquinolones or aminoglycosides can be used as well as, or instead of, parenteral therapy (see Table 95.1).

Diarrhoea can often be treated with fluid therapy and glucose alone, given orally or parenterally (SC or IP), as most causes are self-limiting. Specific treatment for ileus can also be given. It is usually the dehydration and ileus that are life-threatening, rather than the diarrhoea itself. In aged boars, soft faeces can accumulate in a rectal diverticulum and create a foul smell. This material can be easily expressed manually.

Overgrown incisors can be removed entirely or trimmed using a high-speed dental burr. Caries (surprisingly common in Guinea pigs and a cause of anorexia) and periodontal disease are best treated by tooth extraction. Obvious trauma such as leg fractures can either be dealt with by amputation or orthopaedic repair (Guinea pigs tolerate both splinting and external fixators well).

Vitamin C deficiency is treated by supplementation with 100 mg/kg for 7 days then a daily dose of 10 mg/kg for life. As the requirement for vitamin C increases at times of stress or disease, it is wise to treat any sick or injured Guinea pig with extra vitamin C to promote healing and prevent overt deficiency.

Table 95.1 Basic treatments for use in Guinea pigs (this is not a comprehensive formulary).

Drug	Dosage	Route	Frequency	Comment
Antimicrobials				
Enrofloxacin	20 mg/kg	SC	Once daily for up to 6 weeks	Treatment of bacterial infections. Can produce anorexia; not effective against anaerobes; oral treatment less effective
Fenbendazole	20–50 mg/kg	PO	Daily for 3–5 days	Care – toxicity has been suspected even at recommended doses
F10 (an antifungal disinfectant that can be inhaled)	Dilute 1:200	Nebulise for 30 min	1–2 daily for 6 weeks	Combine with relevant oral treatment for bacterial respiratory disease
Gentamicin	5–10 mg/kg	IM	Twice daily for 5 days	Especially *Pseudomonas* pneumonia; maintain hydration status; can be nebulised
Potentiated sulphonamide	30 mg/kg	SC	Twice daily	
Metronidazole	25–50 mg/kg	IM or PO	24 hours for 5 doses	Effective against anaerobes and flagellates

(*Continued*)

Table 95.1   (Continued)

Drug	Dosage	Route	Frequency	Comment
Sulphadimidine	1 g/L drinking water	PO	Continuous for 7 days, stop for 7 days then repeat	Coccidiosis
Itraconazole	10 mg/kg	PO	Once daily for 6 weeks	For Aspergillosis or other fungal respiratory disease, combine with nebulisation for optimum effect
Pain relief				
Meloxicam	0.2–0.4 mg/kg	PO or SC	Once daily	
Buprenorphine	0.05 mg/kg	SC	Every 3–4 hours	As required
Butorphanol	3–4 mg/kg	SC	Every 6 hours	For pre-emptive surgical pain or management of painful conditions
Sedation/anaesthesia				
Hypnorm (fentanyl /fluanisone)	1 ml/kg	SC	Once	Sedation or prior to addition of midazolam for general anaesthesia
Isoflurane	2–4%	Mask, then ET tube	Maintenance of anaesthesia	Swiftly induces anaesthesia, induction and recovery usually within 1 min
Miscellaneous				
Calcium EDTA	25 mg/kg	SC	Every 6 hours for 5 days	To treat lead toxicity
Ivermectin	0.2 mg/kg	SC or IM	Once or repeat weekly × 4 for mites	To treat worms. Toxicity reported with overdosing
Ranitidine	20 mg/kg	PO	1–2 times daily	To treat ulcers and ileus
Metoclopramide	0.5 mg/kg	SC	Twice daily	To treat ileus
Fluid therapy				
Lactated Ringer's	3–5% bodyweight per day	IO or IP	Maintenance of fluid balance	Required if Guinea pig >5% dehydrated or weak. Monitor PCV and urea if possible
Oral fluids	3–5% bodyweight per day	PO	Maintenance	Not if >5% dehydrated or weak. Otherwise, useful in an anorexic Guinea pig

ET = endotracheal tube.

Note: Antibiotics should be used with care in Guinea pigs as they are prone to caecal dysbiosis and clostridial overgrowth if inappropriate drugs, doses and routes are used. In general the parenteral route is safer and often has better pharmacodynamics than the oral route. Few drug dosages are based upon scientific investigation. The drugs listed above are used routinely by the author with clinical success. Note that many drugs are not licensed for this species Oral therapy, unless given directly from a syringe or a piece of favourite food, is rarely taken effectively if placed in water or feed bowls and is not recommended.

What if it doesn't get better?

Very sick Guinea pigs may require intraosseous fluid therapy. For respiratory disease nebulisation therapy may be used as well as parenteral therapy. If an accurate diagnosis has not been established and the Guinea pig fails to respond to appropriate supportive care, further diagnostic evaluation is required. This may entail laboratory work and diagnostic imaging, such as radiography and ultrasonography.

If a Guinea pig is not responding to treatment for a known diagnosis, or diagnostic evaluation is not permitted, euthanasia should be performed. This can be carried out by an intra-hepatic injection of barbiturate (quicker than IP), or induction of general anaesthesia using a gaseous anaesthetic followed by an intracardiac injection of barbiturate.

The low-cost option

Financial limitations may limit the diagnostic and therapeutic options when dealing with Guinea pigs. Clinicians may, therefore, have to prescribe treatment based on a tentative diagnosis, obtained from the history and physical examination alone. Such a diagnosis may not be accurate and clients must be made aware that the prognosis is uncertain. Clinicians should always place the welfare of the Guinea pig first and bear in mind that empirical supportive care may keep a Guinea pig alive when it is actually suffering from a fatal disease, such as terminal renal failure. If the only option permitted by the client is to try supportive care, the Guinea pig should be monitored for a rapid response. Euthanasia should be recommended if there is no improvement within a few hours.

When should I refer?

In many cases, referral of a Guinea pig will not be an option. However, some owners might consider this if there were a specialist within an appropriate distance. Any illness in a Guinea pig would benefit from being diagnosed and treated by a clinician with specific expertise and facilities for dealing with this species.

Sharon Redrobe

There are many species of bird and many reasons why they can get sick. The approach described here is particularly applicable to common pet birds, e.g. budgerigars, parrots, canaries but it is also applicable to other bird species. A major difference between illness in birds and dogs or cats is that birds typically 'hide' signs of disease until they are at a late stage, at which point they can rapidly decompensate. This leads to the impression that birds are weak as they may die 'suddenly' when sick but it should be appreciated they have been masking illness for some time before it is apparent to the owner. Sick birds should therefore always be seen urgently.

Common presentations and conditions affecting birds

- Lethargy, inappetence
  - Chlamydophilosis (psittacosis)
  - Aspergillosis pneumonia/air sacculitis
  - Bacterial pneumonia/air sacculitis
  - Hepatopathies
  - Vitamin A deficiency (usually because it leads to respiratory disease and renal failure)
  - Psittacine beak and feather disease (PBFD) virus
  - Polyomavirus
  - Herpesvirus
- Respiratory disease – bacterial, fungal (aspergillosis)
- Egg binding (particular lovebirds and cockatiels)
- Hypocalcaemic seizures (particularly African Grey Parrots)
- Collapse, weakness – hypoglycaemia, hypocalcaemia, lead poisoning, septicaemia, liver disease, renal disease, heart disease, neoplasia (particularly budgerigars), nutritional hyperparathyroidism and pathological fractures, traumatic fractures
- Feather problems – ectoparasites, stress, systemic disease, feather picking, nutritional deficiencies, PBFD virus, polyomavirus.

100 Top Consultations in Small Animal General Practice, First Edition
By Peter Hill, Sheena Warman and Geoff Shawcross
© 2011 Blackwell Publishing Ltd

Diagnostic approach

Important preliminary information obtained from the owner should include the bird's age (if known), sex (if known), length of time in the owner's possession, details of its husbandry (such as cage location, opportunity to fly), diet (including treats and differentiating what is offered from what is eaten), and whether the owner has any other birds. This information can help to determine if husbandry, nutritional, behavioural or contagious factors could be involved. The symptoms reported by the owner may be vague, but respiratory disease, skin conditions, diarrhoea or musculoskeletal disease may have been specifically noticed. It is also important to determine how long the bird has appeared sick.

It is strongly recommended that sick birds be examined under gaseous (isoflurane) anaesthesia to minimise stress and prevent death from prolonged restraint (Figure 96.1). Over-handling of a conscious sick bird can lead to rapid worsening of clinical signs and death. Clinical examination should quickly establish the body condition of the bird. A prominent keel indicates a thin bird, but overweight birds are also at risk of disease. The nares (nostrils), eyes and beak should be checked for discharges and blockages. The tongue and choana (slit in the roof of the mouth) should be checked for lesions or discharges. The choana should have papillae; loss of these is a sign of chronic sinusitis or vitamin A deficiency. The feathers should be checked for colouration and ability to knit together. Old and discoloured feathers are a sign of chronic disease, whereas chewed feathers may be a sign of ectoparasites. The wings and feet should be examined for injuries, full range of movement or deformities. The cloaca should be everted slightly with a moistened cotton bud to check for papillomata (common in Amazon parrots) and signs of septicaemia indicated by petechiation. Respiratory disease may be suggested by exaggerated tail movement (to assist ventilation when perching), fluffed up appearance, and open-mouthed breathing. The heart and lungs should be auscultated over the dorsum of the bird. Coelomic (the abdominal region of the bird) palpation for eggs and masses is useful. Note that abdominal masses or fluid can compress the air sacs and present as dyspnoea. PBFD may present in adults as feather dystrophy or feather plucking, with eventual white cell depletion and death from secondary infection. Young birds may present with white cell depletion and die before feather changes are evident.

As the clinical signs of illness are not as organ specific as they are in dogs and cats, a minimum database of information is required to make a diagnosis and start useful treatment. This should include a lateral and dorsoventral radiograph, haematology and blood biochemistry. Biochemistry should include uric acid, calcium, phosphorus and glucose as a minimum but preferably also bile acids, CK, AST, albumin and globulin (total protein). A faecal sample should be taken, especially from parrots (including cockatiels and budgerigars) and either submitted for a *Chlamydophila* PCR or saved for testing later should it be necessary (once treatment with a fluroquinolone such as enrofloxacin has started, this test cannot be performed accurately for weeks to months).

Further tests that might be required following the preliminary diagnostic investigations include:

- Bacterial or fungal cultures of respiratory discharges (nasal flush)
- PCR for polyoma and/or PBFD virus
- Aspergillus titre
- *Chlamydophila* serology or PCR
- Endoscopy of airsacs
- Liver biopsy

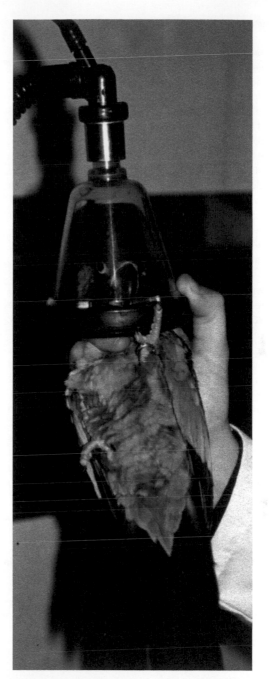

Figure 96.1   Anaesthesia of a bird to facilitate clinical examination

Section 16

Treatment

Very sick birds will benefit from a SC injection of lactated Ringer's solution (see Table 96.1) and isolation in a quiet, warm dark cage. If facilities exist, an incubator at 25–30°C with a relative humidity of 55% is ideal for hospitalisation, as too dry an environment contributes to dehydration and respiratory disease. Birds that appear strong can be crop-tubed (see Table 96.2). This should not be undertaken in birds that are closing their eyes or collapsing in the examination room, as they are likely to collapse and aspirate fluid, leading rapidly to death. Birds may appear brighter within the hour with careful hospitalisation and stabilisation. Diagnostic tests such as blood work and radiography can then be performed.

Respiratory infections in birds are best treated with appropriate systemic antifungal and/or antibacterial agents, and by nebulising with F10 (see Table 96.1). *Chlamydophila* is treated with a six-week course of daily enrofloxacin or weekly doxycycline.

Egg binding is treated by first ensuring the bird is hydrated and not hypoglycaemic. It should be placed in a warm dark area with a high humidity of at least 60%. Medical treatments include prostaglandin gel, which can be applied to the cloaca, or administration of oxytocin, but the use of this drug is controversial. If the bird fails to pass the egg unaided, surgery is indicated.

Vitamin A deficiency is treated by administering a complete, well balanced diet. It is rarely necessary to supplement with additional vitamin A and over-supplementation can result in toxicity leading to renal failure. Treatment of any associated problems, e.g. sinus or respiratory tract infection or nasal plugs may also be required. The return of choanal papillae and roughened feet (often absent in vitamin A deficiency), occur within 6–8 weeks of provision of an adequate diet.

Nutritional hyperparathyroidism is treated by the provision of a nutritionally complete diet. If the bird is suffering from hypocalcaemic tetany, careful parenteral dosing with calcium is required. Otherwise, dietary supplementation with excessive calcium or vitamin D3 is to be avoided as soft tissue calcification can occur. Radiographic evidence of resolution takes 6–8 weeks.

There is no cure for either PBFD or polyomavirus infections. Following a positive PCR test for these conditions, the bird should be isolated and the test repeated after 90 days. Some birds have been known to clear the infection. If a positive test remains after 90 days, the bird may be treated as positive. Many budgerigars live many years with polyoma causing little ill effects or merely the loss of the flight feathers. Likewise, there appears to be a lorikeet-specific PBFD that may cause not harm to the lorikeet but may cause disease in other psittacine birds. In general, therefore, psittacine birds of unknown polyoma or PBFD status should not be mixed together. A polyomavirus vaccine is available in the USA.

Table 96.1 Basic treatments for use in birds (this is not a comprehensive formulary).

Drug	Dosage	Route	Frequency	Comment
Antimicrobials				
Ceftazidime	50 mg/kg	IM/IV	4 × daily	Effective against aerobic and anaerobic bacteria – frequency of treatment makes impractical unless intensive care case
Enrofloxacin	5–15 mg/kg	IM	Once daily for 6 weeks	Treatment for psittacosis and bacterial infections. Can produce anorexia, not effective against anaerobes, oral treatment less effective

Table 96.1 (*Continued*)

Drug	Dosage	Route	Frequency	Comment
Gentamicin	5–10 mg/kg	IM	Twice daily for 5 days	Especially *Pseudomonas* pneumonia; maintain hydration status; can be nebulised
Metronidazole	25–50 mg/kg	IM	24 hours for 5 doses	Effective against anaerobes and flagellates
Itraconazole	10 mg/kg	PO	Once daily for 6 weeks	For aspergillosis; combine with nebulisation for optimum effect
Enilconazole (Imaverol: Janssen)	Dilute 1:10 solution	Nebulise for 30 min	1–2 × daily for 6 weeks	Combine with relevant oral treatment for aspergillosis
Fenbendazole	50 mg/kg once or 20 mg/kg daily for 3 days.	PO	As noted	Care – toxicity has been suspected following small overdose or recommended doses
F10 (an antifungal disinfectant that can be inhaled)	Dilute 1:200	Nebulise for 30 min	1–2 daily for 6 weeks	Combine with relevant oral treatment for aspergillosis or bacterial respiratory disease
Pain relief				
Butorphanol	3–4 mg/kg	IM	Every 6 hours	For pre-emptive surgical pain or management of painful conditions
Sedation/anaesthesia				
Isoflurane	2–4%	Mask, then intubate	Maintenance of anaesthesia	Swiftly induces anaesthesia, induction and recovery usually within 1 minute
Ketamine and medetomidine	Ketamine 5 mg/kg Medetomidine 75 µg/kg	IM	Once	5 mins to maximum effect of deep sedation or anaesthesia, duration up to 2 hours. Intubate and deliver oxygen/isoflurane

(*Continued*)

Table 96.1 (*Continued*)

Drug	Dosage	Route	Frequency	Comment
Miscellaneous				
Calcium gluconate	5–10 mg/kg	IM	Twice daily	As required
Oxytocin	5 IU/kg	IM	Daily or every other day until eggs passed	Can require repeated dosing, administer along with calcium gluconate
Ivermectin	0.1 mg/kg	SC or IM	Once or repeat weekly × 4 for mites	To treat worms. Toxicity with overdosing
Vitamin A (WITH CARE)	Max 12 000 IU/kg	IM	Once, repeat weekly	Often given as part of 'sick bird' regime; diet should also be corrected; fatal toxicity occurs with overdose
Thyroxine	20–100 µg/kg	PO	Once daily for 4 weeks or long-term treatment	To induce moult and treat hypothyroidism
Fluid therapy				
Oral fluids	3–5% bodyweight per day	PO	Maintenance	Useful in an anorexic bird but only if <5% dehydrated
Lactated Ringer's	3–5% bodyweight per day	IO or IV	Maintenance of fluid balance	Required if bird >5% dehydrated. Monitor PCV and urea

Note: This is not a comprehensive formulary. Few drug dosages are based upon scientific investigation. The drugs listed above are used routinely by the author with clinical success. Please note many drugs are not licensed for the species. Oral therapy, unless given via crop tube or a piece of favourite food, is rarely taken effectively by psittacines if placed in water or feed bowls and is not recommended.

Table 96.2 **Oral fluid therapy in birds. Crop tube volumes are approximate and should take into account the condition and size of the bird.**

Species	Volume (ml)	Frequency / day
Budgerigar	2	4
Amazon/African grey parrot	20	3
Macaw	50	3

What if it doesn't get better?

If treatment is being given on the basis of a tentative diagnosis, further diagnostic evaluation is required as described above. Very sick birds may require intra-osseous fluid therapy. If respiratory signs are severe, nebulisation therapy should be instituted, which can be continued at home by nebulising the cage. This allows treatment with minimal handling. If the bird appears to have airway obstruction, placement of an air sac tube can be life-saving. Some conditions in birds (neoplasia, renal failure, heart failure, liver disease) inherently carry a poor prognosis and a full recovery cannot be expected. Euthanasia can be performed by a hepatic injection of barbiturate (taking care not to inject into the airsac or death will occur from drowning) or general anaesthesia and an intrac-ardiac injection of barbiturate.

When should I refer?

Many clinicians now have specialist expertise in the management of bird diseases. Veterinarians who are not confident treating birds should always consider referral to such a specialist, particularly when owner expectations are high. Referral in such cases should be arranged early, and not after the bird has failed to respond to non-specific therapy. As with dogs and cats, referral should also be considered if a diagnosis has not been made following in-house diagnostic investigations and/or the practice does not have the equipment or expertise to perform and interpret more advanced procedures. If treatment has been prescribed, and the bird does not appear to be getting better after 24–48 hours, referral should definitely be offered.

The low-cost option

Empirically prescribed treatment in the absence of a specific diagnosis is unlikely to yield good results in sick birds. Empirical antibiosis (with or without anti-fungal treatment) may be initiated but the prognosis is uncertain and the bird's suffering may be unnecessarily protracted. This approach should really only be taken if a subsequent diagnostic evaluation is likely to yield a definitive diagnosis, allowing a proper drug, dose and treatment course to be prescribed. A prognosis should be established quickly to avoid unnecessary tests and treatment expense (e.g. if the bird has terminal gout as indicated by a very high uric acid level).

If a diagnostic evaluation is not possible due to financial limitations, the welfare of the bird should be paramount. If recovery seems unlikely, euthanasia should be recommended. The risk of zoonotic disease (e.g. chlamydophilosis) being inappropriately treated or not treated at all should also be considered.

Sharon Redrobe

Tortoises require specific care if they are to be kept as pets. Compared to mammalian species, they have very different husbandry and nutritional requirements. As reptiles, they should be kept within the correct temperature ranges for the species and with access to good UV broad-spectrum lighting. The tradition of keeping tortoises in UK gardens has led to many premature deaths because these environmental requirements are not met.

Common presentations and conditions affecting tortoises

The clinical signs of illness in tortoises are not as organ-specific as they are in dogs and cats and the most common presenting signs are anorexia, lethargy, weakness or collapse. These signs are caused most commonly by the following conditions:

- Stomatitis and rhinitis – Commonly caused by Herpes virus or Mycoplasma
- Respiratory disease (pneumonia) – Bacterial, fungal, mycoplasmal or viral infections
- Visceral and/or articular gout – Caused by dehydration leading to high uric acid levels
- Ovarian disease and/or egg binding – Note that the presence of eggs can be a normal finding, and detecting eggs in an anorexic female does not indicate that egg binding is the cause
- Shell problems – Fractures, nutritional osteodystrophy (especially young tortoises)
- Abscesses – Ear, skin
- Cloacal/penile prolapse – Usually secondary to extreme weakness/emaciation or straining because of bladder stones, eggs or (rarely) intestinal nematodes
- Blindness/ocular disease
- Hypoglycaemia, hypocalcaemia
- Lead poisoning
- Septicaemia
- Organ failure – Liver disease, renal disease, heart disease
- Neoplasia.

Post-hibernation anorexia (PHA) is not a diagnosis but a clinical presentation and tortoises should be evaluated for any of the conditions listed above. Uncomplicated PHA (where no disease process is present) may be due to sub-optimum hibernation protocols leading to starvation and/or dehydration. Giving oral glucose and fluids to provide energy and reduce the elevated urea caused by prolonged hibernation, and placing the tortoise under a UV lamp can be sufficient to stimulate appetite.

Diagnostic approach

A tortoise will often have been ill for many weeks or months before presentation so a rapid and accurate diagnosis followed by appropriate treatment is required for a successful outcome. Careful history taking and stabilisation of the patient is important. A detailed history should be obtained from the owner to include:

- Signalment – Age and sex (male tortoises have a longer tail with a vent slit at the end, and tend to walk carrying it tucked to the side; females have a short tail with a vent slit very close to the plastron/shell)
- Duration of the illness
- Diet – Including treats and differentiating between what is offered and what is eaten
- Husbandry – Including housing, substrate, lighting, and maximum and minimum temperatures (estimated if kept outside)
- The presence or absence of other reptiles and when these were introduced.

The first aspect of the clinical examination is to establish the body condition of the tortoise. This is best achieved by palpating the bones of the shoulder or hip region. Prominent bones denote a thin or emaciated condition. The Jackson ratio (body weight to length ratio) provides a crude assessment of the body condition of *Testudo graeca* or *Testudo hermanni* species of tortoises, but it can be misleading. For example, a tortoise may be thin and yet of apparently normal weight due to the presence of eggs, oedema, severe pneumonia, excess coelomic fluid or a large

100 Top Consultations in Small Animal General Practice, First Edition
By Peter Hill, Sheena Warman and Geoff Shawcross
© 2011 Blackwell Publishing Ltd

bladder stone. Hence, the ratio cannot be used as a reliable guide to a tortoise's health and should never be used instead of a full clinical assessment. Further details on measuring this ratio can be found on the Tortoise Trust website.

A full physical examination is more limited in tortoises than it is in dogs and cats because of the shell. The nares (nostrils), eyes and beak should be checked for discharges and blockages. The ear (tympanic membrane) should be checked for swelling (usually due to an abscess, but rarely fluid or neoplasia; Figure 97.1). The tongue and choana (slit in the roof of the mouth) should be checked for lesions or discharges (Figure 97.2). The skin and shell (top = carapace, bottom = plastron), head, legs and feet should be examined for injuries, full range of movement or deformities. The oral mucosa should be checked for signs of septicaemia, indicated by petechiation. The heart and lungs cannot be easily auscultated, and the abdomen cannot be palpated. Diagnosis of diseases of these organs relies upon radiography, ultrasonography and blood tests. The diagnosis of respiratory disease can be challenging in tortoises because radiographic changes in the lungs can indicate acute pneumonia, chronic pneumonia or scarring (Figures 97.3 and 97.4). Definitive differentiation requires a lung biopsy, a procedure that is relatively routine when performed by specialists. Lung lavage is very unlikely to yield a diagnostic sample as the fluid is unlikely to reach the distal areas of the lung and is often merely a tracheal lavage. Eggs or bladder stones may also be seen on radiographs and may or may not be contributing to the current illness as these can be tolerated for years.

Other than conditions such as abscesses, most illnesses in tortoises cannot be diagnosed on history and physical examination alone and further information is required to make a diagnosis and start useful treatment. The minimum requirements include haematology (especially PCV), biochemistry (uric acid, urea, calcium, phosphorus, glucose, CK, AST, total protein, albumin and globulin) and radiography (three standard views: lateral, cranio-caudal and dorsoventral).

Blood samples from tortoises are best obtained from the jugular vein. Alternatively, the dorsal tail vein or subcarapacial vein may be used but both may result in lymph dilution. Restraint for blood sampling or radiography is best achieved by giving a low dose of ketamine IM (3 mg/kg for tortoises weighing up to 3 kg for 20–40 minutes of sedation), or alfaxalone (2 mg/kg IV for tortoises weighing up to 3 kg for 20–40 minutes of anaesthesia) which requires intubation and intermittent positive-pressure ventilation (IPPV).

Specific testing may be required for certain differentials:

- Herpes virus infection – An oral swab or nasal flush submitted for Herpes virus PCR (chelonian Herpes virus)
- Mycoplasma infections – An oral swab or nasal flush submitted for Mycoplasma PCR (*M. agassizi*)
- Aspergillosis – Serum antibody titre, cytology or biopsy for histology
- Intestinal nematodes – Faecal parasitology.

Some tortoises may be suffering from multiple conditions. For example, the common *Testudo graeca* species (known as the Greek or spur-thighed tortoise) or *Testudo hermanni* (known as the Herman's or spur-tailed tortoise) are commonly kept in UK gardens and are often suffering from chronic pneumonia, gout and arthritis (with females also often suffering from ovarian disease; Figure 97.5).

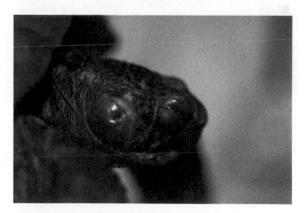

Figure 97.1   Tympanic abscess in a tortoise

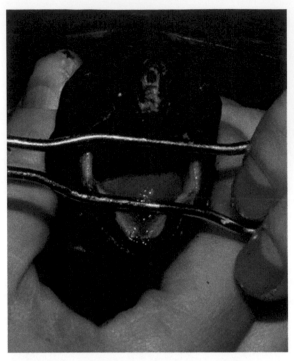

Figure 97.2   Examination of the oral cavity in a tortoise

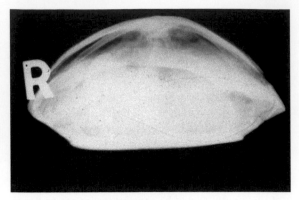

Figure 97.4   Radiograph of a tortoise with pneumonia

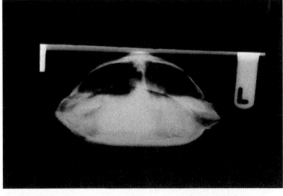

Figure 97.3   Normal radiographic appearance of tortoise lungs

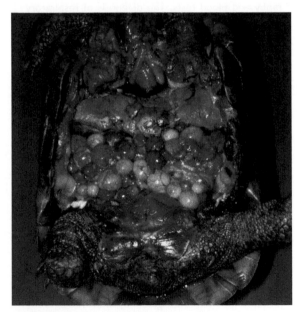

Figure 97.5   Post mortem appearance of a tortoise with follicular stasis

Treatment

Very sick tortoises will benefit from the administration of glucose and saline (see Table 97.1) and isolation in a warm cage or incubator at 25–30°C, with a relative humidity of 55%. Too dry an environment contributes to dehydration and respiratory disease. The provision of a broad-spectrum UV A and B 'reptile' light is essential.

It should be remembered that anorexia (including PHA) is a common presenting sign in tortoises, but this is a symptom and not a diagnosis. The animal needs to be fed (artificially if required) to prevent further starvation but a diagnosis needs to be established. Many anorexic tortoises (providing there is not major disease present) can be encouraged to eat if they are placed under broad-spectrum lighting and in a warmer environment, especially those that have been kept in suboptimal conditions such as a UK garden. If anorexia is persistent, assisted feeding and fluid therapy is required to prevent/reverse hepatic lipidosis and the development of irreversible terminal visceral gout (a consequence of elevated uric acid levels following dehydration). Assisted feeding can be performed in tortoises by repeated stomach tubing (Figure 97.6), although feeding via a pharyngostomy tube can be easier in the long term. Fluid therapy can be given orally, IV (in very sick tortoises, via a jugular catheter), or IO (into the femur or bony bridge between plastron and carapace; Figure 97.7).

Blanket antibiotic and antifungal treatment (see Table 97.1) may be initiated if an infectious disease is suspected, but the diagnosis should be substantiated as soon as possible, so that a disease-specific therapeutic course can be prescribed.

Obvious trauma such as leg or shell fractures requires the same approach to orthopaedic repair as in domestic mammals, with attention to reptile anatomy. Fibreglass repair of shells is no longer recommended because it can trap infection and delay healing. Shell fractures are best managed surgically using screws and wires to stabilise and approximate the fracture pieces and bandaging until healing has sealed the defect. Abscesses require surgical removal because the pus is too thick to allow lancing and drainage, and antibiotics cannot penetrate.

Tortoises require specific management during and after hibernation. Many problems occur at this time, usually in part because the hibernation protocol was suboptimal. Hibernation occurs in response to shortening day length and falling temperatures. For successful hibernation, the tortoise needs to have emptied its intestines, stopped eating and slowed down its metabolism. The hibernation environment needs to be monitored and maintained at 6–10°C. Any higher and the animal can starve during hibernation; any lower and it can suffer frost damage to organs, particularly the retina. This temperature can be achieved in a garden shed or attic, but it is ideally achieved in a designated fridge (a domestic fridge will suffice). The box in which the tortoise is contained should contain some bedding material (shredded paper is ideal) and have adequate air circulation. The tortoise should be checked daily. If the tortoise is awake and moving, it should be offered food and water. In the wild, many tortoise species have short periods of hibernation interrupted by foraging expeditions. Attempting to maintain a prolonged hibernation for 4–6 months is quite unnatural in most species. Hibernation should be monitored and not last longer than 3 months; 6 weeks is usually long enough. On emergence from hibernation, the tortoise should be placed into a shallow bowl of lukewarm water to allow drinking and encourage urination and defecation. This rehydration also serves to reduce the accumulated urea, which suppresses appetite. Tortoises should drink and eat on the day of emergence. Many owners leave the animal for weeks or months without eating before presenting them to the vet. Many of these animals will have severe hepatic lipidosis and are at risk of fatal visceral gout by this stage.

Hibernation places an added stress on sick animals so tortoises that have been sick should be prevented from hibernating. This is achieved by keeping them in a warm, well-lit area. A reptile tank is ideal although many owners manage with a warm kitchen and a UV reptile spotlight. Alternatively, hibernation should be restricted to 3–6 weeks only, under optimal hibernation conditions. The tortoise should then be allowed to awaken by placing it into a shallow bowl of lukewarm water. This should stimulate recovery and prevent another hibernation attempt that season. Pre- and post-hibernation checks should involve a full clinical examination and bodyweight check. There is no value in a 'traditional' one-off multivitamin injection, which may risk hypervitaminosis A if the dosing is not accurate.

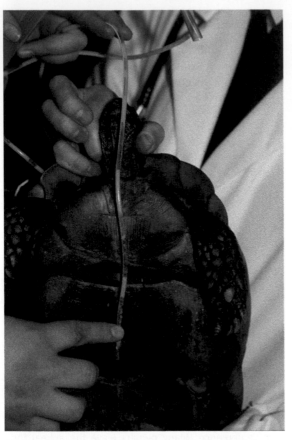

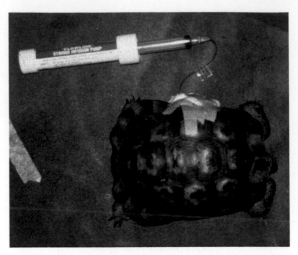

Figure 97.7   Intraosseous fluid therapy in a tortoise

Figure 97.6   Measuring the appropriate stomach
tube length in a tortoise

Table 97.1   Basic treatments for use in tortoises (this is not a comprehensive formulary).

IM injections can be given in the scapular muscles (around the base of the neck; take care not to inject into the neck) or the gluteal muscles (at the rear of the legs). IV injections can be given in the jugular vein, subcarapacial vein or, with more difficulty, into the dorsal tail vein or femoral vein.

Drug	Dosage	Route	Frequency	Comment
Antimicrobials				
Ceftazidime	20 mg/kg	IM	Every 72 h for 10 doses	Effective against aerobic and anaerobic bacteria
Enrofloxacin	5 mg/kg	IM	Every 24–48 h for 10 doses	Can produce anorexia, not effective against anaerobes
Metronidazole	25–50 mg/kg	IM	Every 24 h for 7–14 doses	Effective against anaerobes and flagellates
Gentamicin	5–10 mg/kg	IM	Twice daily for 5 days	Especially *Pseudomonas* pneumonia; maintain hydration status; can be nebulised

Table 97.1 (*Continued*)

Drug	Dosage	Route	Frequency	Comment
Enilconazole (Imaverol, Janssen)	Dilute 1:10 solution	Nebulise for 30 min	1–2 × daily for 6 weeks	Combine with relevant oral treatment for Aspergillosis
F10 (an antifungal disinfectant that can be inhaled)	Dilute 1:200	Nebulise for 30 min	1–2 × daily for 6 weeks	Combine with relevant oral treatment for Aspergillosis or bacterial respiratory disease
Itraconazole	10 mg/kg	PO	Once daily for 6 weeks	For Aspergillosis; combine with nebulisation for optimum effect
Fenbendazole	50 mg/kg once or 20 mg/kg daily for 3–5 days	PO	As noted	Toxicity not yet reported in chelonians but snake toxicity reported following large overdose
Pain relief				
Buprenorphine	0.05	IM	Every 6 h	For pre-emptive surgical pain or management of painful conditions
Sedation/anaesthesia				
Propofol	10–15 mg/kg	IV	For induction of anaesthesia	5 min to maximum effect, lasts approx 20 min
Ketamine	3–5 mg/kg	IM	For sedation; once	20 min to max effect, for sedation to enable gavage or other minor procedures, duration 1 h, usually spontaneous respiration maintained
Ketamine	50 mg/kg	IM	For deep sedation; once	20 min to maximum effect of deep sedation or anaesthesia, duration up to 6 h
Alfaxalone	2–5 mg/kg	IV	For induction of general anaesthesia	Recovery occurs after 20–30 min. Incremental doses every 20–30 min may be used to prolong anaesthesia
Isoflurane	2–4%	ET tube	Maintenance of anaesthesia	Not for induction – tortoises can hold their breath for prolonged periods! Assisted ventilation usually required
Miscellaneous				
Calcium gluconate	5–10 mg/kg	IM	Twice daily	As required
Ivermectin	DO NOT USE IN TORTOISES – FATAL			
Oxytocin	5 IU/kg	IM	Daily or every other day until eggs passed	Can require repeated dosing

(*Continued*)

Table 97.1 *(Continued)*

Drug	Dosage	Route	Frequency	Comment
Vitamin A	Max 12 000 IU/kg	IM	Once	Often given as part of 'sick tortoise' regime; rarely required. Fatal toxicity occurs with overdose
Fluid therapy				
Oral fluids	3% bodyweight per day	PO	Maintenance	Useful in an anorexic tortoise, but only if <5% dehydrated
Parenteral fluids (lactated Ringer's or 1 part Ringer's: 2 parts 2.5% dextrose in 0.45% saline)	3% bodyweight per day	IO or IV	Maintenance of fluid balance	Monitor PCV and uric acid; required if animal >5% dehydrated

Note: Few drug dosages are based upon scientific investigation. The drugs listed above are used routinely by the author with clinical success. Please note, many drugs are not licensed for the species.

What if it doesn't get better?

If treatment is being given on the basis of a tentative diagnosis, further diagnostic evaluation is required as described above. If severe respiratory disease is present, nebulisation therapy should be commenced in addition to parenteral treatment. Very sick tortoises may require intraosseous fluid therapy. Some conditions in tortoises (neoplasia, renal failure, heart failure, liver disease) inherently carry a poor prognosis and a full recovery cannot be expected. Euthanasia can be performed by a hepatic injection of barbiturate or an intracardiac injection of barbiturate. The liver is accessed via the prefemoral fossa, aiming laterally and cranially. Because there is a risk of missing the liver and lacerating the bladder, syringe aspiration before injection is required. Blood in the needle hub confirms organ penetration. The heart is accessed by placing the needle ventral to the head and neck and advancing parallel to the plastron to a distance of two plastral scales (this often requires pre-measurement and a long needle). Death in tortoises can be confirmed by total immobility and lack of a bite response when the glottis or tongue is depressed (a blunt probe should be used for this as a bite from a tortoise is surprisingly strong). Additionally, as glottal closure is under muscular control, if the glottis is open the tortoise is either inspiring (which may take over a minute) or dead. Therefore, the mouth should be opened and the tortoise checked for an open glottis for at least a minute whilst attempting to stimulate glottal closure or a bite by applying light pressure to the tongue or glottis.

The low-cost option

Empirically prescribed treatment in the absence of a specific diagnosis is unlikely to yield good results in sick tortoises. Empirical antibiosis (with or without antifungal treatment) may be initiated but the prognosis is uncertain and the tortoise's suffering may be unnecessarily protracted. A prognosis should be established quickly to avoid unnecessary tests and treatment expense (for example, if the tortoise has terminal gout, as indicated by a very high uric acid and phosphorus level).

Fluid therapy and glucose treatment can be lifesaving in the short term, but non-specific treatment of the anorexic tortoise (feeding, fluids and antibiotics) without a diagnosis should be avoided as the patient may be preserved for many weeks in this condition whilst actually becoming sicker and making a cure less likely.

If a diagnostic evaluation is not possible due to financial limitations, the welfare of the tortoise should be paramount. If a recovery does not seem likely, euthanasia should be recommended.

When should I refer?

Many clinicians now have specialist expertise in the management of tortoise diseases. Veterinarians who are not confident treating tortoises should always consider referral to such a specialist, particularly when owner expectations are high. Referral in such cases should be arranged early, ideally not after the tortoise has failed to respond to non-specific therapy for several weeks. As with dogs and cats, referral should also be considered if a diagnosis has not been made following in-house diagnostic investigations and/or if the practice does not have the equipment to hospitalise a tortoise or the expertise to perform and interpret more advanced procedures. If treatment has been prescribed, and the tortoise does not appear to be getting better after 48–72 hours, referral should definitely be offered.

Section 17
Miscellaneous

Geoff Shawcross

Before any surgery is carried out, it is wise to give the owner a realistic view of what the proposed procedure is likely to achieve, the expected rate of post-operative progress and the potential complications. These comments should be reiterated when the patient is discharged after surgery, and a protocol put in place to monitor post-operative progress. Under no circumstances should an animal be discharged unless the veterinary surgeon is certain that recovery from anaesthesia is complete, that vital signs are satisfactory and stable, and that analgesia is adequate. Pre-existing disease, such as renal disease, diabetes mellitus, hyperadrenocorticism or blood clotting disorders (e.g. Von Willebrand's disease) may increase the risk of post-surgical complications.

Some procedures (e.g. cat castration) may not routinely require a post-operative check-up, particularly if there are no sutures requiring removal. However, it is important to ensure that the owner is aware of the expected recovery rate and how to recognise post-operative complications (usually characterised by general malaise, wound interference and wound swelling). As a guiding principle, it is generally unwise to rely entirely on the owner's view of progress, as owners rarely have the experience to make the correct decisions. Some are overly cautious, while others are apparently oblivious to the most obvious complications. As the practice bears the responsibility for the outcome of the surgery, it is prudent to monitor progress appropriately. To avoid any possible confusion, the owner should be provided with written instructions clearly stating when the animal should be re-examined, the treatment regime to be followed, and signs that could suggest the development of complications.

Surgeons have personal preferences for different skin suture patterns. Interrupted suture patterns (simple or mattress) are commonly used. Mattress sutures are very secure and difficult for the animal to remove but can become embedded if there is significant tissue swelling. The use of a continuous, subdermal suture to close skin wounds has the advantage that suture removal is unnecessary and unintentional removal by the animal is unlikely, but these advantages have to be weighed against the

100 Top Consultations in Small Animal General Practice, First Edition
By Peter Hill, Sheena Warman and Geoff Shawcross
© 2011 Blackwell Publishing Ltd

consequences of total wound breakdown should the suture fail. Some surgeons may also use skin staples. Most skin sutures or staples can be removed 7–10 days postoperatively. However, when dealing with large wounds, especially where some sutures are under tension, staged removal of sutures should be considered.

Dealing with common complications

At a post-surgery check-up, the animal should receive a full physical examination as well as an examination of the wound. Clinical findings need to be interpreted in the context of the type of surgery carried out. The potential for serious complications is much higher following intra-abdominal, thoracic or orthopaedic procedures than following minor, superficial interventions.

- **Malaise** – Lethargy and poor appetite are not uncommon immediately after surgery. This is usually due to an anaesthetic 'hangover' or post-operative pain but should rapidly improve. It is more common in older patients and those that have undergone major surgery. A balanced approach to analgesia, both pre and post-operatively, should minimise problems associated with pain. By 24 hours, all patients should be brighter and showing an interest in their surroundings. If progress is slower than expected the patient should be examined. Body temperature should be checked, assessments for blood loss made, and consideration given to checking for electrolyte disturbances, dehydration, and liver and kidney function.
- **Post-operative haemorrhage** – Haemorrhage is usually apparent in the recovery phase, immediately following surgery, but it can occur a few days post-operatively due to ligature-induced necrosis or wound interference. Haemorrhage from superficial blood vessels is rarely problematic and will resolve with the application of a pressure bandage. The diagnosis of post-operative internal haemorrhage can be difficult but usually the first indication is that the anaesthetic recovery phase is slow. Pale mucous membranes, poor capillary refill and cold extremities are suggestive of blood loss and the decision has to be made whether to re-operate or not. Although conservative management may be successful

(e.g. using a tight abdominal bandage and fluid replacement therapy), the author's view is that valuable time may be lost. Should the animal's condition continue to deteriorate and surgical intervention become essential, the anaesthetic risks are greatly increased.

- **Wound swelling** – It is important to differentiate between hernias, seromas, haematomas and abscesses. Wound swelling can lead to discomfort, which encourages wound interference, and excessive tension on the sutures will predispose to wound breakdown.

- **Herniation** – It should be possible to diagnose herniation through an abdominal incision by careful palpation; the edges of the muscle layer are usually palpable and it should be possible to reduce the contents. However, this is not always straightforward as there may be considerable tissue reaction, early fibrosis and seroma formation, so care must be exercised before dismissing the possibility of a hernia being present. Hernias should always be treated as a matter of urgency as there is a substantial risk of the skin wound breaking down, leading to eventration (protrusion of the intestines through the abdominal wall). The surgical wound should be protected from interference with a dressing or an Elizabethan collar whenever possible, pending surgical repair.

- **Other swellings** – Seromas are fluid-filled sub-cutaneous swellings that occur along the wound line. They are non painful and can usually be easily recognised. Certain types of surgery (e.g. radical mastectomy, removal of large skin tumours) carry a higher risk of seroma formation and wound dehiscence. In these cases the complication rate can be reduced by careful pre-operative planning to ensure that sutures are not placed under too much tension, good surgical technique is used so that tissues are not traumatised unnecessarily, and that drainage tubes are placed. Small seromas and those not putting the skin sutures under too much tension should be left alone as they will resolve spontaneously within a 7–10 day period. Unnecessary interference risks introducing infection and the development of an abscess. Large seromas need to be drained and, whenever possible, a sterile dressing should be applied to prevent wound interference, absorb serum leakage and occlude the subcutaneous dead-space.

If there is uncertainty about the nature of a fluid-filled swelling, it should be aspirated using a sterile needle and syringe (if fluid is not leaking from the incision). This will distinguish between a seroma, haematoma or abscess.

Abscesses should be drained and a swab taken for culture and sensitivity testing; broad-spectrum antibiosis should be instigated pending the laboratory results. Because effective drainage of an abscess is paramount, it may be advantageous to remove one or two sutures. Necrotic tissue and sutures can act as a focus of infection, which may not resolve until the nidus is surgically removed.

Generally, haematomas are best left alone. Drainage by needle aspiration is not usually possible because of blood clots and further disruption of the clot may lead to the haemorrhage restarting. Interference also increases the risk of introducing infection and abscess formation.

- **Wound interference** – Wound interference is an ever-present risk with animals as it is largely in their nature to want to lick wounds. However, interference is much more likely if the wound is uncomfortable because sutures are too tight, infection is present or there is leakage of serum from the wound. When interference is likely, wounds should be protected by either a dressing or the use of an Elizabethan-type collar.

- **Wound breakdown** – Wound breakdown can occur for various reasons such as excessive tension, inadequate blood supply, skin necrosis, infection or self-trauma. The clinician needs to make a decision as to how a wound breakdown is best managed. Removal of sutures by the animal is best treated by re-suturing. Replacement of one or two sutures can be achieved by passing a 21-gauge needle through both sides of the wound edges, and then passing a piece of suture material through the bore. When the needle is removed, the suture can be held in place and tied. More extensive suture loss may require re-suturing under general anaesthesia. Wound breakdowns due to infections, skin necrosis or inadequate blood supply should not be re-sutured as further failure is inevitable. Infections should be managed medically and the wound left to heal by secondary intention until the infection is cleared. A decision can then be made as to whether further surgical intervention would speed up the healing process. Wound breakdowns due to inadequate blood supply or skin necrosis should either be left to heal by secondary intention, or treated with more advanced surgical techniques, such as skin grafts or flaps.

- **Surgical errors** – When unexpected complications arise, the clinician should always consider the possibility that a surgical error has been made. This might include leaving in swabs, use of inappropriate suture material, inadequate ligation of vessels, damage to previously healthy structures (e.g. accidental ligation of a ureter) or inappropriate dosing of drugs. Such errors should be recognised as soon as possible and the appropriate remedial action taken.

- **Meticillin-resistant infections** – Strains of *Staphylococcus aureus* or *pseudintermedius* that are resistant to multiple antibiotics have become common in human hospitals and are increasing in prevalence in veterinary facilities. If what appears to be a routine post-operative wound infection does not respond to appropriate treatment, a swab should be submitted for culture and sensitivity to see if antibiotic resistance is a problem. Identification of meticillin-resistant strains needs to be taken very seriously because they can cause infections in multiple patients once they become established in a hospital. Guidelines on dealing with such infection can be found on the BSAVA website.

Managing dressings

Dressings may be used to protect a wound from interference, provide support during repair, hold medication in place, or absorb discharges. The function of the dressing will dictate the way it is managed.

Leg dressings are the most common and can be used for support or protection of a wound. As treatment may last several weeks, the dressings will need to be renewed at frequent intervals and care must be taken in their application. Padding needs to be placed between the toes and over bony prominences to prevent pressure necrosis of the skin. Bandages applied too tightly to limbs or the tail can act like a ligature, cutting off the blood supply and leading to extensive necrosis that may necessitate amputation. The ligature effect may also occur if a leg dressing does not include the foot. If the foot is left exposed, there is the possibility that it will swell and become painful, which in turn, will lead to chewing at the dressing/foot and possibly necrosis. Leg dressings are best replaced at 5-day intervals when covering a wound. When splints or casts are used, they should be checked every 5–7 days to ensure they have not slipped, and are secure and comfortable.

Care must be exercised when applying a head dressing as it is very easy to apply one too tightly, which will cause breathing difficulties. Whenever possible, one pinna should be left out of the dressing as this helps keep the dressing in place. Initially, the dressing should be changed at 2–3-day intervals if ear canal surgery has been carried out, as these wounds tend to weep, resulting in a wet dressing that becomes uncomfortable very quickly. As the wound heals, the interval between redressing can be extended up to 5 days. When the pinna is included in the dressing, it should be folded over the top of the head and well padded under the earflap to avoid ulceration.

When applying elasticated bandages, they should be unrolled a short distance and then 'applied' over the padded layer; this prevents the bandage from being applied too tightly.

Owners must be advised to keep the dressing dry at all times and that it must be replaced if it gets too wet. A plastic bag over the dressing will provide temporary protection from moisture but it must be removed as soon as possible. When an animal tries to remove a dressing, it is sensible to presume that it is uncomfortable and the dressing should be checked or replaced (this is particularly true when the previous dressing was well tolerated). Only when the clinician is satisfied that the animal is being mischievous should the dressing be protected by additional constraint, such as an Elizabethan collar.

Monitoring progress

With a substantial number of surgical cases, the need for post-operative monitoring ends when sutures are removed (neutering, benign skin lesions) but for some procedures, return to full function takes longer than simply the time taken for the surgical wound to heal. Many orthopaedic procedures (e.g. cruciate repair, fracture repair, total hip replacement/femoral head arthroplasty) can be expected to take many weeks to resolve and should be checked at 10–14 day intervals for the first 6–10 weeks, followed by less frequent rechecks until the animal has returned to the expected level of function. Improvements should be steady and the owner can be advised about appropriate levels of exercise or physiotherapy during these visits. The owner should be warned that any sudden deterioration needs to be evaluated at the earliest opportunity.

Sue Shaw

Increased mobility of dogs and cats over long distances and through different bioclimatic areas has resulted in the relatively rapid appearance of infectious diseases in areas where they were previously absent. The major zoonotic disease of concern in travelling animals is rabies, although the risk is low if licensed vaccination regimes are used as recommended by the manufacturer, and if the risk of exposure from wild or feral sources is minimal. The most commonly diagnosed illnesses in travelling companion animals are vector-transmitted diseases in dogs. Cats are less likely to travel over long distances and appear to be less susceptible to major vector-borne diseases. Dogs travelling from countries bordering the Mediterranean, or central, eastern and Northern Europe, have been the source of increasing reports of diseases previously considered as 'exotic', and establishment of these infections in local vector and/or dog populations is occurring. Any history of travel in an animal's history is important; disease within a few days/weeks of travel may be easy to associate with exposure to unusual infections but those with sub-clinical infection may develop disease months/years after exposure if immunologically compromised (e.g. by surgery, immunosuppressive therapy, systemic illness, or neoplasia).

Common differential diagnoses

- **Babesiosis (piroplasmosis)** – Caused by tick-transmitted protozoan parasites that are adapted to red blood cells. In dogs, infection occurs throughout the world in temperate and tropical countries. The species most frequently causing disease in dogs are *Babesia canis* and *Babesia gibsoni*, although several new species have been identified in the past 10 years. Feline babesiosis (*B. felis*) is primarily seen in cats that have travelled from southern African countries. The common Babesia species affecting dogs and cats have minimal zoonotic significance
- **Ehrlichiosis and anaplasmosis** – Caused by tick-transmitted bacteria that invade circulating white cells or platelets (depending on the ehrlichial species). The most commonly diagnosed are monocytic ehrlichiosis caused by *Ehrlichia canis* and cyclic thrombocytopenia caused by *Anaplasma platys*. Both have a similar distribution in tropical and temperate areas of the world as they share the same species of tick vector. Ehrlichiosis is rare in cats. The common ehrlichial species have negligible zoonotic implications but some rarer species diagnosed in the Americas are considered zoonotic
- **Leishmaniosis** – Caused by sand fly-transmitted protozoan parasites of the *Leishmania* genus. *Leishmania infantum* is the most common species affecting dogs. Infection is widespread in countries bordering the Mediterranean. The parasites invade tissue macrophages not only causing chronic local granulomatous inflammation but also widespread dissemination of infection in susceptible dogs. Feline *Leishmania* infection may occur in areas where the canine disease is prevalent but it is still considered to be rare. Leishmaniosis is a zoonotic disease, and dogs are the main reservoir host for *L. infantum* but direct infection from infected dogs to humans without the vector has not been reported. Even so, close contact between infected dogs and humans who could be immunosuppressed should be discouraged
- **Dirofilariosis (heartworm)** – Caused by the mosquito-transmitted nematode parasite *Dirofilaria immitis,* which has a worldwide distribution in tropical and temperate areas with warm summers. Intermediate stages of *D. immitis* migrate to the pulmonary artery where they mature. Feline heartworm disease is less common and cats are accidental hosts for infection. *D. immitis* can also be accidentally transmitted to humans resulting in pulmonary and ocular granuloma formation, but this is extremely rare and occurs only in areas of high prevalence.

100 Top Consultations in Small Animal General Practice, First Edition
By Peter Hill, Sheena Warman and Geoff Shawcross
© 2011 Blackwell Publishing Ltd

Diagnostic approach

These conditions may cause overlapping clinical signs so they need to be considered as a group if a pet presents with non-specific symptoms. Common presenting signs seen with these conditions include:

- **Babesiosis (piroplasmosis)** – Fever, lethargy, weakness, red urine (haemoglobinuria) and collapse in severe cases. Later, severe anaemia, jaundice and multiple organ failure can occur. Further clinical and clinicopathological examination reveals further consequences of haemolytic anaemia and spenomegaly
- **Ehrlichiosis** – Fever, lymphadenopathy, bleeding (petechiation, haematuria, epistaxis, retinal haemorrhage). Thrombocytopenia is the most common finding on further clinicopathological examination. Chronic infection may be associated with splenomegaly, weight loss, panophthalmic disease, other signs of immune-mediated disease and bone marrow hypoplasia with cytopenias. The latter is reportedly more common in German Shepherd dogs and related breeds
- **Leishmaniosis** – Skin lesions (alopecia, scaling, ulceration, and nodules), lymphadenopathy, weight loss, muscle atrophy, epistaxis and panophthalmitis. Further clinicopathological investigation may reveal splenomegaly, glomerulopathy and polyarthritis
- **Dirofilariosis (heartworm)** – Dogs: exercise intolerance, coughing, weight loss, and occasionally death. The onset of disease is usually slow (months to years) unless the dog has been exposed to a large number of infected mosquitoes at the same time. Cats: more rapid onset of disease and increased severity compared to dogs. Signs are dominated by sudden-onset lethargy, exercise intolerance, coughing and sudden death. In areas of high prevalence, up to 20% of cats may be infected but few worms reach maturity in the pulmonary artery.

For all these conditions, full haematological, biochemical and urinalysis is required, not only to aid diagnosis, but also to evaluate organ dysfunction and provide baseline values to use in assessing therapeutic response. Thoracic imaging may reveal characteristic pulmonary artery changes with Dirofilariosis, but it is also recommended to assess cardiopulmonary function prior to therapy.

Diagnosis of the specific organism involved may involve multiple tests and owners should be advised that a single test may not provide the answer. The following tests can be valuable:

- Blood smears may demonstrate *Babesia* and *Ehrlichia* organisms, and occasionally *Leishmania* or microfilaria
- Cytology of lymph node, bone marrow or splenic aspirates may be used for *Leishmania* or ehrlichial infection. However, more sensitive and specific tests are available commercially
- PCR-based methods are widely available to identify (and in many cases quantify) *Babesia*, *Ehrlichia*, *Leishmania* (and in some countries *Dirofilaria*) DNA in blood, bone marrow, lymph node aspirates, conjunctival swabs or biopsies
- Antigen serology testing is widely available for diagnosis of *D. immitis* infection
- Serological tests looking for antibody responses to infection are available but have varying sensitivity and/or specificity. It is advisable to contact your local diagnostic laboratory for interpretation
- Histopathology of skin or lymph node biopsies may be useful for *Leishmania* diagnosis although both sensitivity and specificity are limited.

Treatment

Treatment and monitoring of these diseases involves time and expense. Clinical response to appropriate treatment is usually good in cases diagnosed early and without significant organ dysfunction. However, some animals may remain sub-clinically infected. The availability of licensed products may be limited and importation of drugs may be required. Several of the drugs used have side-effects and referral should be considered in animals with severe disease or where there is limited practice capacity for regular monitoring of treatment response.

- **Babesiosis** – Treatment for shock and anaemia may be required in severe cases. For *Babesia canis* species, injectable imidocarb dipropionate is the drug of choice. A repeat injection is given either 2 weeks or, less commonly, 48 hours later. A rapid clinical response (within 48 hours) should be expected. Small *Babesia* species (e.g. *B. gibsoni*) require more complex therapy such as the anti-malarial drug, ataquavone, in combination with azithromycin. Treatment response can be monitored using PCR. If clinical or haematological response is poor, or if a small *Babesia* species is suspected, referral for further investigation or treatment /management should be considered.

- **Ehrlichiosis –** The treatment of choice is oral doxycycline for 28 days. Full haematology with a manual platelet count should be monitored every 7–14 days, depending on the dog's clinical condition. Treatment response can be monitored using PCR. Most dogs respond well but if clinical response is poor, platelet counts remain sub-normal or if anaemia or low white cell counts are present, a further 28-day course of doxycycline can be used. However, referral or a bone marrow investigation should be planned.

- **Leishmaniosis –** Treatment protocols are complex and it is difficult to determine the prognosis. Owners must be advised that specific treatment is aimed at lowering parasite load and that subsequent recovery is dependent on the dog's individual immune response. Some susceptible dogs will require long-term (perhaps life-long) therapy. Haematology, biochemistry (especially blood urea nitrogen, creatinine and albumin/globulin) and urinalysis including urine protein:creatinine (UPC) ratio are essential prior to therapy. Dogs with relatively minor abnormalities can be started with a combination of oral allopurinol and either injectable meglumine antimonate or oral miltefosine for a 28-day period. Treatment with allopurinol is continued until dogs are clinically normal, have a globulin and UPC values within the reference range, a negative PCR and quantitative *Leishmania* serology ≤1:50. In successful cases, this may take 9–12 months. In animals with severe organ dysfunction, the prognosis is poor to guarded and these cases commonly require supportive therapy for renal failure before specific therapy can be considered for the leishmaniosis.

- **Dirofilariosis (heartworm) –** Treatment is complex and potentially dangerous due to the risk of thromboembolism associated with dead or dying worms. Dirofilaria like other filarial worms, contain symbiotic bacteria (*Wolbachia*). Release of these bacteria and their products when worms die may play a major role in side-effects associated with adulticide therapy. Consequently, treatment with doxycycline for 28 days should be started prior to specific treatment for adult nematodes. Doxycycline also decreases the viability of microfilaria by killing the symbiotic *Wolbachia*. In dogs, injectable melarsomine and less commonly thiacetarsemide are used as adulticides, and the protocols vary with disease severity. Neither drug is appropriate for cats. Animals should be hospitalised during adulticide therapy to monitor drug-associated side-effects. Supportive therapy, including oxygen, should be available in severe cases. Anti-inflammatory doses of glucocorticoids can be used prior to adulticide therapy if there is evidence of severe peri-bronchiolar disease. Animals should have house rest for 4–6 weeks post-adulticide therapy. Treatment response can be monitored using antigen-based serology. Treatment for circulating microfilariae can be started 6 weeks post adulticide therapy using moxidectin, milbemycin or ivermectin. These drugs have some adulticidal activity when given over several months and may be used in cats as well as dogs that do not tolerate the more effective but more toxic adulticides.

What if it doesn't get better?

With the possible exception of ehrlichiosis, treatment may be associated with complications, particularly in those dogs that have significant pre-existing organ dysfunction. Owners should be made aware of this possibility. Clinical response to the correct treatment protocol when it is started early in the course of disease, is good to excellent in most cases. However, although parasite numbers may be greatly reduced by drug therapy, complete parasiticidal cure will not occur unless there is also an effective anti-parasite immunological response by the dog. Most young healthy dogs with *Babesia canis* infection and ehrlichiosis are effectively 'cured' after the treatment course. However, exceptions are dogs with babesiosis due to *B. gibsoni* infection in which treatment is only partially effective and relapses are common, and German Shepherd dogs with monocytic ehrlichiosis that have a predisposition for severe bone marrow disease, irrespective of treatment.

Dogs with leishmaniosis are often asymptomatic or greatly improved after a month of combined treatment, but long-term treatment with the static drug allopurinol is necessary to maintain control of parasitic load. Even so many of these dogs enjoy long periods of remission and some dogs in non-endemic areas can discontinue therapy if PCR and serological results are negative after a year.

Treatment for heartworm is complex and involves several stages over several months. Clinical response is good to excellent in the majority of cases and even if adulticide therapy is not fully effective, any remaining adults are often disabled and die later as a result of subsequent microfilaricide therapy in combination with host response.

The low-cost option

These conditions are typically expensive to diagnose, treat and monitor. In particular, optimum treatment of *Babesia gibsoni* infection, leishmaniosis and dirofilariosis is likely to incur significant costs. When funds are limited and the dog does not have serious organ damage that warrants euthanasia, some less-effective treatment protocols could be used to control clinical disease in the short term. These could include imidocarb dipropionate for *B. gibsoni*, allopurinol alone for leishmaniosis and a microfilaricide with doxycycline followed by preventative therapy for heartworm disease. However, owners must be aware that this is a compromise and that even though clinical improvement may occur, there is considerable risk that it may not be maintained.

When should I refer?

Most of these conditions would benefit from the input of an internal medicine specialist for both the diagnostic and therapeutic phases of management.

Geoff Shawcross

This is a common procedure that requires technical expertise to perform efficiently, and often takes considerable tact and understanding when dealing with the client.

Reasons for euthanasia

- Chronic illness that is resulting in intractable pain or suffering
- Acute illnesses or injuries that are assessed to be untreatable
- Financial constraints which prevent appropriate treatment from being given
- Behavioural problems that cannot be resolved satisfactorily despite appropriate advice/treatment (e.g. aggression, noise, inappropriate elimination)
- Changes in owner's circumstances (housing, job, separation, bereavement).

When welfare is the primary issue, euthanasia is usually a mutual decision between the clinician and owner, although sometimes the clinician may have to be proactive and suggest to the owner that euthanasia is the best treatment option. In this situation, the commonly used phrase 'If he were my dog. ...' can be helpful. The clinician may have personal objections to euthanising an apparently healthy animal but needs to be understanding of the owner's situation. Once an owner has decided on euthanasia, alternatives should only be suggested if they have a realistic chance of success.

Permission for euthanasia

Written consent to euthanise a pet should be obtained whenever possible. Such permission avoids any ambiguity regarding what is going to happen to the animal, and also provides a reasonable defence if there is a threat of litigation at a later date. A signed consent form should always be obtained in the following circumstances:

- Where the animal is presented for euthanasia by someone other than the owner
- Where the animal is accepted for euthanasia by the practice lay-staff and not via a consultation

100 Top Consultations in Small Animal General Practice, First Edition
By Peter Hill, Sheena Warman and Geoff Shawcross
© 2011 Blackwell Publishing Ltd

- Where the client is new to the practice and euthanasia is the only request.

Minors cannot sign a euthanasia consent form (or any other consent form), even if they claim to be the animal's owner.

A clinician may euthanise an animal on welfare grounds even if the owner is not immediately available, for instance following an RTA where the injuries are severe. To avoid litigation, however, it is prudent to attempt to stabilise the patient pending the decision of the owner. With advancing veterinary expertise at referral centres, and veterinary medical insurance, there are fewer cases where euthanasia is an imperative. Under no circumstances should an animal be admitted for euthanasia and then rehomed without the express permission of the owner.

Techniques for euthanasia

The most common method of euthanasia is by the IV injection of a barbiturate solution through the cephalic vein. The procedure requires a competent IV injection technique and is best carried out in the practice, where experienced help and proper facilities are available. The lateral saphenous vein can be used if the cephalic veins are unavailable but, although this vein is easy to visualise, it is quite difficult to stabilise during venipuncture and often requires a shorter, narrower gauge needle to enter it successfully. Ideally, there should be a separate room for euthanasia as this allows the owner time in private with their pet without adversely affecting a busy consulting session.

Clinicians should ensure that all materials are to hand before starting. When a syringe larger than 2 ml is required, one with an eccentric nozzle should be used; 21-gauge needles are appropriate for most dogs and 23-gauge needles are suitable for cats and very small dogs. Note that a narrow-gauge needle makes it difficult to deliver the solution rapidly, especially if it is viscous. At least two syringes should be prepared, with needles attached and filled with the euthanising solution, as there may be a need to discard one if the first attempt at venipuncture is unsuccessful. Although electric clippers are both quick and efficient, some animals, particularly cats, can be upset by the noise and, on these occasions, it may be better to use blunt pointed 'curved on flat' scissors to remove the hair from over the vein. The site should be swabbed, not to sterilise the skin, but to emphasise the vein. Enough solution to result in a rapid loss of consciousness should be injected quickly. It is sometimes easier to use two smaller syringes in quick succession rather than one large syringe, which can be cumbersome.

Owner involvement in euthanasia consultations

It is important to try to understand the owner's perception of what the process entails: some owners are totally detached from the event, some are very upset but put on a brave face, and some are devastated by the loss of their pet. In all cases, however, they will be left with a lasting impression that will have an impact on the reputation of both the clinician and the practice.

Many owners feel obliged to stay with their pet during euthanasia, feeling that they should not desert their pet in its final moments. However, they should always be given a tactful excuse in case they do not want to stay. This is especially true when children are present, who can become very upset. Often owners are satisfied if they see their pet after it has been euthanised, rather than having watched the entire process. An owner may want to hold their pet during the procedure but they are rarely capable of doing it properly. It is better to let a nurse hold the animal and let the owner just comfort the head. If the owner wants to be present when a hospitalised patient is euthanised, an IV catheter should be pre-placed before their arrival and flushed with a heparinised solution to ensure it remains patent. Owners should be sensitively advised that the eyes remain open after death and that their pet may urinate and/or defaecate as the sphincter muscles relax. They should also be forewarned that agonal gasping may occur, and possibly spastic extension of the limbs and neck: it can be disconcerting for owners to see and they will often question if their pet is actually dead.

It is quite common for an owner to request a domiciliary visit when their pet has to be euthanised, feeling that it is less stressful than travelling to the surgery. Euthanasia in the home does pose additional problems for the veterinary surgeon, which must be taken into consideration. Animals, far from being relaxed in their own home, can be protective or nervous of strangers. Lighting is often poor, and the veterinary surgeon often has to work kneeling on the floor. Whenever possible, a nurse experienced in dealing with difficult animals and situations should accompany the veterinary surgeon. It should be confirmed that all equipment is serviceable, and that there is an ample supply of drugs, before arriving at the house. It also helps if reception staff ascertain when the request is made whether the owner will be disposing of the body, or whether it will be taken back to the practice.

Euthanasia of aggressive dogs

The safety of all involved in the procedure is paramount and the veterinary surgeon is likely to be held legally responsible if anyone gets injured. There is no legal obligation for a veterinary surgeon to euthanise an aggressive dog, and it should not be attempted if there is a significant risk of personal injury. Whenever possible, these cases should be dealt with at the practice where there are adequate facilities, equipment and competent staff to deal with the situation. Personnel not strictly required to carry out the procedure should not be allowed in the vicinity, and that could include the owner. Domiciliary visits should be discouraged because of the lack of facilities, and the fact that most dogs are more confident and protective on their own territory.

If the owner has sufficient control of the dog, they should be asked to apply a muzzle and a choke chain with a long lead attached. Muzzles should be of the Baskerville or leather, box type. Owners should not be asked to apply a tape muzzle as they are unlikely to be able to do it effectively. A choke chain or slip-lead should be used, rather than relying on a leather collar, as it is harder for the dog to escape and gives an additional level of control/ restraint. It may not be practical to attempt an IV injection even when the dog is muzzled because it can be difficult to keep the dog still enough. In such circumstances, high doses of a potent sedative (such as medetomidine) should be injected IM and given time for it to act fully, preferably in a quiet room. Oral sedation, with drugs such as acetylpromazine tablets, is generally unreliable. A member of staff should be given the responsibility of frequently checking that all safety equipment used (muzzles, dog catcher, leads, etc) is serviceable, strong and reliable.

Euthanasia of aggressive or feral cats

All potential escape routes (doors, windows, vents, etc.) should be secured before any attempt is made to remove the cat from its carrier or trap. The cat should be transferred to a crush cage, using a cat catcher if necessary. Gloves that are thick enough to give protection from being bitten are usually too cumbersome to make it possible to grasp the cat securely. Once constrained, a sedative can be given IM, or the euthanising solution injected intraperitoneally. Once the cat is sedated sufficiently, it can be removed from the crush cage and euthanised by an IV or intracardiac injection.

Euthanasia when no help is available

Occasionally, a situation arises where there is no competent help available. In such situations, dogs should be heavily sedated with a potent IM agent (e.g. medetomidine). Once sedated, the forelimb can be clipped and swabbed as usual. The cephalic vein can be raised by the application of a makeshift tourniquet made from a bandage applied above the elbow; alternatively, a rubber band held in place by mosquito forceps can be used. If sedation is profound, the euthanising solution can be injected directly into the heart. Cats can also be sedated prior to intracardiac or intra-renal injection. The intercostal approach for intracardiac injection can be painful and is not recommended without prior sedation. In cats it is also possible to pass a 21-gauge 1.5 inch needle anteriorly into the heart from just behind the xiphoid.

After the event

Death should always be confirmed before the animal is prepared for disposal or released to the owner. Time and care should be taken to ensure that all reflexes are abolished, there are no respiratory movements and there has been no heartbeat for several seconds. The use of a stethoscope helps to reassure the owner that death has been confirmed.

Owners want to feel that their pet will be treated with respect after it has been euthanised. It is, therefore imprudent to bundle the body into a polythene bag in the owner's presence. At the practice, the body should be covered with a blanket if the owner is going to spend a little time alone with their pet. If the body is to be removed following a domiciliary visit, it should be wrapped neatly in a sheet or blanket and if necessary, a stretcher should be used to take it from the house. Once wrapped, a cat should be placed in a cat carrier that is large enough for it to be laid out fully. Once at the practice premises, the body can be transferred to a polythene bag, to comply with waste-disposal regulations.

The practice should be able to arrange, or supply the names of agencies that will organise, the burial or individual cremation of pets for those owners who would prefer this to mass cremation. For some owners, the grieving process may be particularly difficult and they may benefit from being tactfully referred to a bereavement counsellor.

It is imperative that all reminders for vaccinations, dental appointments, etc., should be removed from the pet's records. Long-standing clients of the practice often appreciate a condolence card or a letter, but these should always be hand-written to give a personal touch, and never appear to be 'computerised'.

Section 18
Appendices

Sheena Warman

This appendix provides guidance regarding commonly used oral antibiotics in first opinion practice. For further guidance regarding parenteral treatment of life-threatening infections, the reader is guided to critical care and emergency medicine textbooks.

Antibiotics are used frequently in veterinary medicine, often without the benefit of culture and sensitivity testing. In many situations inexpensive, 'first-line' antibiotics will be effective. In general, drugs such as fluoroquinolones and second or third generation cephalosporins should be reserved for life-threatening, severe, or recurrent problems, and should ideally only be used following results of culture and sensitivity testing. Rational use of antibiotics is essential for the following reasons:

1. To ensure that the antibiotic is appropriate for the organism likely to be causing the infection
2. To ensure that the antibiotic is likely to reach the site of infection
3. To minimise the development and spread of antibiotic resistance.

Rational antibiotic use can be achieved by paying attention to the following questions.

Are the animal's clinical signs likely to be caused by a bacterial infection?

There are many circumstances in which the clinician can make a reasonable assumption that an animal's signs are caused at least in part by a bacterial infection. Examples include pyoderma, abscesses, pyometra, kennel cough and canine lower urinary tract infections. However, there are other circumstances where routine antibiotic use is not indicated. For example, acute, self-limiting vomiting and diarrhoea does not require treatment with antibiotics, and lower urinary tract signs in cats are rarely caused by bacterial infections. It is important to remember that pyrexia has many other potential causes besides bacterial

infections (see Chapter 7). Similarly, neutrophilia is common in many ill animals as part of a stress leukogram, and does not necessarily indicate a bacterial component to the disease.

Which antibiotic will be effective?

The important question to ask is which antibiotic will be effective against the likely cause(s) of infection in particular organ systems, and whether it will achieve therapeutic concentrations in the target tissue. There are many circumstances in which culture and sensitivity testing is unlikely to be performed prior to initiation of treatment, due to financial or practical limitations. In these cases, antibiotic therapy must be chosen empirically, based on knowledge of the organisms likely to be responsible. Antibiotic concentration at the site of infection is affected by factors such as local blood supply, lipid barriers, local inflammation and pH. Lipid barriers prevent many antibiotics from reaching the eye, CNS, bronchial lumen, prostate and mammary glands; some drugs are more able to cross lipid barriers and are more likely than others to achieve therapeutic concentrations in these tissues (see Table A1.1).

- Respiratory system – Appropriate initial choices for respiratory infections include oxytetracycline, doxycycline, amoxicillin/clavulanic acid or potentiated sulphonamides. Fluoroquinolones should be reserved for life-threatening infections or following culture and sensitivity testing of organisms resistant to other medications
- Urinary tract – Many antibiotics are excreted renally and therefore achieve high concentrations in the urine. Common organisms include staphylococci, streptococci, and *E. coli*. Useful first-line antibiotics include amoxicillin, ampicillin, amoxicillin/clavulanic acid and potentiated sulphonamides. In patients with recurring or relapsing infections culture and sensitivity testing should be performed
- Prostate – Although many antibiotics penetrate the acutely inflamed prostate gland, few penetrate in chronic prostatitis. The most effective drugs in this circumstance are highly lipophilic and weak bases, for example doxycycline, potentiated sulphonamides and fluoroquinolones

100 Top Consultations in Small Animal General Practice, First Edition
By Peter Hill, Sheena Warman and Geoff Shawcross
© 2011 Blackwell Publishing Ltd

Table A1.1 Properties of commonly used oral antibiotics.

	Spectrum of activity					Ability to cross cellular/lipid barriers	Bactericidal or bacteriostatic	Optimal absorption if given with or without food	Relative cost of licensed preparations
	Gram-positive aerobes	Gram-negative aerobes	Penicillinase-producing *Staphylococcus* spp.	Obligate anaerobes	Additional activity				
Amoxicillin, ampicillin	++	+	-	++	-	Poor	Bactericidal	Ampicillin – without food Amoxicillin – with food	£/££ (varies depending on brand)
Amoxicillin/clavulanic acid	++	+(+)	++	++	-	Poor	Bactericidal	With food	££/£££ (varies depending on brand)
Cefalexin	++	+	++	+	-	Poor	Bactericidal	Either	££ (low dose), £££ (high dose)
Oxytetracycline	++	+	+	+	*Mycoplasma, Chlamydia*	Moderate	Bacteriostatic	Without food	£

Antibiotic									
Macrolides (e.g. erythromycin) and lincosamides (e.g. clindamycin)	++	-	+	++	Toxoplasma (clindamycin)	Moderate	Bacteriostatic	Without food	Erythromycin £ Clindamycin £££
Trimethoprim-potentiated sulphonamides	+	+	+	+	Toxoplasma, Neospora, Coccidia and Isospora	Moderate	Bactericidal	Without food	£
Fluoroquinolones	++	++	++	-	Mycoplasma, Chlamydia, Rickettsia and Mycobacterium spp.	Good	Bactericidal	Without food	£££
Metronidazole	-	-	-	++	Protozoa	Good	Bactericidal	With food	£

Section 18

- Skin – Staphylococcal pyoderma is treated using antibiotics that are effective against gram-positive, beta-lactamase producing cocci. Appropriate choices include cefalexin, amoxicillin/clavulanic acid, clindamycin or potentiated sulphonamides
- Bone – Antibiotics used should be effective against beta-lactamase producing staphylococci and anaerobes, for example amoxicillin/clavulanic acid, cefalexin or clindamycin
- Gastrointestinal disease – Acute vomiting and diarrhoea are usually self-limiting and do not generally require treatment with antibiotics. Patients with haemorrhagic gastroenteritis should receive broad-spectrum antibiotics such as amoxicillin/clavulanic acid to reduce the risk of bacteraemia caused by translocation of bacteria across the intestinal wall. Enteric-coated erythromycin is the drug of choice for symptomatic *Campylobacter* infections. Oxytetracycline is often used in the treatment of chronic antibiotic-responsive diarrhoea. Metronidazole is sometimes used in treatment of inflammatory bowel disease for both its antibacterial and immunomodulatory properties
- Hepatic/biliary disease – Appropriate initial choices for treatment of liver/biliary infections include ampicillin, amoxicillin or amoxicillin/clavulanic acid. Other drugs which penetrate well include cephalosporins, fluoroquinolones, metronidazole, and clindamycin.

Further details regarding antibiotic use in specific conditions are found throughout this text.

What patient factors might influence the choice of antibiotic?

Bactericidal antibiotics may be more effective than bacteriostatic drugs in immunocompromised patients (Table A1.1). Concurrent diseases or drugs may influence drug choice or dosage due to increased risk of toxicity. Pregnant or neonatal patients require special care with drug choices; data sheets and formularies should be consulted. Most drugs have some potential for side-effects. Those commonly associated with antibiotics are listed in Table A1.2. In particular, owners must be made aware of the risk of oesophageal strictures in cats following administration of doxycycline tablets or clindamycin capsules, and taught to syringe water orally after pilling their cat. Attention must also be paid to compliance with local prescribing laws such as the cascade system that is used in Europe.

Patient and owner compliance will also influence choice of drugs. It is essential that time is spent advising owners effective means of administering tablets to their pets. Whilst some drugs are better given without food, a small amount of soft food to disguise the tablet may be necessary to ensure compliance. Some antibiotics require more frequent administration than others (see below).

How long a course should be given?

For most simple, first-time infections, a 5–7 day course is adequate (apart from staphylococcal pyoderma which usually requires a 2–3 week course). Treatment is usually continued for at least 2 days after resolution of the clinical signs. If the infection is chronic, recurrent, involves bony tissue, is in an immunosuppressed patient, or involves granulomatous lesions, then a longer course is recommended, ideally based on culture and sensitivity results. In these circumstances treatment is usually continued for 1–2 weeks beyond clinical cure, often resulting in a 4–6 week course of treatment.

What route and frequency of administration should be used?

Oral administration is appropriate in most circumstances, but it is important that time is taken to ensure that the owner is able and willing to administer the medication. In severe or life-threatening infections, or in patients unable to tolerate oral medication (e.g. those with vomiting or regurgitation) a few days of parenteral antibiotic administration is appropriate until oral medication is possible. In well-hydrated patients, SC injections are often appropriate. With severe or life-threatening infections, antibiotics should be administered by the IV route.

Frequency of administration depends on the type of antibiotic (this information is found in drug data sheets and formularies). Some antibiotics, such as penicillins and cephalosporins, are 'time-dependent', meaning that clinical efficacy is dictated by the length of time for which the concentration remains above the minimum inhibitory concentration for the pathogen. These antibiotics usually need to be administered at least twice daily. Other antibiotics, such as aminoglycosides and fluoroquinolones, are 'concentration-dependent'; their efficacy depends on achieving high plasma concentrations relative to the minimum inhibitory concentration of the pathogen. These antibiotics often have prolonged post-antibiotic effects, allowing for once-daily dosing.

Some antibiotics can be formulated as long-acting injectables. One form involves incorporating the drug into a depot suspension that is slowly absorbed from the injection site providing up to 48 hours of cover (e.g. long-acting ampicillin or amoxicillin). A newer drug is the long-acting cephalosporin cefovecin. This drug has a novel pharmacokinetic profile that provides efficacy against many

Table A1.2 Potential side-effects of commonly used antibiotics (*common).

Antibiotic	Side-effect/precautions
Aminoglycosides	*Renal failure *Ototoxicity Neuromuscular blockade
Cephalosporins	Vomiting, immune-mediated disease
Chloramphenicol	Aplastic anaemia (especially cats) Inhibition of drug metabolism (impairment of hepatic cytochrome P450-dependent enzymes)
Clindamycin	*Oesophagitis or strictures in cats given clindamycin capsules – administer water by syringe immediately after administering capsule
Erythromycin	*Vomiting – enteric-coated preparations may be useful
Metronidazole	Neutropenia CNS toxicity
Penicillins	Immune-mediated disease
Fluoroquinolones	*Abnormal cartilage development in growing animals *Retinal toxicity in cats (enrofloxacin) Potentiation of seizures (reported in humans, particularly when used in conjunction with NSAIDs)
Sulphonamides	Dogs – Vomiting, cholestasis, thrombocytopenia, polyarthritis, *keratoconjunctivitis sicca, suppression of thyroid function Cats – Drowsiness, anorexia, leukopenia, anaemia, hypersalivation
Tetracyclines	*Doxycycline – Oesophagitis or strictures in cats – administer water by syringe immediately after administering tablet; vomiting and diarrhoea Oxytetracycline – Renal tubular disease, cholestasis, pyrexia (cats) *Staining of teeth in young animals

causes of skin, soft tissue and urinary tract infections for up to 14 days. Whilst this may be convenient for many owners, thought should be given as to whether use of a cephalosporin is justified in individual situations.

What cost is involved?

Antibiotics vary enormously in price. In many clinical situations, inexpensive antibiotics will be appropriate in terms of spectrum of activity and efficacy (see Table A1.1).

Peter Hill

Indications

Glucocorticoids are widely used drugs in small animal practice. They are potent immunomodulatory drugs and can be indicated for the treatment of a variety of conditions including:

- Pruritic skin conditions caused by allergies or certain parasites, e.g. atopic dermatitis, flea allergy dermatitis, sarcoptic mange
- Allergic and inflammatory disorders affecting the respiratory tract or intestines, e.g. feline asthma, chronic non-infectious bronchitis, inflammatory bowel disease
- Immune-mediated disorders, e.g. sterile granulomatous meningoencephalitis
- Auto-immune diseases affecting the skin, blood, joints, liver or kidneys, e.g. pemphigus, lupus, immune mediated haemolytic anaemia, immune mediated thrombocytopenia
- Certain neoplastic conditions, e.g. lymphoma
- Certain ocular conditions, e.g. conjunctivitis, uveitis
- Otitis externa.

Glucocorticoids can be used as a specific treatment for a particular condition (e.g. an auto-immune disease) or as an adjunctive treatment (e.g. to treat the pruritus in a dog that is being treated for sarcoptic mange).

In general, glucocorticoids are contraindicated in animals suffering from bacterial, viral or fungal infections, unless such treatment is deemed to be life-saving. Glucocorticoids are also contraindicated in dogs suffering from demodicosis.

Glucocorticoids should only be used after an accurate diagnosis has been made. For example, they should not be used to treat pruritus in a dog unless a cause for that pruritus has been established.

Potency and formulations

Different glucocorticoids vary in their potency, ranging from most to least potent as follows: dexamethasone / betamethasone > triamcinolone > prednisolone > hydrocortisone. Various preparations are also available and they can be administered by mouth, injection or topically.

100 Top Consultations in Small Animal General Practice, First Edition
By Peter Hill, Sheena Warman and Geoff Shawcross
© 2011 Blackwell Publishing Ltd

- Oral glucocorticoids are used most commonly and are indicated for any condition in which treatment for longer than 3 days is required
- Short-acting injectable glucocorticoids are best reserved for hospitalised patients, animals that are not eating, or patients that require immediate but short-term treatment (e.g. bee sting reactions)
- Long-acting glucocorticoid injections (e.g. methyl prednisolone acetate, Depo-Medrone, Pfizer) provide sub-optimal control of dosage regimes and are rarely indicated. They may occasionally be indicated for intra-articular or intra-bursal use to treat severe localised degenerative or inflammatory joint disease. For long-term anti-inflammatory treatment, they should only be considered in a patient that refuses to take tablets under any circumstances
- Topical glucocorticoids are indicated for the treatment of certain skin conditions such as atopic dermatitis and hot spots; otitis externa; and some ocular conditions.

Anti-pruritic and anti-inflammatory therapy

Glucocorticoids can have either anti-inflammatory or immunosuppressive effects, depending on the dose given. For anti-inflammatory or anti-pruritic therapy, the most appropriate drug is prednisolone. **A starting, anti-inflammatory dose of prednisolone is 0.5–1 mg/kg daily,** depending on severity.

For parasitic skin diseases and hot spots, a short course of prednisolone lasting 5–7 days is indicated. With such short courses, there is no need to taper the dose at the end of the course, although giving half the dose for the last two days allows the dose given to be titrated against the reducing severity of pruritus.

If longer term use is considered, such as when treating atopic dermatitis on a limited budget, or conditions such as inflammatory bowel disease, the aim should be to give the 'minimally effective dose' and try to establish 'alternate-day therapy'. Both of these will minimise the prevalence of adverse effects and reduce adrenal suppression. Typically, an anti-inflammatory dose of prednisolone is given until the condition is under control and the dog is then converted to alternate-day therapy. The dose given on the alternate days is then reduced to the minimum level that will keep the dog's signs under an acceptable degree of control. Note that there is no point in using alternate-day therapy to taper a short course of glucocorticoids. In some cases, alternate-day therapy does not keep the symptoms under control. In such cases, the clinician needs to balance the benefit of ongoing daily therapy against the risk of adverse effects.

In cats with severely pruritic skin diseases, it is sometimes necessary to use higher starting doses of prednisolone than those stated above (2 mg/kg daily).

An alternative to prednisolone for anti-inflammatory therapy is methyl prednisolone (Medrone, Pfizer Animal Health). This drug produces less mineralocorticoid effects than prednisolone, so there is reduced tendency for polydipsia and polyuria. When methyl prednisolone is used, a 4-mg tablet can be regarded as being equivalent in potency to a 5-mg prednisolone tablet.

Clinicians should always be aware of the alternatives to glucocorticoid therapy. For many conditions, especially when long-term treatment is required, there are other treatment options that have fewer adverse effects.

Immunosuppressive therapy

Immunosuppressive therapy is used to treat auto-immune and immune-mediated diseases. These conditions are uncommon in general veterinary practice, and require considerable expertise to manage them appropriately. Inexperienced clinicians should consider referral of such patients for specialist management. As with anti-inflammatory therapy, prednisolone is the initial drug of choice in most cases. **A starting, immunosuppressive dose of prednisolone is 2–4 mg/kg daily**, depending on severity. Because of this high starting dose, the dose needs to be gradually tapered towards either a maintenance regime or cessation of the drug. Usually the high dose is maintained until the condition is under control (usually within 2 weeks). Then, the doses are gradually tapered over a few weeks until the patient is receiving 1–2 mg/kg daily. At this stage, an attempt can be made to convert the patient to alternate-day therapy. Some clinicians may recommend a gradual reduction in the dose given on the second day, rather than suddenly stopping it. This avoids the immediate dosage reduction of 50% which occurs when treatment is changed from daily to alternate-day dosing. This clinical decision is based on experience of the conditions and is more of an art than a science. Once the patient is receiving alternate-day therapy, further dosage reductions should be attempted to establish the minimal effective dose.

Patients receiving immunosuppressive therapy need to be carefully monitored. Animals should be re-inspected after 7 days, 14 days and then every 2 weeks until the clinician is happy with the progress (usually for the first 6–8 weeks). After that, the frequency of re-inspections can be gradually reduced to monthly and then every 2–3 months. Due to the nature of the drugs being prescribed, it is preferable to continue monitoring the animal every 3–6 months, even if the condition is completely stable. Routine haematology and biochemistry profiles are indicated at these time points to monitor for organ damage, although it should be remembered that a stress leukogram and elevations in serum ALKP would be expected in patients receiving glucocorticoids.

Other drugs are available for immunosuppressive therapy (e.g. ciclosporin, azathioprine, cyclophosphamide, chlorambucil). The use of one or more of these drugs can be indicated in patients with auto-immune or immune-mediated disease, either to improve the efficacy or to reduce the glucocorticoid requirements. Familiarity with these medications and their adverse effects is required for safe use.

Adverse effects of glucocorticoids

Corticosteroids are known to exert a wide range of side-effects. Short-term use of systemic glucocorticoids can lead to polydipsia, polyuria, polyphagia, panting and behaviour changes. Prolonged use of glucocorticoids can lead to signs of iatrogenic Cushing's disease (muscle wastage, pot belly, hepatomegaly, fat redistribution, osteoporosis, calcinosis cutis, alopecia, poor wound healing, recurrent pyoderma, generalised demodicosis, comedones, silent urinary tract infections, pyelonephritis, cataracts, insulin-resistant diabetes mellitus). These adverse effects are less common in cats, even though they may need higher doses for certain conditions. Some corticosteroids cause sodium and water retention, and hypokalaemia with long-term use. In the presence of a viral infection, steroids may worsen or hasten the progress of the disease. Glucocorticoids have caused gastro-intestinal ulceration, especially in patients receiving concurrent NSAIDs. Glucocorticoids may also predispose to pancreatitis, although this is considered controversial. Sudden withdrawal of glucocorticoids after prolonged therapy can lead to an Addisonian crisis (adrenal insufficiency). Glucocorticoids should be avoided in animals with pre-existing renal disease, diabetes mellitus or congestive heart failure. In cats, high doses of glucocorticoids have been reported to precipitate congestive heart failure. Glucocorticoids should not be given to pregnant animals as they can cause foetal abnormalities and abortion. Administration is contra-indicated where corneal ulceration is present. Glucocorticoids may lead to a sub-optimal response following vaccination. Glucocorticoid injections can cause focal areas of cutaneous atrophy and hair loss.

Appendix 3 – General principles of non-steroidal anti-inflammatory drug (NSAID) use for the treatment of musculoskeletal pain

Martin Owen

Indications

In healthy dogs, any of the NSAIDs shown in Table A3.1 can be used for the control of musculoskeletal pain due to traumatic injury, joint inflammation, osteoarthritis, vertebral column pain, or musculoskeletal pain following excessive activity. **In cats, great care should be taken to ensure that a drug licensed for this species is used, to avoid potential toxicity**. Some NSAIDs are also licensed for the control of intraoperative and/or postoperative pain.

General treatment principles

For the initial management of a painful musculoskeletal condition, a short course (5–7 days) of NSAID should be prescribed. If there is a satisfactory response to treatment and if the painful condition is predicted to be chronic, the NSAID treatment should be continued for two to four weeks to allow inflammation to subside. After this period, when clinical signs are controlled, withdrawal of medication should be attempted, since many patients with chronic musculoskeletal disease do not require persistent long-term NSAID therapy. If drug withdrawal precipitates return of clinical signs, a chronically painful condition is likely to be present and long-term NSAID treatment may be required. Drugs licensed for long-term administration should always be used. The efficacy of pain control should be assessed by regular patient review and side-effects should be investigated by taking a careful history and by performing a clinical examination. Routine blood and urine tests may be helpful to monitor for evidence of organ dysfunction. If a switch of NSAID is planned for patients receiving long-term NSAID therapy, a 'wash out' period of at least 5 days should be observed before introducing an alternative NSAID, in order to minimise the chance of NSAID toxicity.

Adverse effects

General adverse effects associated with the use of NSAIDs include:

- Nausea
- Vomiting and/or diarrhoea due to gastrointestinal irritation
- Haematemesis and/or melaena due to gastrointestinal ulceration
- Acute renal failure due to papillary necrosis, particularly if there is hypotension, dehydration or if other nephrotoxic drugs are used concurrently
- Impairment of haemostasis (rarely a clinical problem)
- There is a theoretical risk of precipitation of congestive heart failure in patients with underlying cardiac disease, although this is rarely seen in practice.
- For PLT tablets (Novartis), additional adverse effects may be seen due to the glucocorticoid component (see Appendix 2 for further details).

NSAIDs should not be used if gastrointestinal disease/ulceration is present or suspected, in haemorrhagic syndromes, in hypovolaemic or hypotensive patients, or in patients with renal or hepatic insufficiency. NSAIDs are generally not licensed for use in pregnant animals.

NSAIDs should not be used concurrently with corticosteroids because of the increased risk of gastro-intestinal ulceration. Care should be taken when using NSAIDs in patients with heart failure, in particular those on diuretics, because of increased risk of nephrotoxicity and the slight risk of worsening heart failure. Some NSAIDs are highly protein-bound and can displace other protein-bound drugs, increasing risk of toxicity.

NSAIDs should be discontinued in animals that experience signs of toxicity. Acute signs of toxicity are normally vomiting and diarrhoea. If there is evidence of gastric ulceration, administration of gastric protectants is prudent until clinical signs are controlled.

The use of NSAIDs licensed for humans but not small animals (e.g. ibuprofen) is not recommended because such drugs can be toxic.

100 Top Consultations in Small Animal General Practice, First Edition
By Peter Hill, Sheena Warman and Geoff Shawcross
© 2011 Blackwell Publishing Ltd

Table A3.1 – Some commonly used NSAIDs.

Availability of drugs varies in different countries. Clinicians should check the drug's data sheet for precise dosing instructions before prescribing.

Active agent	Trade names	Formulations	Oral dosing schedules
Carprofen	Rimadyl (Pfizer) Carprogesic (Pfizer) Rimifin (Vetoquinol) Carprodyl (CEVA) Canidryl (Chanelle) Dolagis (Alstoe)	Tablet Injection	*Dogs only* 4 mg/kg/day for up to 7 days May reduce to 2 mg/kg/day for longer term use
Meloxicam	Metacam (Boehringer) Meloxidyl (CEVA) Flexicam (Dechra) Meloxicam (Janssen) Rheumocam (Chanelle)	Oral suspension Tablet Injection	*Dogs* 0.2 mg/kg/day on day 1 0.1 mg/kg/day subsequently *Cats* 0.1 mg/kg/day on day 1 0.05 mg/kg/day subsequently
Tepoxalin	Zubrin (Intervet/Schering Plough)	Tablet	*Dogs only* 10 mg/kg/day
Firocoxib	Previcox (Merial)	Tablet	*Dogs only* 5 mg/kg/day
Robenacoxib	Onsior (Novartis)	Tablet	*Dogs and cats* 1–2 mg/kg/day
Mavacoxib	Trocoxil (Pfizer)	Tablet	*Dogs only* 2 mg/kg on day 1 Repeat after 7 days Repeat monthly Maximum of 7 doses in all
Deracoxib	Deramaxx (Novartis)	Tablet	*Dogs only* 1–2 mg/kg/day
Tolfenamic acid	Tolfedine (Vetoquinol)	Tablet Injection	*Dogs and cats* 4 mg/kg/day for 3 days *Dogs only* May be repeated for 3 days out of every 7
Ketoprofen	Ketofen (Merial)	Tablet Injection	*Dogs and cats* 1 mg/kg/day for up to 5 days *Dogs only* 0.25 mg/kg/day for longer term
Etodolac	Etogesic (Fort Dodge)	Tablet	*Dogs only* 10–15 mg/kg/day
Cinchophen Prednisolone	PLT (Novartis)	Tablet	*Dogs only* ½ tablet per 8 kg twice daily
Paracetamol Codeine phosphate	Pardale V (Dechra)	Tablet	*Dogs only* 1 tablet per 12 kg every 8 hours (maximum 5 days)

Sheena Warman

Obesity is a common problem, with surveys suggesting that 25–40% of dogs and cats presented to veterinary clinics are overweight. The presence of obesity has an impact on many organ systems and makes clinical signs associated with other disease processes far more severe (e.g. arthritis, cardiovascular problems and respiratory disease). It can also lead to exercise intolerance, an increased risk of diabetes mellitus, hepatic lipidosis, feline lower urinary tract disease, urinary incontinence and dermatitis, as well as increasing surgical and anaesthetic risks.

Obesity is caused, in simple terms, by excessive calorie consumption compared to calorie expenditure. Calorie requirements and the tendency to weight gain are influenced by neuter status, age and activity levels. Neutered and older pets require fewer calories, and since neutering often happens at a time of a natural reduction in calorie requirements in the young dog, it is essential that appropriate advice is given to owners to prevent weight gain developing at a young age. Some breeds are more prone to weight gain, suggesting a genetic association. Commercial diets are designed to be highly palatable, which can lead to over-feeding particularly in pets fed *ad libitum*. There are also human social and behavioural issues that can lead to overfeeding; food is often an important part of the human–animal bond, with excessive feeding of treats and human food being a very common occurrence. Dogs value food as a social commodity, although this is not the case with cats. Owners frequently misinterpret common feline behaviours as 'begging' for food, which can lead to overfeeding.

Other conditions can predispose to obesity (e.g. hypothyroidism, hyperadrenocorticism, insulinoma, administration of phenobarbitone, progesterones or glucocorticoids), but these cases represent a very small minority of obese patients.

Diagnosis

Diagnosis of obesity is straightforward and is based on body weight and body condition scoring (see Table A4.1). Patients that are greater than 20–25% over their ideal bodyweight are generally considered to be obese. Owners often do not realise that their pet is overweight, and it helps to explain how you are assessing their body condition score. Various 5- and 9-point scoring systems have been developed, and a new algorithm designed specifically for owners to use is also available online (SHAPE body condition scoring system; Royal Canin).

Further diagnostic testing may be appropriate in patients with additional clinical signs of endocrinopathy, and alternative treatments may be considered in patients where medication is thought to be playing a role.

Table A4.1 **An example of a 5-point scoring system for Body Condition Score (BCS) in dogs and cats.**

Score	Description	Clinical findings
1	Thin	Underweight; no obvious body fat
2	Lean	Skeletal structure visible; little body fat; obvious waist and abdominal tuck
3	Optimum	Ribs easily palpable but not visible; moderate body fat; waist and abdominal tuck visible
4	Overweight	Ribs barely palpable; excessive fat palpable; waist and abdominal tuck may not be visible
5	Obese	Ribs not palpable; large amount of body fat causing physical impairment; waist and abdominal tuck absent; abdomen distended

100 Top Consultations in Small Animal General Practice, First Edition
By Peter Hill, Sheena Warman and Geoff Shawcross
© 2011 Blackwell Publishing Ltd

Management

Effective management of obesity relies firstly on ensuring the owners recognise the problem and are committed to addressing it. Good client compliance is essential. They should be made aware of the possible consequences of obesity as outlined above, and of the improvement in the pet's quality of life that can be expected if a healthy weight is reached. Weight loss can be achieved by a combination of reducing caloric intake, and increasing energy expenditure with exercise and play. The client should be warned that weight loss is a long-term commitment and that it may well take 3–6 months or longer to achieve the target weight.

How much to feed?

There are two approaches to this: a simple, practical approach which may work well in many cases, and a more structured, scientific approach which may result in better compliance with some clients (see below). With either approach, a target weight should be initially identified for the pet. If this requires a greater than 15% weight loss, then this should be done in a step-wise fashion, aiming at 15% reduction as the initial target weight. This helps the owners feel a sense of achievement when the initial target is reached, and prevents an excessive rate of weight loss if the 'high-tech' approach described below is being used. The aim is to achieve 1–2% weight loss/week in dogs, and 1% weight loss/week in cats.

The 'low-tech' approach

The owners are asked to weigh and record the animal's dietary intake for a week, without making any changes. The owners are then advised to cut out the most calorific 'titbits' and reduce the remainder by a small percentage. The diet can be 'bulked out' with additional vegetables (but not potatoes). The pet is then weighed on a weekly basis and further adjustments made until an appropriate rate of weight loss is achieved.

The 'high-tech' approach

The owner is again asked to keep an accurate diary of the pet's food intake for a week. This can then be used to calculate current calorie intake. Caloric content of commercial dog foods is usually available from resources supplied by the pet food companies, and caloric content of other foods/titbits can be sourced online. An approximation can be achieved using the nutritional details on packaged foods and the formula below:

Formula for calculating approximate nutritional content of pet foods:

Protein and carbohydrate both contain 3.5 kcal/g; fat contains 8.5 kcal/g.

Protein and fat content are usually listed on the nutritional panel on the packaging. Carbohydrate can be approximated by subtracting the percentage of protein, fat and water from 100% and assuming the rest of the content is carbohydrate. Kcal/100 g are then calculated by:

$$Kcal/100\,g = 3.5\,(\%\ protein + \%\ carbohydrate) + 8.5\,(\%\ fat)$$

Divide by 100 to calculate kcal/g. For dry food this is usually 3–4 kcal/g; for canned diets this is usually 1–1.5 kcal/g.

The calorie requirement that would be expected to achieve appropriate weight loss is generally 60% of the maintenance energy requirement (MER) for the **target** weight in dogs, and 75% of the MER for the target weight in cats (see Table A4.2). The weight of dried or wet diet required for this should be calculated for the client, who must be advised to weigh the food accurately at each mealtime.

As all individuals vary and some will gain weight more easily than others, on occasion the calculated calorie requirement may actually be more than what the pet is currently consuming. If this is the case, then feeding 80% of the current calories is a sensible starting point.

What to feed?

It is convenient for many owners to feed one of the veterinary prescription diets designed to achieve weight loss. This reduces day to day variation in caloric provision, may help with compliance, and also ensures that the correct balance of proteins, vitamins and minerals will still be fed despite the reduced calories. However if finances or other factors preclude the use of prescription diets, ordinary or home-made diets can be used if necessary. Treats and snacks should be avoided; if this meets with resistance from the client, they can be advised to use some of the daily allowance as treats (easier with dry food), or to replace up to 10% of the allowance with commercially available low-calorie treats or alternatives such as raw carrots or even ice-cubes, which some dogs enjoy. It often helps compliance to feed the animal several small meals a day, rather than one large one.

Multi-cat households can present difficulties in achieving weight loss in an individual cat. Ideally, cats should be

Table A4.2 Calculation of energy requirements in dogs and cats.

	Canine	Feline
Resting energy requirement (for target weight) in kcal (RER)	[30 (Target Wt) + 70]	
Neutered adult MER in kcal (normal activity level)	RER × 1.6	RER × 1.2
Intact adult MER in kcal (normal activity level)	RER × 1.8	RER × 1.4
To achieve weight loss, feed:	60% of MER	75% of MER
Example: neutered bitch with target weight of 10 kg	BER = 30(10) + 70 = 370 MER = 370 × 1.6 = 592 60% of MER = 355 kcal/day	

MER = maintenance energy requirement.

fed separately but this is not always possible. Alternatives include feeding healthy cats on an elevated surface (as many overweight cats cannot jump), or feeding healthy cats in an overturned cardboard box with a hole cut in the side through which the overweight cat cannot fit.

Weight-loss drugs

Recently, dirlotapide (Slentrol, Pfizer) and mitratapide (Yarvitan, Janssen Animal Health) have been licensed for dogs (NOT cats due to the risk of hepatic lipidosis) to aid in weight loss. These inhibit microsomal triglyceride transfer proteins, reducing fat absorption from the intestine and decreasing the dog's appetite. Side-effects can include vomiting and diarrhoea. They should only be used in conjunction with a calculated weight-loss diet, and owners should be counselled that dietary control must be maintained once the dog has lost weight and is no longer being treated with the medication. Whilst medication is unlikely to be necessary in managing the majority of obese dogs, it may be useful in dogs where owner compliance is poor or the dog constantly appears hungry.

Increased activity

Clients should also be encouraged to increase their dog's exercise. This can be achieved through longer, more frequent walks and/or through increased play. Increased activity levels are important in cats as well, and can be achieved with the help of interactive cat toys. Increased play opportunities also help fill any perceived 'gaps' in the owner–animal relationship created by dietary restriction.

Follow-up

The pet should be weighed fortnightly. Some practices run weight-loss clinics which help with client motivation. Clients often feel better supported if they have a named member of the nursing or lay staff who helps them weigh their pet and chart their progress, with further nursing or veterinary advice sought if satisfactory weight loss is not achieved. If inadequate weight loss is achieved, then calories should be restricted by a further 10%. If the pet loses >2% weight a week, then calories should be increased by 10%.

Once the pet has reached its final target weight, it must be emphasised that good eating and exercise habits need to be maintained. Food should continue to be weighed. The weight-loss diet can be continued at slightly increased quantities to maintain a stable weight, or the pet can be switched to an adult maintenance 'light' diet. Regular weigh-ins at 2–3 month intervals are recommended.

Peter Hill and Sheena Warman

Haematology (complete blood count)

Routine haematology can be used to diagnose diseases that affect the number or appearance of circulating blood cells. It also provides information on the severity of certain diseases and can be used to monitor the effects of treatment. Haematology can provide valuable information in any patient with non-specific illness and, along with biochemistry and urinalysis, it should form part of the 'minimum database' in the initial investigation of any sick animal for which a cause cannot be determined on history and physical examination. It is particularly indicated in the following circumstances:

- In a pale animal, to determine whether or not anaemia is present and to characterise this further
- When endocrine, neoplastic or inflammatory diseases are suspected
- Prior to and during immunosuppressive or cytotoxic therapy.

Haematological examination provides information about red cells, white cells and platelets. Table A5.1 shows the parameters that usually appear in a haematology profile (complete blood count). In addition to these values, a haematology report will normally include comments about the appearance of the cells. In some laboratories, abnormal values will be indicated with an asterisk or similar mark. However, clinicians should always examine all the parameters carefully.

Haematology profiles are interpreted by determining if the values are in the normal range, elevated or decreased. The significance of the various changes can then be assessed, but clinicians should note that considerable variation occurs both in healthy and sick animals, and the expected changes in all parameters are not always present. Clinicians should also be aware that values can be outside the normal range in approximately 5% of healthy animals.

100 Top Consultations in Small Animal General Practice, First Edition
By Peter Hill, Sheena Warman and Geoff Shawcross
© 2011 Blackwell Publishing Ltd

Decreased red cell parameters (anaemia)

- Haemorrhage
- Haemolysis
- Non-regenerative anaemias, e.g. anaemia of chronic disease, bone marrow disorders, myelosuppressive effects of some drugs.

Increased red cell parameters

- Dehydration
- Erythrocytosis (polycythaemia) – in response to hypoxia, excessive erythropoietin production or bone marrow disorder.

Changes to MCV and MCHC

MCV and MCHC are usually assessed together in relation to a diagnosis of anaemia. The main abnormalities seen are:

- High MCV / low MCHC (macrocytic–hypochromic anaemia) – regenerative anaemia in which immature red cells (reticulocytes) are being produced. Reticulocytes are larger than normal red cells and contain less haemoglobin
- Normal MCV and normal MCHC (normocytic–normochromic anaemia) – non-regenerative anaemia, or sudden-onset anaemia before there has been a bone marrow response
- Low MCV / low MCHC – iron deficiency, resulting in small red cells which contain inadequate amounts of haemoglobin.

Increased total WBC count (leukocytosis) / Increased neutrophil count (neutrophilia)/ Increased monocyte count (monocytosis)

- Acute or chronic inflammation / infection
- Stress response
- Hyperadrenocorticism
- Steroid therapy

Increased eosinophil count (eosinophilia) / Increased basophil count (basophilia)

- Parasitic infestations
- Allergic inflammation
- Hypoadrenocorticism (eosinophilia)
- Hypereosinophilic syndromes.

Increased lymphocyte count (lymphocytosis)

- Chronic infection
- Viral infection
- Immune-mediated disease
- Leukaemia.

Decreased neutrophil count (neutropenia)

- Sepsis

- Bone marrow disorders
- Cytotoxic drug therapy.

Decreased eosinophil count (eosinopenia) / Decreased lymphocyte count (lymphopenia)

- Some viral infections (lymphopenia)
- Stress response
- Hyperadrenocorticism
- Steroid therapy.

Table A5.1 Components of a haematology profile (the normal ranges are only provided for guidance. Clinicians should always use the normal ranges provided by their own laboratory).

Parameter	Normal range		Units
	Dog	Cat	
Red cell parameters			
Packed cell volume (PCV)	37–55	24–45	%
Total red blood cell count (RBC)	5.5–8.5	5.0–10.0	$\times 10^{12} / L$
Haemoglobin concentration (Hb)	12–18	8–15	g/dl
Mean corpuscular volume (MCV)	60–77	39–55	fl
Mean corpuscular Hb concentration (MCHC)	32–36	30–36	%
White blood cell parameters			
Total white blood cell count (WBC)	6.0–17.0	5.5–19.5	$\times 10^9 / L$
Neutrophil count	3.6–12.0	2.5–12.5	$\times 10^9 / L$
Band neutrophil count	0	0	$\times 10^9 / L$
Lymphocyte count	0.7–4.8	1.5–7.0	$\times 10^9 / L$
Eosinophil count	0–1.0	0–1.5	$\times 10^9 / L$
Monocyte count	0–1.5	0–0.8	$\times 10^9 / L$
Basophil count	Rare	Rare	$\times 10^9 / L$
Differential white blood cell count			
Neutrophils	40–80	35–75	%
Band neutrophils	0–3	0–3	%
Lymphocytes	12–30	20–55	%
Eosinophils	2–10	2–12	%
Monocytes	3–10	1–4	%
Basophils	Rare	Rare	%
Platelets			
Platelet count	200–500	300–600	$\times 10^9 / L$

The stress leukogram

The stress leukogram is a collection of haematological changes that are seen in association with stress, hyper-adrenocorticism or steroid therapy. A stress leukogram comprises leukocytosis, neutrophilia, eosinopenia, lymphopenia and possible monocytosis.

The left shift

A left shift occurs when increased numbers of immature (band) neutrophils are seen in the circulation. A left shift is a characteristic sign of inflammation, especially with infections.

Decreased platelets (thrombocytopenia)

* Immune-mediated destruction
* Cytotoxic drugs
* Bone marrow disorder
* DIC.

Biochemistry (clinical chemistry)

Routine serum biochemical analysis can be used to diagnose diseases that affect the function of various internal organs. It also provides information on the severity of certain diseases and can be used to monitor the effects of treatment. Biochemistry can provide valuable information in any patient with non-specific illness and, along with haematology and urinalysis, it should form part of the 'minimum database' in the initial investigation of any sick animal for which a cause cannot be determined on history and physical examination. It is particularly indicated when renal, hepatic, endocrine or other metabolic conditions are suspected.

Most laboratories offer a range of biochemical tests to assess various aspects of internal organ function. Instead of performing these tests individually, they are usually grouped together to produce a standard biochemistry profile. This profile is designed to provide information about most of the common organ dysfunctions. The components of a standard biochemistry profile vary from laboratory to laboratory. This depends to some degree on cost. However, if clinicians want additional tests they can usually be specifically requested from the laboratory.

Table A5.2 shows the parameters that often appear in standard biochemistry profiles. When these results are reported, many laboratories highlight the values that have fallen outside the normal range with an asterisk or similar marker. Clinicians should not fall into the trap of looking only for these marked results. This tends to distract attention from the other results which may also contain diagnostically useful information.

When interpreting biochemistry profiles, clinicians should look at each parameter in turn and ask the following questions:

* Is it in the normal range?
* Is it at the top or the bottom of the normal range?
* If the value is elevated, what conditions may have caused the elevation?
* If the value is decreased, what conditions may have caused the decrease?

The significance of the various changes can then be assessed, but clinicians should note that considerable variation occurs both in healthy and sick animals, and the expected changes in all parameters are not always present. Clinicians should also be aware that values can be outside the normal range in approximately 5% of healthy animals. Erroneous results can be obtained if samples are not taken and stored appropriately.

ALT and AST – markers of hepatocellular damage

ALT is liver-specific whereas AST is also released from damaged muscles. Mild to moderate elevations are common in many pets with systemic illness due to secondary hepatic damage (e.g. endocrinopathies, sepsis). Some drugs, in particular glucocorticoids and phenobarbitone, invariably cause mild-moderate elevations of liver enzymes. Moderate–severe elevations are more likely to reflect an acute hepatic insult (e.g. toxin, infection, hypoxia, hepatotoxic drug) or chronic hepatic disease (e.g. chronic hepatitis).

ALKP and GGT – markers of cholestasis

ALKP and GGT are elevated by intra- or extra-hepatic cholestasis. ALKP is also increased in response to increased endogenous or exogenous cortisol (steroid isoenzyme – dog not cat), bone growth (in animals less than 8 months of age) or bone damage (bone isoenzyme). GGT measurement is particularly useful in cats as it tends to be elevated in cholangitis but not in hepatic lipidosis.

Bile acids (pre- and post-prandial) – markers of liver function

The measurement of bile acids in a 12-hour fasted serum sample and then 2 hours after ingestion of a fatty meal can be used to assess hepatic function. Increased pre and/ or post-fasting bile acids are associated with hepatic insufficiency (e.g. chronic hepatitis, cirrhosis, neoplasia, portosystemic shunt). If fasting bile acids are markedly elevated there is little point in obtaining a post-prandial sample. Since bile acids are excreted in the biliary tract, there is little value in performing bile acid assays in patients with severe cholestasis, as they will inevitably be elevated.

Table A5.2 Useful components of a biochemistry profile (the normal ranges are only provided for guidance. Clinicians should always use the normal ranges provided by their own laboratory).

Parameter	Normal range		Units
	Dog	Cat	
Alanine aminotransferase (ALT)	15–60	15–60	IU/L
Aspartate aminotransferase (AST)	20–35	0–20	IU/L
Gamma-glutamyl transferase (GGT)	0–15	0–2	IU/L
Alkaline phosphatase (ALKP)	20–60	10–100	IU/L
Fasting bile acids	0–7.0	0–7.0	µmol/L
Total bilirubin	0–6.8	0–6.8	µmol/L
Urea	1.7–7.4	2.8–9.8	mmol/L
Creatinine	30–90	26–118	µmol/L
Glucose	3.0–5.0	3.3–5.0	mmol/L
Cholesterol	3.8–7.0	2.0–3.4	mmol/L
Triglycerides	0.57–1.14	0.57–1.14	mmol/L
Total protein	58–73	69–79	g/L
Albumin	27–37	27–41	g/L
Globulin	21–50	22–56	g/L
Amylase	13–53	28–51	µmol/L
Lipase	13–200	0–83	U/L
Creatinine kinase (CK)	50–200	50–200	IU/L
Calcium	2.3–3.0	2.1–2.9	mmol/L
Inorganic phosphate	0.9–1.2	1.4–2.5	mmol/L
Sodium	139–154	145–156	mmol/L
Chloride	99–115	117–140	mmol/L
Potassium	3.6–5.6	4.0–5.0	mmol/L

Bilirubin

Increased total bilirubin is usually associated with haemo-lytic disease or hepatic disease. Causes include:

- Pre-hepatic disease – Haemolysis, e.g. immune-mediated haemolytic anaemia, *M. haemofelis* infection in cats
- Hepatic disease – Hepatitis, cholangitis, neoplasia, lipidosis, FIP, cirrhosis, sepsis
- Post-hepatic disease – Pancreatitis or pancreatic tumour, biliary duct neoplasia, biliary rupture.

Urea and creatinine

The measurement of blood urea and creatinine is usually used to assess renal function. Increased urea and creati-nine can be caused by pre-renal, renal and post-renal factors. Urea in particular can be increased by pre-renal factors such as dehydration, hypovolaemia, a high protein meal or gastrointestinal bleeding. Dehydrated or hypovol-aemic patients without renal insufficiency will have con-centrated urine (USG > 1.030 in dogs and >1.035 in cats) unless there is another reason for an inability to concen-trate urine (e.g. hypercalcaemia, or treatment with drugs such as furosemide or glucocorticoids). Post-renal causes of azotaemia include urinary tract obstruction or rupture.

Decreased urea may be seen with chronic hepatic insufficiency or severe polydipsia and polyuria.

Glucose

The measurement of blood glucose is usually used to detect the presence of diabetes mellitus. Blood glucose can be increased by stress (particularly in cats), diabetes mellitus, glucocorticoids, hyperadrenocorticism or acute pancreatitis. Hypoglycaemia can be caused by insulin overdose, insulinoma, hepatic failure, sepsis, hypoadrenocorticism, neoplasia or lack of reserves (neonates, hunting dogs).

Cholesterol

Increased cholesterol in a fasting sample can be seen with:

* Hypothyroidism
* Hyperadrenocorticism
* Diabetes mellitus
* Steroid therapy
* Cholestasis
* Nephrotic syndrome
* Idiopathic hyperlipidaemia.

Hypocholesterolaemia can be seen with:

* Protein-losing enteropathy
* Severe gastrointestinal disease (maldigestion/ malabsorption)
* Hepatic disease.

Triglycerides

Increased triglycerides in a fasting sample can be seen with:

* Hypothyroidism
* Diabetes mellitus
* Hyperadrenocorticism
* Acute pancreatitis
* Primary hyperlipidaemia (e.g. Miniature Schnauzer).

Decreased triglycerides are not thought to be significant.

Total protein, albumin and globulin

Total protein can be decreased by reductions in albumin, globulin or both. Likewise, increased total protein can be caused by elevations in albumin, globulin or both.

Reductions in both albumin and globulin suggest haemorrhage, exudation from severe skin lesions or protein losing enteropathy.

Hypoalbuminaemia alone is usually due to decreased production (liver disease or rarely, dietary deficiency or malabsorption), sequestration (body cavity effusions or vasculopathy) or increased loss (acute haemorrhage, protein-losing enteropathy or nephropathy). Hypoglobulinaemia is usually caused by acute haemorrhage or protein-losing enteropathies.

Hyperalbuminaemia is usually due to dehydration. A combination of mild hypoalbuminaemia with mild hyperglobulinaemia is frequently seen in acute inflammation. A moderate to severe hyperglobulinaemia should prompt a request that serum protein electrophoresis is performed. This indicates whether a polyclonal or monoclonal gammopathy is present. Causes of a polyclonal gammopathy include infections (in particular bacterial disease, *Leishmania* or FIP), immune-mediated disease (e.g. systemic lupus erythematosus, IMHA) or neoplasia (especially lymphoma). Causes of a monoclonal gammopathy include multiple myeloma, lymphoma, *Leishmania*, or rarely FIP.

Amylase and lipase

The measurement of amylase and lipase is often used to assess diseases of the pancreas but neither is very sensitive nor specific, particularly in cats. They can be helpful in dogs presenting with acute signs consistent with pancreatitis if markedly elevated (more than three times the top of the reference range), but are not considered useful in cats. If pancreatitis is suspected, pancreatic lipase immunoreactivity testing should be performed.

CK and AST

The measurement of CK and AST is used as a crude indicator of muscle damage, although it has poor sensitivity and specificity for spontaneous muscle disease.

Calcium and inorganic phosphate

Many conditions can lead to alterations in blood calcium and phosphate concentrations. By far the commonest cause of hypercalcaemia is neoplasia (humoral hypercalcaemia of malignancy, HHM), in particular with lymphoma and anal sac adenocarcinomas. HHM and primary hyperparathyroidism usually lead to elevated calcium and decreased phosphate. Some cases of renal failure, Vitamin D toxicity, granulomatous inflammatory diseases and Addison's disease can lead to elevations in both calcium and phosphate.

Hypocalcaemia can be caused by eclampsia, acute pancreatitis, primary hypoparathyroidism, renal failure, ethylene glycol toxicity, hypoalbuminaemia, intestinal

Section 18

malabsorption, nutritional secondary hyperparathyroidism, or be iatrogenic following bilateral thyroidectomy (cat).

Hyperphosphataemia is most commonly associated with renal failure, but can also be seen in young animals, osteolytic diseases, and in conjunction with hypercalcaemia as indicated above. Hypophosphataemia is rare but can be observed with HHM, primary hyperparathyroidism, eclampsia, or insulin therapy.

Sodium, chloride and potassium

Hypernatraemia can be seen with pure water loss (adipsia, inadequate access to water, heat stroke, pyrexia) or hypotonic fluid losses due to intestinal disease, renal failure or diuretic therapy. Hyponatraemia can also be associated with losses due to gastrointestinal disease, diuretics or renal failure; fluid retention due to congestive heart failure; hypoadrenocorticism; or 'third spacing', e.g. abdominal or pleural effusions.

Hyperchloraemia can be caused by small intestinal diarrhoea, fluid therapy or renal failure. Hypochloraemia is most commonly associated with vomiting of gastric contents or aggressive diuretic therapy.

Hyperkalaemia can be caused by hypoadrenocorticism, acute renal failure or urinary rupture/obstruction. Hypokalaemia can be caused by gastrointestinal losses, anorexia, chronic renal failure, diuretics, or insulin therapy.

ACE inhibitors	angiotensin-converting enzyme inhibitors	EFA(s)	essential fatty acid(s)
ACP	acepromazine	ELISA	enzyme-linked immunosorbent assay
ACT	activated clotting time	ET	endotracheal tube
ACTH	adrenocorticotrophic hormone (adrenocorticotropin)	FART	fragment arthroscopic retrieval treatment
ADH	adrenal-dependent hyperadrenocorticism	FCE	fibrocartilaginous embolus
		FCGS	feline chronic gingivitis/stomatitis syndrome
AGP	alpha-1 acid glycoprotein	FCoV	feline coronavirus
AI	aortic insufficiency	FCV	feline calicivirus
ALKP	alkaline phosphatase	FDA	Food and Drug Administration (US)
ALT	alanine transaminase (alanine aminotransferase)	FeLV	feline leukaemia virus
		FHV	feline herpes virus
APTT	activated partial thromboplastin time	FIC	feline idiopathic cystitis
AS	aortic stenosis	FIP	feline infectious peritonitis
AST	aspartate transaminase	FIV	feline immunodeficiency virus
AZT	azidothymidine	FSH	follicle-stimulating hormone
BID	twice a day	GDV	gastric dilaattion and volvulus
bpm	beats per minute	GGT	gamma glutamyl transferase
BUN	blood urea nitrogen	GI	gastrointestinal
CAV-1	infectious canine hepatitis	GME	granulomatous meningoencephalitis
CCL(I)	cranial cruciate ligament (insufficiency)	GnRH	gonadotropin-releasing hormone
CDRM	canine degenerative radiculomyelopathy	HAC	hyperadrenocorticism
CHF	congestive heart failure	HCM	hypertrophic cardiomyopathy
CK	creatine kinase	HGE	haemorrhagic gastroenteritis
CNS	central nervous system	HHM	humoral hypercalcaemia of malignancy
COX inhibitors	cyclo-oxygenase inhibitors	ICA	immunochromatographic assay
CRT	capillary refill time	IFA	immunofluorescence antibody
CSF	cerebrospinal fluid	IM	intramuscular(ly)
CT	computed tomography	IMHA	immune-mediated haemolytic anaemia
CVD	central vestibular disease	IO	intra-osseous(ly)
DDAVP	1-deamino-8-D-arginine vasopressin (desmopressin)	IPPV	intermittent positive-pressure ventilation
DIC	disseminated intravascular coagulation	IV	intravenous(ly)
DM	diabetes mellitus	KCS	keratoconjunctivitis sicca
ECG	electrocardiogram	LDDS	low-dose dexamethasone suppression (test)
EDTA	ethylenediaminetetra-acetic acid		
		LH	luteinising hormone
		LMN	lower motor neuron
		LUTD	lower urinary tract disease
		MCH	mean corpuscular haemoglobin

100 Top Consultations in Small Animal General Practice, First Edition
By Peter Hill, Sheena Warman and Geoff Shawcross
© 2011 Blackwell Publishing Ltd

MCHC	mean corpuscular haemoglobin concentration	PS	pulmonary stenosis
MCV	mean corpuscular volume	PT	prothrombin time
MER	maintenance energy requirement	PUO	pyrexia of unknown origin
MRI	magnetic resonance imaging	PUPD	polyuria and polydipsia
MVD	mitral valve disease	PVD	peripheral vestibular disease
NSAID(s)	nonsteroidal anti-inflammatory drug(s)	RBC(s)	red blood cell(s)
NT pro-BNP	N-terminal pro-B-type natriuretic peptide	RT-PCR	reverse-transcriptase polymerase chain reaction
PBFD	psittacine beak and feather disease	S-AME	S-adenosyl methionine
P:C ratio	protein:creatinine ratio	SARD	sudden acquired retinal degeneration
PCR	polymerase chain reaction	SC	subcutaneous(ly)
PCV	packed cell volume	SI	small intestinal
PDA	patent ductus arteriosus	T3	triiodothyronine
PDH	pituitary-dependent hyperadrenocorticism	T4	thyroxine
PHA	post-hibernation anorexia	TID	three times a day
PIVKA	proteins induced by vitamin K antagonism	TLI	trypsin-like immunoreactivity
		TRH	thyrotropin-releasing hormone
PLI	pancreatic lipase insufficiency	TSH	thyroid-stimulating hormone
PMI	point of maximal intensity	TVD	tricuspid valve disease
PO	per os	UDCA	ursodeoxycholic acid
PRA	progressive retinal atrophy	UMN	upper motor neuron
		USG	urine specific gravity
		VSD	ventricular septal defect

Index

100 Top Consultations in Small Animal General Practice, First Edition
By Peter Hill, Sheena Warman and Geoff Shawcross
© 2011 Blackwell Publishing Ltd

Cardiac arrhythmia 214, 216, 217
Cardiac disease
  as a cause of collapse 42
  as a cause of retching 138, 139
Cardiac tamponade 46
Caries 133, 134
Carprofen 405
Castration 20–2
Cat-bite abscess 109–10
Cat flu 207, 208, 209
Cataracts 234–6
  as a cause of blindness 237, 238
Cefalexin 398
  for infected skin lesions in cats 65
  for treatment of acral lick dermatitis 89
  for treatment of cat flu 208
  for treatment of deep hot spots 87
  for treatment of otitis interna 324
  for treatment of pyoderma 81
Cefovecin
  for infected skin lesions in cats 65
  for treatment of deep hot spots 87
  for treatment of pyoderma 81
Cellulitis 109
Central vestibular disease 322, 323, 324
Cerebrovascular disorder, as a cause of central vestibular
    disease 322
Cervical lymphadenitis in Guinea pigs 127
Cervical spondylopathy 319
  as a cause of spinal pain 194
Chalazion 224, 225
Chemical burns 297
Chemical neutering 21
Chemotherapy 304, 305, 306
Cheyletiella 67, 68, 70, 71, 72
  dermatitis as a cause of pruritus 59, 63, 64
Cheyletiella parasitovorax
  in Guinea pigs 127
  in rabbits 126
Chirodiscoides caviae, in Guinea pigs 127
Chitosan 253
Chlamydophila
  as a cause of conjunctivitis 227, 228
  secondary to FIV 51
Chlamydophilosis 368, 369, 370
Chloride 412, 414
Chlorphacinone poisoning 347
Chocolate poisoning 342
Cholangiohepatitis 40, 152
Cholesterol 412, 413
Chondroitin sulphate 188
CHOP protocol, for lymphoma 311
Chorioretinitis 237, 238
  with FIP 54

Chronic active hepatitis 151
Chronic bronchitis 201, 202, 203, 204
Chronic interstitial nephritis 253
Chronic renal failure as a cause of PUPD 29, 30
Chronic superficial keratitis 227
Chronic tracheobronchial syndrome 206
Chylothorax 218
Ciclosporin 84, 102
Cimetidine 142, 144
Cinchophen 405
Cirrhosis 151, 152, 153
  as a cause of jaundice 39, 40, 41
Claw injuries 177, 180, 289
Claw-bed tumours 99
Clindamycin 399, 400, 401
  for treatment of deep hot spots 87
  for treatment of periodontal disease 136
  for treatment of pyoderma 81
Clinical examination 1–9
Cloacal prolapse, in tortoises 374
Clomipramine
  for separation anxiety 334
  for treatment of acral lick dermatitis 89
Cloprostenol 262
Clostridia, as a cause of diarrhoea 143
Clostridium perfringens 146
  as a cause of colitis 148, 149
Clotrimazole as a treatment for otitis 97
Cnemidocoptes pilae 127
Coagulopathy, as a cause of haemorrhagic gastroenteritis 146
Coat brushings for ectoparasites 68
Cobalamin deficiency in Border Collies and Giant
    Schnauzers 37
Codeine phosphate 405
Colitis 143, 148–50
Collapse 42–4
Colotomy/colectomy 165
Colour dilution alopecia 120
Colposuspension 251
Comedones 74
Compartment syndrome 297
Congenital alopecia 120, 121, 122
Congenital mitral valve disease 210
Congenital tricuspid valve disease 210
Congestive heart failure 214
Conjunctivitis 227–9
Constipation 162–5
Consultation process 1–9
Contact dermatitis, as a cause of pododermatitis 99
Contact dermatitis, as a cause of pruritus 59, 60
Contact lenses 231, 232
Coombs' test 37, 39
COP protocol, for lymphoma 311
Corn 99